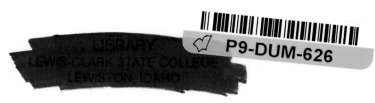

A Dictionary *of* Epidemiology

A
Dictionary
of
Epidemiology

Sixth Edition

Edited for the
International Epidemiological Association
      by
Miquel Porta
Professor of Preventive Medicine & Public Health,
School of Medicine, Universitat Autònoma de Barcelona
Senior Scientist, Hospital del Mar Institute of Medical Research – IMIM
Barcelona, Catalonia, Spain
Adjunct Professor of Epidemiology, Gillings School of Global Public Health
University of North Carolina at Chapel Hill, USA

Associate Editors
Sander Greenland
Miguel Hernán
Isabel dos Santos Silva
John M. Last

Assistant Editor
Andrea Burón

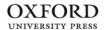
OXFORD
UNIVERSITY PRESS

OXFORD

UNIVERSITY PRESS

Oxford University Press is a department of the University of
Oxford. It furthers the University's objective of excellence in research,
scholarship, and education by publishing worldwide.

Oxford   New York
Auckland   Cape Town   Dar es Salaam   Hong Kong   Karachi
Kuala Lumpur   Madrid   Melbourne   Mexico City   Nairobi
New Delhi   Shanghai   Taipei   Toronto

With offices in
Argentina   Austria   Brazil   Chile   Czech Republic   France   Greece
Guatemala   Hungary   Italy   Japan   Poland   Portugal   Singapore
South Korea   Switzerland   Thailand   Turkey   Ukraine   Vietnam

Oxford is a registered trademark of Oxford University Press
in the UK and certain other countries.

Published in the United States of America by
Oxford University Press
198 Madison Avenue, New York, NY 10016

Library of Congress Cataloging-in-Publication Data
A dictionary of epidemiology. — Sixth edition / edited for the International Epidemiological
Association by Miquel Porta; associate editors, Sander Greenland, Miguel Hernán, Isabel dos Santos
Silva, John M. Last; assistant editor, Andrea Burón.
p. ; cm.
Includes bibliographical references.
ISBN 978–0–19–997672–0 (hbk. : alk. paper) — ISBN 978–0–19–997673–7 (pbk. : alk. paper)
I. Porta, Miquel S., editor.   II. Greenland, Sander, 1951–, editor.   III. Hernán, Miguel, editor.
IV. dos Santos Silva, Isabel, editor.   V. Last, John M., 1926–, editor.   VI. International
Epidemiological Association, sponsor.
[DNLM: 1. Epidemiology — Dictionary — English. WA 13]
RA651
614.403 — dc23
2014001686

3 5 7 9 8 6 4
Printed in the United States of America
on acid-free paper

Foreword

....

TO WRITE A DICTIONARY IN ANY SCIENTIFIC DISCIPLINE IS A RISKY ENDEAVOR, BECAUSE scientists often disagree. The nature of science is not to reach consensus but to advance our knowledge by bringing conflicting ideas to critical examinations. That is true also for how we define the concepts we use. No dictionary will ever be able to satisfy all, nor should it try to.

The aim of the International Epidemiological Association (IEA) in cosponsoring this dictionary in its more than 30 years' history has been to facilitate communication among epidemiologists—to develop a "common language" to the extent that this is possible. We need a common language when we write papers, teach, and communicate findings to the public.

This "common language" changes over time, as anybody can see by reading the successive editions of this dictionary. The language changes because our understanding of the concepts changes over time and new research options bring forward new concepts.

From the IEA, we want to thank John Last for his tremendous achievements as former editor of the dictionary, and Miquel Porta as the editor since the fifth edition. Miquel continues the IEA's long-standing tradition of collaborating with leading epidemiologists worldwide to ensure that our dictionary reflects the current state of the art in our rapidly evolving discipline.

Cesar Victora, Neil Pearce, and Jørn Olsen
Current and past presidents,
International Epidemiological Association
www.ieaweb.org

Foreword to the Fourth Edition, 2001

....

IF I HAD TO LIMIT MY PROFESSIONAL BOOKCASE TO A SINGLE VOLUME, I WOULD choose this dictionary. With many new entries, updates, and other refinements in the fourth edition, the dictionary has grown from the original slim pocket book into a mature and substantial volume. John Last and his collaborators must be congratulated for their extraordinary devotion and productivity over the past 20 years, from which epidemiologists around the world have benefited.

The dictionary's authority stems from its international recognition. It is an immediate source for students and practitioners to verify their understanding of the increasing number of technical words in epidemiologic practice. It clarifies concepts that may not have been understood in class, fills many gaps in anyone's education, and jogs the memory of near-forgotten terms. It has no equal in the field of epidemiology.

The International Epidemiological Association is proud to have had such a long-standing association with the dictionary. We all hope this relationship will continue indefinitely in the future, even though John Last, being mortal, will not. He has set a high standard for his successors. We are grateful that he has prepared the way so well to ensure that the dictionary remains of contemporary relevance in the coming decades.

Charles du V. Florey
President, 1999–2002
International Epidemiological Association
www.ieaweb.org

Preface

....

WHO KNOWS TOMORROW: "ERAS"—I HEARD—ARE NO LONGER WHAT THEY USED TO BE. But, right now, we do live an era of unprecedented progress in the speed and scope of access to information and cognitive devices, and in the nature and scale of the access to data, information, and knowledge, and millions of us often enjoy knowledge sources of high quality. (Of course, nothing is perfect, and too much is rubbish or hidden.) Such devices and sources obviously affect and include dictionaries and most other reference sources—yes, many, of high *quality*.[1] If you think that this is essentially true, and in particular if your personal experience pretty much agrees with such statements, then I believe you may also find it remarkable that to offer you this preface I had only to revise slightly the preface to the previous, fifth edition, written in early 2008. That was yesterday —seemingly, decades ago—, before the *first* iPhones and iPads came out, before WhatsApp (of which there are currently over 440 million users), before Dropbox, Instagram, Android (over 1,000 million such devices activated),[2] before AppStore, GooglePlay, the one billion monthly users of Facebook, or the common scanning and storage of petabytes of data. Not to mention rating agencies and "Inside job" or the "genomic bubble." [1-5] In the few years since the fifth edition was published we've suffered—and many still suffer—a systemic financial crisis, as well as a no less systemic economic and environmental crisis, with enormous effects on the determinants of public and global health. Of significance for us, users of dictionaries and related sources, during the past few years we've also witnessed symbolic events as the closure of the Encarta digital multimedia encyclopedia published by Microsoft, the last print edition of *Encyclopædia Britannica*, the purchase of *The Washington Post* by the owner of Amazon, the end of many newspapers, a radical change in the nature of all others, the uncertain search for sustainable business models, and a permanent, breathtaking sense of sailing into stunning, unknown seas. All this and much more[1] happened around us and inside us while the previous, fifth edition of this book was born, lived, and "retired," so to speak. And yet here we are, with a profoundly renovated sixth edition.

How we search and where we search for meaning has changed and continues to change deeply, beautifully. Some other things, of course, never change.

Indeed, in the meantime our nature, values, beliefs, and needs, the fundamental approach, methods, and aims of this dictionary, did not change much or not at all. If something, in the midst of the storm of petabytes, the role and functions of this dictionary became more crucial than ever. Yet, the purpose and challenges when making it remained unaltered: to seek and capture the proper, true, accurate *meaning* of words; to quietly and critically listen and read, think, and discuss with highly knowledgeable, modest, scientifically productive, and wise colleagues; to think beyond ourselves—beyond our personal experiences and interests—, and to *select* terms, meanings, and definitions with open minds and ears, critical sense, common sense, intellectual rigor, creativity, flexibility, and craftsmanship.

Remember, there was virtually no Google, and no Wikipedia then, centuries ago, when the fourth edition of this dictionary came out—in 2001. No smartphones, no apps, no wifi. Fingers did nothing on a screen just two editions ago. And of the respected dictionaries, very little was "posted on the Internet." Hard to believe. How did we manage, how could we ever have worked? But we did, we surely did: with open minds, critical sense, intellectual rigor, feet on earth. No *google* or *wiki* or information technology (IT) whatsoever will change that. The need to do the epidemiological work, the scientific work, the clinical or public health work with "that": open minds, critical and common sense...

Now we have thousands of webs and blogs with millions of articles and scientific papers, definitions, and discussions regarding terms—all at our very fingertips. Many sources, authors, and texts are truly authoritative. You'll find them—a few, selected—duly referenced at the end of this book. Yes, to write this book we googled and used Wikipedia, "surfed," and "visited" many remote, beautiful places. To surf, to post—whew, these terms will soon be obsolete, won't they? Maybe not.

We continue to seek, appraise, and find *meaning*: in some articles in PubMed/Medline and elsewhere, in some online textbooks, in some websites. In some books. Some. And within parts of the main dictionaries, which we often read again while writing this new edition, and which I hope you will always use in case of doubt or simply to enrich the definitions that we offer here (See pages 301–306 and 307–343). At and through "places" such as HighWire, ResearchGate, ScienceDirect, Scopus, SciELO, ISI Web of knowledge, and countless other platforms and digital publishing businesses, what yesterday was an unthinkable utopia—did anybody predict its magnitude, really?—has become an "achievable utopia," in millions of places almost all over the world actually achieved daily: the infinite library, and with it the unlimited dictionary too. I wish Borges were alive to enjoy it, if not actually to see it, since he was blind. Long life to the "The Library of Babel."

So what sense does it make today to craft a dictionary? What are such crucial roles and functions? Simple: in a radically new way, the "IEA dictionary," "Last's dictionary" can be more relevant and useful than ever before because nowadays we suffer from an unprecedented level of "data pollution," "noise," and potential confusion. Never have we been exposed to so many erroneous and misleading definitions. Which is why we again critically listened and read, thought, discussed, and *selected* terms, definitions, and complementary comments. With "that": open minds, critical sense, common sense, intellectual rigor, creativity, flexibility, craftsmanship. Because with more "data pollution" and "noise" than ever in history, sifting, decanting—selection with "that"—is more necessary and valuable than ever before. To explain, educate, orientate, stimulate. To help increase the validity and relevance of scientific research in the health sciences, to advance knowledge and practice.

* * *

You will judge, but writing this dictionary confirmed to me that it was perfectly feasible to achieve a normative purpose and an informative one.[6] With help of the highest possible academic level from many colleagues (duly acknowledged later), I tried to integrate two approaches to dictionary making: expert-opinion-based prescription (to aid production) and corpus-based description (to aid decoding). Meanings of scientific terms need to be proposed—and may occasionally be imposed—on the basis of expert advice; yet experts and specialists can also keep an ear for actual usage, from which meanings must also be extracted. When we were choosing terms and meanings, we not only kept epidemiological theory and general logic in mind, but usage as well, and often attested explicitly the different uses of polysemic terms. The word "dictionary" is itself notoriously polysemic.[6] This book shows how comfortable the coexistence of diverse meanings of "dictionary" can be. More importantly, it also shows a healthy "micropolysemic" variation[6] in the terms and definitions.

Indeed, like all previous editions, this edition also reflects how diverse and plural—scientifically, professionally, culturally, ideologically—epidemiologists globally are. Take a broad look at the whole population of outstanding epidemiologists, and at the even wider population of users of epidemiologic knowledge in so many disciplines and professions worldwide. I am sure you see the diversity of views and practices about health, science, methods, society, values—the legitimate, necessary, inevitable, and enriching diversity. Such variety is crystal clear in the topics and issues that textbooks of epidemiology choose to cover: just take a look at the tables of contents and indexes of a few textbooks and you'll see an amazing diversity.[7]

Even old controversies can be constructively overcome if the ethics and personality of the contenders has sufficient height and high-mindedness:

"At one time or another we have all seen reasonable people talk past each other because they use the same terms with different definitions attached, or because they do not stand willingly in their opposite's shoes to view the other side of the discussion with intellectual empathy. We support reasoned debate, but we wish to avoid the unproductive debate that characterizes conversations that slide past each other without meaningful discourse."[8]

It makes little sense to pretend that one's views and the ideology of some close colleagues is the only correct way to view and practice the discipline. Look at the terms included in the following pages, read the definitions, please. There often is more than one right option and choice (should this term be included? should it be defined just in this way or also in this other way?). There is not just one valid view, not one truth. This is science. A scientist cannot be dismissive about the views of other scientists, as we sometimes see, for instance, toward clinicians or environmental scientists. The fact that someone in science is rigid, dogmatic, dismissive, or narrow-minded is a pathological sign: something is wrong (too much economic dependence on obsolete industries, perhaps? a peculiar character or personal history?). As always, these issues must not be analyzed only at the individual level: the context and upper levels of organization are essential as well (e.g., the academic culture of a Department or School, their positive links with institutions, authorities, companies, and citizens organizations). Narrow demarcations of epidemiology and related epistemic closures are wrong for the most essential reasons: ethics, science, culture, democracy, history, effectiveness. This issue is particularly important to remember when assessing a dictionary to which a wide collegium of professionals worldwide has contributed for three decades. This book is by no means "Porta's dictionary." It is not even exclusively "IEA's dictionary." Even more relevant: What is sketched in this paragraph is important to keep in mind when assessing a dictionary that rather different types of professionals worldwide will *use* in rather different tasks and settings: foremost, epidemiologists and public health professionals, but also very commonly physicians and students of medicine; other professionals in the health, life, and social sciences; undergraduate students; citizens in daily life.

John Last's outstanding first four editions were the result of a highly comprehensive and inclusive process of selection of terms and definitions. A truly global process, when "global" was much less in vogue. The heritage, the legacy—the contemporary, sharp, accurate tool that we can now enjoy, this edition—stems from over 30 years of fantastic collaborative work by several hundred contributors, since the early 1980s. The six editions are an extraordinary "record"—a DVD, if you wish and remember what that was, an mp4, a list in Spotify,[9] you choose—of the evolution of epidemiology and related sciences during the last quarter century. I suppose these editions are also excellent materials for a sociology of epidemiology.[10]

Therefore, as we continued the process started with the first edition and revised the last edition, we kept well in mind several types of reader, most with (un)imaginable resources, smart, "IT-wise." Surely, you are cordially invited to navigate inside the book, to click or pull the many strings that the book holds by simply reading and turning its pages with your mouse or fingers (odd and familiar as this may at once seem) (fingers on the paper page or on the screen?). Fingers, eyes, brain, heart... in any case, in each case.

No matter how, no matter what, please remember: I assumed that these pages were just *part* of your experience, a stop on your journey today. Perhaps after you physically visited your library (unlikely). Or perhaps after you spent a lot of time (should we still say virtually, really?) reading and thinking at a digital library or publisher's server, the Oxford Reference Online or *The Lancet*. More likely: after you skimmed through a few web pages, article pdfs, and digital books. And maybe such *experiences* happened right before you next go to The Cochrane Library, the *International Journal of Epidemiology, Nature...* or yes, sure, it's a blog in *The Guardian...*Of course, of course. Who could know? You know. In any case, and

I care quite a lot about this: I expect you to hear here in this book, if you care to listen, a music whose quality and texture will be unmatched. Unique. Unlike any other experience with any other cognitive device. But... see, the thing is that only you can finally achieve that. Only some unique and antique cognitive, rational, and emotional process between these pages and *you* can make the experience complete, fulfilling, relevant, and happy.[11-14] I trust you will make it happen.

How we think and act while we search for meaning has also changed slightly, and yes, beautifully. Not only can you always expand, deepen, and progress on what you find here, we know you can always assess, contrast, verify. Quite a responsibility for an editor of a dictionary. This duty is not new; but it surely works on an immensely different scale nowadays. It is now so easy to find that my fellow editors and I were wrong, narrow-minded, off beam, too punctilious. But I love the responsibility, the challenge, the work it entailed. And I am deeply happy with the huge benefits, with what I believe are huge human, scientific, and professional benefits that the galaxy of ITs is making reality daily worldwide.[9]

And also in the meantime, the ancestral book and our beloved libraries have not died. Fantastic. Neither did the scientific journal. They only changed a bit: radically, profoundly, dramatically. It's just been a revolution, a big bang. Yes, a monument must be erected to the "pdf." Right beside the statue to the best craftsmen of the very antique art of typography. Sure, nobody knows precisely how journals will look on screens next decade, next year. But fundamentally, in what really matters, news of the death of academic journals and books—merrily proclaimed by some colleagues in the early years of this, the long-awaited twenty-first century—were...premature. We therefore may hope that the contents of this *book* will again find a place in your mind and be close to your heart. No matter in which format you read it, think through it, skim it. If it's in your smartphone, that's more than fine, of course, what else? If you read this book bound in old fashioned *paper*, you will enjoy its light weight, its pages will easily welcome your handwriting, your very own, and you will comfortably enjoy it out there in the sunlight—batteries are not needed. Maybe at the same time, the same smartphone, a "network receiver" or a vinyl record will be playing Coltrane, Reed, Wainwright, or Bach in the background. Anyway, anyhow, enjoy. (Uhm, does good old Rufus have anything on vinyl? Answer: yes, he does!).

* * *

Our call for contributions to this sixth edition was widely disseminated worldwide, beginning in May 2012—prominently, in the *International Journal of Epidemiology* and the Newsletter of the International Epidemiological Association (IEA), the global scientific organization that has nurtured all editions. We organized a specific website for contributions from any interested individual worldwide, and we also accepted contributions directly from selected colleagues. We received over 400 contributions, most of which (71%) were suggestions to include new terms; a change in the existing definition was suggested by 17% of the contributions, only

4% suggested the removal of an existing term, and 8% made other proposals and comments.

Slightly over 84% of the contributors reported to have "some to extensive training in epidemiology, and to currently work or have professional experience as an epidemiologist"; the rest declared that "while my main job is not as an epidemiologist, I often use epidemiologic knowledge, methods or reasoning in my work."

Over three quarters of the contributors (79%) reported using the fifth edition, the remaining were using other editions, and only three people declared that they had never used the Dictionary. Contributors to this sixth edition and to the previous two are mentioned in pages xxv-xxx.

Through its president, Cesar Victora, the IEA Council suggested over a dozen names of epidemiologists of high scientific standing, whom I duly invited to contribute at their leisure, and from whom I obtained excellent proposals and solutions (please see below). I also asked advice from other colleagues worldwide, and the names of those who contributed relevant contents are also gratefully acknowledged in pages xxv-xxx. The core editorial tasks were the responsibility of the associate editors and myself.

We trust the process of revision of the past edition was wide open, and that everybody who was capable and willing to take part had a channel to do so through the specific website, the IEA, and the editors.

* * *

Is this dictionary an attempt to *demarcate* epidemiology neatly? I don't think so. Or I'd rather think it is not, to the extent that a dictionary can—or needs to— avoid demarcating a discipline.[15] Yet like many other scientists, every now and then epidemiologists engage in boundary-making endeavors and disciplinary demarcation. And then, as usual in other disciplines, epidemiologists assert or reclaim contested epistemic authority and may claim jurisdiction over areas of public health, medicine, statistics, methods, or science. These efforts evolved in the course of the twentieth century while epidemiology developed as a very diverse, eclectic—and foremost, *integrative*—field of practice and scientific discipline.[15-24] And so will they evolve as the societies of the twenty-first century continue developing. There is nothing wrong with that, it is the *natural* thing.

Is this dictionary an epistemic space? Well, of course it is, in the broadest sense: a space of knowledge. Does it belong to an epistemic community or to more than one? Both answers are true. It belongs to one very diverse community of knowledge—epidemiologists around the globe. And to a lesser but no less important extent, the dictionary pertains also to the many communities of knowledge that interact and cooperate with epidemiology, or with which epidemiology cooperates, or that simply use epidemiological reasoning, knowledge, methods, or techniques.

No matter how many mistakes we may have committed (eventually, they are all my responsibility), I would like to think that in making this new edition we again practiced a high level of intellectual rigor in two opposite and complementary directions: (1) in selecting and defining terms that are at the ontological, epistemological, and methodological core of epidemiology, and (2) in selecting and defining terms that are near or within disciplines with which epidemiology maintains vital interactions—vital for epidemiology, the other disciplines, science, and society.

These I take to be facts: today research methods with strong epidemiological roots, dimensions, and properties are fruitfully applied "within" and "outside" epidemiology.[7,23-25] A positive blurring of the boundaries of epidemiological research methods occurred in the last decades of the last century; for example, the integration of population thinking and group comparison into clinical and public health research.[7,10] The expansion of this influence toward other research areas remains a significant—and in my view highly attractive—challenge for many scientists. Such an expansion of influence will not be identical to what occurred via clinical epidemiology and, later, evidence-based medicine (and today evidence-based health care). The nature of the hypotheses at stake is often quite different in clinical medicine than in, say, molecular biology or proteomics. Largely because of this ontological fact, because biotechnologies generate different types and amounts of information and research, and for other reasons, today epidemiological thinking continues to create new approaches, research designs, strategies of analysis, and ways to assess causality for such microbiological disciplines.[26] Thus the influence of epidemiology continues. The potential to improve the health of citizens is there. In fact, the rationale for task (2) mentioned above also includes the relevance of epidemiological methods for research on the public health problems that are best tackled by blending the reasoning and tools of epidemiology and of some of the social sciences. Therefore, this new edition aims at being useful again not only to classic epidemiological and clinical research, but would also like to continue favoring the integration of epidemiology into "microbiological" and "macrosocial" health research and practice. I am confident that much of this is already happening, and thus feel this book is rather in harmony with most of the contemporary scientific world: wide open and interconnected—much more creative, relevant, efficient, and interesting because of the porousness and plasticity of the disciplines than because of the putative higher mission or language of their leaders and disciples.[24,27-29]

In short, if you live in a foreign land and have come to visit this book from "outside" epidemiology, be welcome. If you are an epidemiologist on the eve of a "trip" to a foreign discipline, please take this book with you. And, again, if you mostly work "inside" epidemiology, please keep it at hand: this is your territory—yet I hope you will here discover new landscapes of unsuspected beauty.

Miquel Porta
Barcelona and Ransol
January 2014

Acknowledgments

···

IT IS A PLEASURE AND A PRIVILEGE TO THANK EACH AND ALL INDIVIDUALS throughout the world who volunteered to contribute terms, definitions, or other ideas for this dictionary: I immensely enjoyed such a large, diverse, and creative group of coauthors. Thanks! I trust you will understand that we could not always make all your scientific, linguistic, and lexicographic dreams come true. I very much hope you will have fun skimming and thinking through the pages that follow.

It is equally a joy and an honor to thank all members of the International Epidemiological Association (IEA) and, in their name, past presidents Rodolfo Saracci, Charles du V. Florey, Chitr Sitthi-Amorn, Jørn Olsen, Neil Pearce, and Cesar Victora for their intellectual stimulus, personal encouragement, and institutional support in editing this book. Our warm memories and gratitude are also with and for Patricia Buffler, whose academic legacy is also part of this book, and whose brightest students at Berkeley feature among the contributors of this edition thanks to Pat.

Also sadly deceased at a young age during the making of this book was Rosa Colomer, whose world-level work in terminology from TermCat[30] was a precious inspiration, and highly useful technically—thanks to Jordi Bover as well.

I also feel extremely fortunate that John Last (University of Ottawa), Sander Greenland (UCLA), Miguel A. Hernán (Harvard), and Isabel dos Santos Silva (London School of Hygiene and Tropical Medicine) accepted the invitation to act as associate editors: a lot in this volume is due to Isabel, Miguel, Sander and John. It is also my pleasure to thank the following colleagues for their thoughtful intellectual and practical contributions, some made speedily and when it seemed impossible to achieve further clarity for particularly complex or new terms: Mauricio Barreto, Xavier Basagaña, George Davey-Smith, Charles du V. Florey, Matthias Egger, Caroline Fall, John Ioannidis, Daniel Kotz, Esa Läärä, Ricard Meneu, Alfredo Morabia, Jørn Olsen, Neil Pearce, Ezra Susser, Jan Vandenbroucke, Tyler VanderWeele, Cesar Victora, Ester Villalonga, Vasya Vlassov, and Chris Wild. Many of the ideas on and actual drawings of the new figures of this edition are due to Mati Rahu and Jordi Blanch, to whom I also express my appreciation. For what I have made of the advice of all contributors, and for any errors, I alone am responsible.

A huge amount of highly complex and fragile editorial material was sensitively and efficiently handled by Andrea Burón, whose intelligence, skill, kindness, and *alegría* I have seldom found in my professional life: *moltes gràcies*, Andrea.

Excellent editorial assistance was also provided by Tomas Lopez, Magda Gasull, Jose Pumarega, Sergio Sanz, and Yolanda Rovira; I am grateful for their daily patience and hard work. I am also happy to express my gratitude to Maria Dolors and Jaume Calvó i Casal from Ca'n Soldevila up in Els Plans; they know why. Some operational costs of this edition were absorbed in our budget at the Hospital del Mar Institute of Medical Research (IMIM) and at the Universitat Autònoma de Barcelona, for which I am also obliged.

Like countless other human beings for centuries, I continue to treasure a love —both emotional and practical— for books. I am thus happy to acknowledge the professionals at Oxford University Press, who with their outstanding editorial competence and wisdom also *made* this book. I dedicate it to the youngest generation of health scientists and advocates. And to Júlia, Joan, and Anna, with deep gratitude, admiration, and love.

M. P.

....

Alphabetical Listing

The alphabetical listing is a guide to the placement of entries and follows a letter-by-letter sequence of headwords without regard to word spacing, hyphens, or apostrophes. For example:

Case classification
Case-cohort study
Case collateral
Case-comparison study
Case-control study
Case-crossover study
Case definition
Case fatality rate

Headwords

Headwords (terms) are in **BOLD SMALL CAPITALS**. If there are several varieties of a concept, such as *bias*, all are listed alphabetically under the headword **BIAS**; but when customary epidemiological usage places an adjective before the headword, the alphabetical listing is usually a cross-reference to the entry where the definition is to be found. Thus **BIAS, CONFOUNDING** leads the reader to the definition under **CONFOUNDING BIAS**. However, terms on the periphery of epidemiology are mostly located together under the pertinent headword. For example, most of those associated with *costs* appear under **COST**. When several logical options were feasible, we avoided the automatic "solution" and chose the one we deemed most practical for the reader's mind and needs.

Compound Phrases

Epidemiology has many compound phrases, not all of which have an obvious headword. Thus *rare-disease assumption* is found under **RARE-DISEASE ASSUMPTION**, not under disease.

Bibliographic Citations

In the previous, fifth edition all citations of articles and books made in the definitions and comments on terms were moved to the back of the book, and this is again the case now (see pages 307–343). This decision allows to avoid repetition—most books and articles are cited several times—, and to present the definition and comments without the interference of the full references.

Importantly, most citations are just meant to invite or help the reader follow up on some of the other meanings, dimensions, levels, or implications of the definition and related ideas. They just aim to *evoke* or *suggest* further avenues of thought. Bibliographic citations need not be, cannot be, and are not exhaustive. None is meant to endorse the definition or the comment. No citation is meant either to imply that an article or book is the original or most authoritative source on the issue. Many cited books will offer additional ideas on the term and on related terms and concepts; this is particularly the case for definitions of terms on epidemiological methods. Some fundamental, auxiliary, or advanced books are cited either in the term definition (and then appear in the References, pages 307–343) or in the Bibliography (please see pages 301–306). Once again, it would be impossible and illogical to pretend to cite *all* books that might be relevant to a definition or comment. While we trust that the books, articles, and websites cited are indeed relevant, we are sure that many which are also relevant could not be cited, for obvious reasons.

Cross-References

Often, a definition—or part of the text commenting a TERM—includes a cross-reference to another term to be found elsewhere in the dictionary: such cross-references are in nonbold small capitals. Cross-references are again just meant to *suggest*—to invite the reader to take a look elsewhere in the book. If a highly related term is nearby (i.e., because of alphabetic order), the text is unlikely to mention it in nonbold small capitals; the eye will catch it (wide visual scopes: an undervalued strength of the printed book in expert hands). Cross-references need not be exhaustive and could never be so; if they were they'd become a nightmare labyrinth, not a seductive suggestion. They are not exhaustive: a term may have a definition in the book and yet not be marked in nonbold small capitals in the definition of another term; the two most common reasons for that are to avoid a baroque or visually confusing sentence, and, foremost, to elude *gardens of forking paths*. For the same intellectual, cognitive, aesthetic, and practical reasons, cross-references should never be automatically marked, not even as hyperlinks in a digital medium. To mark all cross-references and to do so automatically would be equally easy as wrong.

Other important words and phrases mentioned in a definition are sometimes italicized to draw attention to their special significance in relation to that particular term or to signify the absence of a cross-reference.

Definitions and Discussions

A brief definition generally appears at the beginning of each entry. This usually follows dictionary conventions and is a statement of the meaning rather than an explanation. An explanation will often follow, and then some remarks, a brief discussion, and, occasionally, illustrative examples and a comment on the provenance of the term. Explicit admonitions and cautionary notes about use and abuse of terms have been kept to a minimum.

Acronyms

There is no generally agreed way to pronounce or print acronyms, but some usages are commonly agreed. Thus, for instance, WHO is always spelled out in pronunciation ("W-H-O"), never pronounced "Hoo." By contrast, AIDS is always pronounced "Aids" and never spelled out. Acronyms can be made up of the initial letters of the words on which they are based, such as NIOSH (National Institute for Occupational Safety and Health, pronounced "Ny-osh"), or on parts of words or abbreviations, such as QUANGO (quasi-autonomous nongovernmental organization). Acronyms can survive after the organization they signify has changed names; for example, UNICEF originally stood for United Nations International Children's Emergency Fund. This UN agency is now called the United Nations Children's Fund, but the acronym is unchanged. Generally, all the letters of an acronym are upper case, even when not all the letters are initial letters of individual words; so, ANOVA (analysis of variance) is spelled as here, not AnOVa, although Anova is sometimes seen.

During the past 20 years the Internet has increasingly allowed to reliably identify the meaning of many acronyms. Hence, in the present edition we suppressed almost all acronyms included in previous editions. Thus, for instance, SER was suppressed; in some previous editions it referred to the Society for Epidemiologic Research (www.epiresearch.org). SEER (Surveillance, Epidemiology and End Results, a program of the U.S. National Cancer Institute) was also deleted. Similarly, ACE (American College of Epidemiology, http://acepidemiology.org) was also removed. By the way, with Sander Greenland we also decided against mentioning that ACE also refers to a statistical method called *Alternating Conditional Expectations*, since we did not wish to burden the dictionary with entries for every special statistical technique. Many such choices had to be made to avoid a too extensive, expensive, and specialized book. We hope we struck a balance most of the time. Acronyms and full names of studies (e.g., NHANES, Framingham Study) were also deleted in this edition. We did retain and update acronyms of guidelines of worldwide importance (e.g., CONSORT; PRISMA; STROBE; TREND).

Evolving Language and Changing Usage

English and its common, technical, and scientific varieties are rapidly evolving, as now do many societies, cultures, and epistemic communities worldwide — foremost, perhaps, the Internet and the virtual / real *global society*. A simple example: the meaning of *E-book* in the first five editions (from 1983 to 2008: 25 years) became obsolete; it is no longer a method of recording encounters used in primary medical care (but do let me preserve the 55-year-old article for us all: "organized curiosity").[31] And, of course, a completely new meaning emerged with electronic publishing. In addition to *E-book, Hollerith cards, punch card, spreadsheet*, and *jargon* are also examples of words that we deleted to make place for terms more current, relevant, and closely related to epidemiology.

Speaking of which, and of some human leanings that never change much, I am afraid the definition of *jargon* by Edmond Murphy, reproduced by John Last in the preface of earlier editions of this dictionary, is still worth keeping in mind:

"Obscure and/or pretentious language, circumlocutions, invented meanings, and pomposity delighted in for its own sake."[32]

I hope we avoided much of this.

Words such as *gay, computer,* and *Internet* were still defined in the fourth edition (of 2001), but no longer in the fifth (2008). We did not remove *PLAs* (persons living with AIDS). We aimed at respecting all scientific, democratic, and reasonable sensitivities, and we found no major difficulties in doing so while at the same time maximizing precision and minimizing ambiguity.

Scope

A couple of additional remarks on the scope of this work. Epidemiology continues to expand and bud off subspecialties, each of which has, in part, its own vocabulary, creating its own neologisms. Epidemiology regularly absorbs, transforms, embodies, codes for, and expresses terms from other fields: as a living organism, it actively metabolizes language. We have tried to capture and present the essential terminology of clinical, environmental, social, genetic, and molecular epidemiology as well as core terms from subspecialties of epidemiology such as pediatric epidemiology, pharmacoepidemiology, and some others. Of course, we did not wish to lengthen the book too much, as mentioned. Thus, the reader seeking definitions of highly specialized terms will need to go to the specialty books, articles, and websites.

As mentioned in several term entries below, epidemiology studies *all types* of diseases, health-related events, and health determinants in populations; hence, this dictionary includes just some examples of definitions for a few disease-based branches or subspecialties of epidemiology.

Some common everyday words are defined and discussed because they often occur in epidemiological articles with a distinct meaning, because they are particularly relevant to conducting health research, or because their sense is not always clear in these contexts to people whose first language is not English. Words and expressions from disciplines that overlap or interact with epidemiology are defined here for the same reasons.

What Is New?

Thorough as all past revisions have been, this sixth edition contains the most profound changes that the dictionary ever experienced. The fundamental reason is that a methodological "revolution" is ongoing. It is deeply changing how we conceive epidemiological and clinical research, and how we assess the validity of findings, to say the least. It is having an immense impact on the production of scientific evidence in the health sciences, and on most policies, programs, services, and products in which such evidence is used, affecting thousands of institutions, organizations, and companies, and millions of people.

There is no quick way to explain this. But a real way to understand what is happening is to read the fundamental changes that this book contains, and if you wish, to keep on reading the suggested references. The new ideas partly or completely change basic concepts such as, for example, risk, rate, risk ratio, attributable fraction, bias, selection bias, confounding, residual confounding, interaction, cumulative and density sampling, open population, test hypothesis, null hypothesis, causal null, causal inference, Berkson's bias, Simpson's paradox, frequentist statistics, generalizability, representativeness, missing data, standardization, or overadjustment. They are also reflected in recent and new terms as collider, M-bias, causal diagram, backdoor (biasing path), instrumental variable, negative controls, inverse probability weighting, identifiability, transportability, positivity, ignorability, collapsibility, exchangeable, g-estimation, marginal structural models, risk set, immortal time bias, Mendelian randomization, nonmonotonic, counterfactual outcome, potential outcome, sample space, or false discovery rate.

The scope of this sixth edition has also broadened with definitions of methods for clinical research, public health practice, genetics, and the social sciences. There are new terms from biostatistics, clinical epidemiology, preventive medicine, health promotion, and behavioral sciences; environmental, life course, and social epidemiology; genetic and molecular epidemiology; health economics; and bioethics. In addition, scientific terms relevant to professionals in clinical medicine, public health, and the other health, life, and social sciences are included.

Pledge

We have tried to be highly rigorous intellectually and formally, clear, stimulating, systematic, thorough, and to a reasonable extent explicit and transparent. Yet, when necessary, these goals gave precedence to the primary objective: that the dictionary should be accurate, practical, and plural, and that it should encourage critical and creative thinking. I will amend any errors that are brought to my attention, and I will be glad to consider with all respect any suggestions that are rigorous, relevant, constructive, and potentially useful to most readers.

M. P.

Contributors to the Fourth, Fifth and Sixth Editions

PREBEN AAVITSLAND
  Kristiansand, Norway
IBRAHIM ABDELNOUR
  Damascus, Syria
THEO ABELIN
  Berne, Switzerland
AMAN-OLONIYO ABIMBOLA
  Abuja, Nigeria
VICTOR ABRAIRA
  Madrid, Spain
JOE ABRAMSON
  Jerusalem, Israel
ANDERS AHLBOM
  Stockholm, Sweden
NEAL ALEXANDER
  London, England, UK
MOHAMED FAROUK ALLAM
  Córdoba, Spain
ÁLVARO ALONSO
  Minneapolis, Minnesota, USA
JORDI ALONSO
  Barcelona, Catalonia, Spain
DOUGLAS ALTMAN
  London, England, UK
JANET BYRON ANDERSON
  Rocky River, Ohio, USA
KUNIO AOKI
  Nagoya, Japan
ONYEBUCHI ARAH
  Los Angeles, USA
HAROUTUNE ARMENIAN
  *Baltimore, Maryland, USA,
  and Yerevan, Armenia*
SHABNAM ASGHARI
  St. John's, Canada
MARY JANE ASHLEY
  Toronto, Ontario, Canada
ALEKSEI BABURIN
  Tallinn, Estonia

JOHN BAILAR III
  Chicago, Illinois, USA
MICHAEL BAKER
  Wellington, New Zealand
MAURICIO BARRETO
  Salvador, Bahia, Brazil
ALUÍSIO J. D. BARROS
  Pelotas, Brazil
XAVIER BASAGAÑA
  Barcelona, Catalonia, Spain
OLGA BASSO
  Aarhus, Denmark
RENALDO BATTISTA
  Montreal, Quebec, Canada
ROBERT BEAGLEHOLE
  Auckland, New Zealand
STELLA BECKMAN
  Berkeley, California, USA
SOLOMON BENATAR
  Cape Town, South Africa
FERNANDO G. BENAVIDES
  Barcelona, Catalonia, Spain
YOAV BEN-SHLOMO
  Bristol, England, UK
ROGER BERNIER
  Atlanta, Georgia, USA
SILVINA BERRA
  Córdoba, Argentina
RAJ BHOPAL
  Edinburgh, Scotland, UK
NICHOLAS BIRKETT
  Ottawa, Ontario, Canada
JORDI BLANCH
  Girona, Catalonia, Spain
DANKMAR BÖHNING
  Berlin, Germany
JEAN-FRANÇOIS BOIVIN
  Montreal, Quebec, Canada

FRANCISCO BOLÚMAR
  Madrid, Spain
DAVID BONIFACE
  London, England, UK
KNUT BORCH-JOHNSEN
  Horsholm, Denmark
RIC BOUVIER
  Kew, Victoria, Australia
ANNETTE BRAUNACK-MAYER
  Adelaide, South Australia, Australia
CLIVE BROWN
  Port of Spain, Trinidad and Tobago
ROSS BROWNSON
  St. Louis, Missouri, USA
JIM BUTLER
  Canberra, ACT, Australia
LEE CAPLAN
  Atlanta, Georgia, USA
IAIN CHALMERS
  Oxford, England, UK
YUE CHEN
  Ottawa, Ontario, Canada
BERNARD CHOI
  Ottawa, Ontario, Canada
STELLA CHUNGONG
  Geneva, Switzerland
MIKE CLARKE
  Oxford, England, UK
TAMMY CLIFFORD
  London, Ontario, Canada
ALISON COHEN
  Berkeley, California, USA
PHILIP COLE
  Birmingham, Alabama, USA
DEBORAH COOK
  Hamilton, Ontario, Canada
DOUG COYLE
  Ottawa, Ontario, Canada
ANDREW CREESE
  Geneva, Switzerland
GIOVANNA CRUZ
  Berkeley, California, USA
NANCY CZAICKI
  Berkeley, California, USA
GEORGE DAVEY SMITH
  Bristol, England, UK

SILVIA DECLICH
  Rome, Italy
DEL DE HART
  Saginaw, Michigan, USA
JULIA DEL AMO
  Madrid, Spain
N. S. DEODHAR
  Pune, India
BOB DOUGLAS
  Canberra, ACT, Australia
GERARD DUBOIS
  Amiens, France
JOHN DUFFUS
  Edinburgh, Scotland, UK
KATE DUNN
  Keele, Newcastle, UK
SHAH EBRAHIM
  London, England, UK
MATTHIAS EGGER
  Bern, Switzerland
EMON ELBOUDWAREJ
  Berkeley, California, USA
MARK ELWOOD
  Melbourne, Victoria, Australia
LEON EPSTEIN
  Jerusalem, Israel
CAROLINE H.D. FALL
  Southampton, England, UK
ALVAN FEINSTEIN
  New Haven, Connecticut, USA
CHARLES DU V. FLOREY
  Sidmouth, England, UK
STEPHEN FRANCIS
  Berkeley, California, USA
ERICA FRANK
  Atlanta, Georgia, USA
RAYNER FRETZEL-BEHME
  Bremen, Germany
GARY FRIEDMAN
  Oakland, California, USA
ANA M. GARCIA
  Valencia, Spain
B. BURT GERSTMAN
  San Jose, California, USA
MILENA GIANFRANCESCO
  Berkeley, California, USA

ALAN GIBBS
  Manchester, England, UK
PHILIPPE GRANDJEAN
  Odense, Denmark
NICOLA GRANDY
  Paris, France
SANDER GREENLAND
  Los Angeles, California, USA
DUANE GUBLER
  Atlanta, Georgia, USA
CHARLES GUEST
  Canberra, ACT, Australia
TEE GUIDOTTI
  Washington, DC, USA
GORDON GUYATT
  Hamilton, Ontario, Canada
MATTI HAKAMA
  Tampere, Finland
TIMO HAKULINEN
  Helsinki, Finland
PHILIP HALL
  Winnipeg, Manitoba, Canada
PHILIP HANNAFORD
  Aberdeen, Scotland, UK
SUSAN HARRIS
  Boston, Massachusetts, USA
MAUREEN HATCH
  New York, New York, USA
BRIAN HAYNES
  Hamilton, Ontario, Canada
MIGUEL A. HERNÁN
  Boston, Massachusetts, USA
ILDEFONSO HERNÁNDEZ
  Maó, Menorca, and Alacant, Spain
SONIA HERNÁNDEZ-DIAZ
  Boston, Massachusetts, USA
ANDREW HERXHEIMER
  Edinburgh, Scotland, UK
BASIL HETZEL
  Adelaide, South Australia, Australia
ALAN HINMAN
  Decatur, Georgia, USA
WALTER HOLLAND
  London, England, UK
MARÍA-GRACIELA HOLLM-DELGADO
  Montreal, Quebec, Canada

D'ARCY HOLMAN
  Perth, Western Australia, Australia
ERNEST HOOK
  Berkeley, California, USA
JEFFREY HOUSE
  San Francisco, California, USA
JOHN P. A. IOANNIDIS
  Stanford, California, USA, and
  Ioannina, Greece
MASAKO IWANAGA
  Tokyo, Japan
KONRAD JAMROZIK
  Perth, Western Australia, Australia
MOHSEN JANGHORBANI
  Isfahan, Iran
TOM JEFFERSON
  Camberley, England, UK
MILOS JENICEK
  Rockwood, Ontario, Canada
ROSE KAGAWA
  Berkeley, California, USA
DEB KARASEK
  Berkeley, California, USA
WILFRIED KARMAUS
  Columbia, South Carolina, USA
SURAJ KHANAL
  Norfolk, USA
MUSTAFA KHOGALI
  Beirut, Lebanon
DANIEL KIM
  Boston, Massachusetts, USA
MAURICE KING
  Leeds, England, UK
TORD KJELLSTRÖM
  Auckland, New Zealand
ROSEMARY KORDA
  Canberra, ACT, Australia
DANIEL KOTZ
  Maastricht, Netherlands
DAN KREWSKI
  Ottawa, Ontario, Canada
NINO KÜNZLI
  Basel, Switzerland
DIANA KUH
  London, England, UK

ESA LÄÄRÄ
Oulu, Finland

CHANDRAKANT LAHARIYA,
New Delhi, India

STEPHEN LAMBERT
Melbourne, Victoria, Australia

HENK LAMBERTS
Amsterdam, Netherlands

RON LAPORTE
Pittsburgh, Pennsylvania, USA

JOHN LAST
Ottawa, Ontario, Canada

DIANA LAUDERDALE
Chicago, Illinois, USA

DUK-HEE LEE
Daegu, Korea

ABBY LIPPMAN
Montreal, Quebec, Canada

IRVINE LOUDON
Oxford, England, UK

TAPIO LUOSTARINEN
Oulu, Finland

SHI LUYAN
Wuhan, China

OUTI LYYTIKÄINEN
Helsinki, Finland

JOHAN MACKENBACH
Rotterdam, Netherlands

AHMED MANDIL
Alexandria, Egypt

ARTURO MARTÍ-CARVAJAL
Valencia, Venezuela

JOHN McCALLUM
Canberra, ACT, Australia

IAN McDOWELL
Ottawa, Ontario, Canada

ROBERT McKEOWN
Columbia, South Carolina, USA

RICK McLEAN
Melbourne, Victoria, Australia

TONY McMICHAEL
Canberra, ACT, Australia

CURTIS MEINERT
Baltimore, Maryland, USA

RICARD MENEU
Valencia, Spain

JUAN MERLO
Lund, Sweden

JAIME MIRANDA
Lima, Perú

DAVID MOHER
Ottawa, Ontario, Canada

ALFREDO MORABIA
New York, New York, USA

SALAH MOSTAFA
Cairo, Egypt

KIUMARSS NASSERI
Santa Barbara, California, USA

ANA NAVAS-ACIEN
Baltimore, Maryland, USA

NORMAN NOAH
London, England, UK

PATRICIA O'CAMPO
Baltimore, Maryland, USA

JØRN OLSEN
Aarhus, Denmark

NIGEL PANETH
Ann Arbor, Michigan, USA

TONI PATAMA
Helsinki, Finland

SKIP PAYNE
Tiffin, Ohio, USA

NEIL PEARCE
London, England, UK, and Wellington, New Zealand

SUSANA PEREZ-GUTTHANN
Barcelona, Catalonia, Spain

DIANA PETITTI
Sierra Madre, California, USA

AILEEN PLANT
Perth, Western Australia, Australia

MIQUEL PORTA
Barcelona, Catalonia, Spain

EERO PUKKALA
Helsinki, Finland

HEDLEY QUINTANA
Stockholm, Sweden

ZORAN RADOVANOVIC
Belgrade, Yugoslavia

MATI RAHU
Tallinn, Estonia

GLORIA RAMIREZ
Santiago de Chile, Chile

ARINDAM RAY
New Delhi, India

JOSE RIGAU
  Atlanta, Georgia, USA
CHRIS RISSELL
  Sydney, New South Wales, Australia
STEFAN RÖDER
  Leipzig, Germany
ALFONSO RODRIGUEZ-MORALES
  Pereira, Colombia
KEN ROTHMAN
  Boston, Massachusetts, USA
MICHAEL RYAN
  Geneva, Switzerland
LUCIE RYCHETNIK
  Sydney, New South Wales, Australia
RODOLFO SARACCI
  Lyon, France, and Pisa, Italy
SEPPO SARNA
  Helsinki, Finland
DAVID SAVITZ
  New York, New York, USA
PATHOM SAWANPANYALERT
  Bangkok, Thailand
SABINE SCHIPF
  Hamburg, Germany
FRAN SCOTT
  Hamilton, Ontario, Canada
PIPPA SCOTT
  Bern, Switzerland
ANDREU SEGURA
  Barcelona, Catalonia, Spain
JACK SIEMIATYCKI
  Laval, Quebec, Canada
GUSTAVO A. SILVA
  Geneve, Sweden
ISABEL DOS SANTOS SILVA
  London, England, UK
CHITR SITTHI-AMORN
  Bangkok, Thailand
BJÖRN SMEDBY
  Uppsala, Sweden
ROBBIE SNYDER
  Berkeley, California, USA
CYNTHIA SONICH-MULLIN
  Paris, France
COLIN SOSKOLNE
  Edmonton, Alberta, Canada

BOB SPASOFF
  Ottawa, Ontario, Canada
HANS STORM
  Copenhagen, Denmark
DAVID STREINER
  Hamilton, Ontario, Canada
EZRA SUSSER
  New York, New York, USA
MERVYN SUSSER
  New York, New York, USA
KAZUO TAJIMA
  Nagoya, Japan
JOSÉ A. TAPIA
  Ann Arbor, Michigan, USA
MICHEL THURIAUX
  Geneva, Switzerland
AURELIO TOBÍAS
  Barcelona, Catalonia, Spain
BERNARD TOMA
  Maisons-Alfort, France
KAREN TROLLOPE-KUMAR
  Hamilton, Ontario, Canada
ELENA TSCHISHOWA
  Berlin, Germany
JAN VANDENBROUCKE
  Utrecht, Netherlands
TYLER VANDERWEELE
  Boston, Massachusetts, USA
FRANK VAN HARTINGSVELD
  Amsterdam, Netherlands
HECTOR VELASCO
  *Baltimore, Maryland, USA, and
  Cuernavaca, Mexico*
SALLY VERNON
  Houston, Texas, USA
CESAR G. VICTORA
  Pelotas, Brazil
ESTER VILLALONGA
  *Maó, Menorca, Spain, and
  Boston, Massachusetts, USA*
PAOLO VINEIS
  London, England, UK
ANNA-MAIJA VIRTALA
  Helsinki, Finland
VASILY VLASSOV
  Moscow, Russia

DIVYA VOHRA
Berkeley, California, USA
DOUGLAS L. WEED
Salt Lake City, Utah, USA
PAUL WESSON
Berkeley, California, USA
DENISE WERKER
Ottawa, Ontario, Canada
CLAES-GÖRAN WESTRIN
Uppsala, Sweden
AMANDA WHEELER
Berkeley, California, USA
FRANK WHITE
Karachi, Pakistan
KERR WHITE
Charlottesville, Virginia, USA
MARTIN WHITE
Newcastle, *UK*
P. AUKE WIEGERSMA
Groningen, Netherlands

DON WIGLE
Ottawa, Ontario, Canada
ALLEN WILCOX
Research Triangle Park, North Carolina, USA
CHRISTOPHER P. WILD
Lyon, France
KATHLEEN WINTER
Berkeley, California, USA
MICHAEL WOLFSON
Ottawa, Ontario, Canada
CAROLINE WOOD
London, England, UK
HIROSHI YANAGAWA
Jiichi, Japan
KUE YOUNG
Winnipeg, Manitoba, Canada

References

1. Berkman Center for Internet & Society at Harvard University. Internet Monitor 2013. Reflections on the Digital World. Boston, December 11, 2013. http://cyber.law.harvard.edu/publications/2013/reflections_on_the_digital_world

2. http://en.wikipedia.org/wiki/Android_%28operating_system%29#Market_share; http://blogs.wsj.com/corporate-intelligence/2014/02/19/facebooks-whatsapp-price-tag-19-billion; http://investor.fb.com/releasedetail.cfm?ReleaseID=821954.

3. Evans JP, Mesliin EM, Marteau TM, et al. Genomics: deflating the genomic bubble. Science 2011; 331: 861–862.

4. Porta M, Hernández-Aguado I, Lumbreras B, et al. "Omics" research, monetization of intellectual property and fragmentation of knowledge: can clinical epidemiology strengthen integrative research? J Clin Epidemiol 2007; 60: 1220–1225.

5. Trouble at the lab: unreliable research. The Economist 2013 (Oct 19). http://www.economist.com/node/21588057/comments.

6. Norman G. Description and prescription in dictionaries of scientific terms. Int J Lexicography 2002; 15: 259–276.

7. Porta M, Vandenbroucke JP, Ioannidis JPA, et al. Trends in citations to books on epidemiological and statistical methods in the biomedical literature. PLoS ONE 2013; 8(5): e61837.

8. Rothman KJ, Stein Z, Susser M. Rebuilding bridges: what is the real role of social class in disease occurrence? Eur J Epidemiol 2011; 26: 431–432.

9. Porta M. Las quiero a morir. Claves de Razón Práctica [Madrid] 2013(226): 172–179.

10. Porta M, Fernandez E, Bolúmar F. The "bibliographic impact factor" and the still uncharted sociology of epidemiology. Int J Epidemiol 2006; 35: 1130–1135.

11. Kahneman D. Thinking, Fast and Slow. New York: Farrar, Straus and Giroux; 2011.

12. Gould SJ. The Hedgehog, the Fox and the Magister's Pox. Mending and Minding the Misconceived Gap Between Science and the Humanities. London: Vintage; 2004.

13. Manguel A. A History of Reading. New York: Penguin Putnam; 1996.

14. Porta M. Do we really need "real" epidemiological scientific meetings?. Eur J Epidemiol 2003; 18: 101–103.

15. Amsterdamska O. Demarcating epidemiology. Science Technology & Human Values 2005; 30: 17–51.

16. Rothman KJ, Greenland S, Lash TL, eds. Modern Epidemiology. 3rd. ed. Philadelphia: Lippincott-Raven; 2008.

17. Miettinen OS. Theoretical Epidemiology. Principles of Occurrence Research in Medicine. New York: Wiley; 1985.

18. Greenland S, ed. Evolution of Epidemiologic Ideas. Annotated Readings on Concepts and Methods. Chestnut Hill, MA: Epidemiology Resources; 1987.

19. Susser M, Stein Z. Eras in Epidemiology. The Evolution of Ideas. New York: Oxford University Press; 2009.

20. Almeida-Filho N. La Ciencia Tímida. Ensayos de Deconstrucción de la Epidemiología. Buenos Aires: Lugar; 2000.

21. Morabia A. A History of Epidemiologic Methods and Concepts. Basel: Birkhäuser / Springer; 2004.

22. Holland WW, Olsen J, du V Florey C, eds. The Development of Modern Epidemiology. Personal Reports from Those Who Were There. New York: Oxford University Press; 2007.

23. Porta M, Alvarez-Dardet C. Epidemiology: bridges over (and across) roaring levels [Editorial]. J Epidemiol Community Health 1998; 52: 605.

24. Bolúmar F, Porta M. Epidemiologic methods: beyond clinical medicine, beyond epidemiology. Eur J Epidemiol 2004; 19: 733–735.

25. Fine P, Goldacre B, Haines A. Epidemiology—a science for the people. Lancet 2013; 381: 1249–1252.

26. Geneletti SG, Gallo V, Porta M, et al. Assessing causal relationships in genomics: From Bradford-Hill criteria to complex gene-environment interactions and directed acyclic graphs. Emerg Themes Epidemiol 2011; 8: 5. http://www.ete-online.com/content/8/1/5

27. Rockström J, Steffen W, Noone K, et al. A safe operating space for humanity. Nature 2009; 461: 472–475.

28. Feinberg AP. Phenotypic plasticity and the epigenetics of human disease. Nature 2007; 447: 433–440.

29. Gluckman PD, Hanson MA, Bateson P, et al. Towards a new developmental synthesis: adaptive developmental plasticity and human disease. Lancet 2009; 373: 1654–1657.

30. http://www.termcat.cat/en.

31. Eimerl TS. Organized curiosity. A practical approach to the problem of keeping records for research purposes in general practice. J Coll Gen Pract 1960; 3: 246-252; and J Coll Gen Pract 1961; 4: 628-636.

32. Murphy EA. The Logic of Medicine. Baltimore: Johns Hopkins University Press; 1976. p. 16.

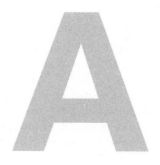

ABATEMENT The process of reducing or minimizing public health or other types of dangers and nuisances, usually supported by regulation or legislation; e.g., noise abatement, pollution abatement.

ABC APPROACH "Abstinence, Be faithful, use Condoms." ABC strategies are promoted to combat, foremost, infection with HIV and the HIV / AIDS PANDEMIC, as well as other sexually transmitted diseases. Pragmatic sex education policies that aim at balancing abstinence-only sex education by including education about safe sex and birth control methods. Excessive emphasis on ABC strategies may marginalize broader, integrated programs. See also CNN APPROACH.

ABORTION RATE The estimated annual number of abortions per 1000 women of reproductive age (usually defined as ages 15–44).

ABORTION RATIO The estimated number of abortions per 100 live births in a given year.

ABSCISSA The distance along the horizontal coordinate, or x axis, of a point P from the vertical or y axis of a graph. See also AXIS; GRAPH; ORDINATE.

ABSENTEEISM Habitual failure to appear for work or other regular duty. Contrast with SICKNESS ABSENCE and PRESENTEEISM.

ABSOLUTE EFFECT The effect of an exposure (expressed as the difference between rates, proportions, means), of the outcome, etc., as opposed to the ratio of these measures.[1-3] See also RISK DIFFERENCE.

ABSOLUTE POVERTY LEVEL Income level below which a minimum nutritionally adequate diet plus essential nonfood requirements is not affordable.[4] The amount of income a person, family, or group needs to purchase an absolute amount of the basic necessities of life. See also RELATIVE POVERTY LEVEL.

ABSOLUTE RATE See RATE.

ABSOLUTE RISK (AR) The probability of an event (usually adverse, but it may also be beneficial) in a CLOSED POPULATION over a specified time interval. The number of events in a group divided by the total number of subjects in that group.[1,5-8] This usage presumes the population is a COHORT. AR is not a synonym of ATTRIBUTABLE FRACTION, EXCESS RISK, or RISK DIFFERENCE. See also RISK.

ABSOLUTE RISK INCREASE (ARI) The absolute risk of adverse events in the exposed or treatment group (ART) minus the absolute risk of events in the control group (ARC): ARI = ART–ARC. Same as RISK DIFFERENCE. Also, the proportion of treated persons who experience an adverse event minus the proportion of untreated persons who experience the event. See also NUMBER NEEDED TO HARM.

1

ABSOLUTE RISK REDUCTION (ARR) The absolute risk of events in the control group (ARC) minus the absolute risk of events in the exposed or treatment group (ART): ARR = ARC–ART. The negative of the RISK DIFFERENCE. Also, the proportion of untreated persons who experience an adverse event minus the proportion of treated persons who experience this event.

The reciprocal of the ARR is the NUMBER NEEDED TO TREAT (NNT). The ARR is one measure of the strength of an association. It varies with the underlying risk of an event; e.g., it becomes smaller when event rates are low. The ARR is higher and the NNT lower in groups with higher absolute risks.[9,10] See also HILL'S CONSIDERATIONS FOR CAUSATION; MEASURE OF ASSOCIATION; PROBABILITY OF CAUSATION; RELATIVE RISK REDUCTION.

ACCELERATED FAILURE-TIME MODEL A model for survival analysis that models the relation between exposure (or treatment) and survival time. For example, if the probability of being alive at time t is $S_0(t)$ under no exposure, then the probability for exposed individuals is

$$S(t) = S_0(t / \gamma)$$

where γ quantifies how much the survival expands (or contracts) under exposure. Thus, if γ is 0.25, the survival time would be four times longer than under conditions of nonexposure. Contrast with PROPORTIONAL HAZARDS MODEL, which models the relation between exposure and the hazard.[1,7,11]

ACCEPTABLE RISK Risk that appears tolerable to some group. Risk that has minimal or long-term detrimental effects or for which the benefits outweigh the hazards.[12-14] See also CLINICAL DECISION ANALYSIS; HEALTH TECHNOLOGY ASSESSMENT.

ACCEPTANCE SAMPLING (Syn: stop-or-go sampling) Sampling method that requires division of the "universe" population into groups or batches as they pass a specified time point (e.g., age) followed by sampling of individuals within the sampled groups.

ACCESS Potential and actual utilization of HEALTH CARE services.[15] The usage of health services, influenced by predisposing factors (e.g., age, health beliefs), enabling factors (e.g., family support, health insurance), and need (perceived and actual need for health care services).[16-19] The perceptions and experiences of people as to their ease in reaching health services or health facilities in terms of location, time, and ease of approach. See also GATEKEEPER; HEALTH EQUITY; SICKNESS "CAREER."

ACCESSORY RESERVOIR A reservoir that contributes to the maintenance of a pathogen in nature but is not the primary reservoir for such agent.[20-22] See also RESERVOIR OF INFECTION.

ACCIDENT An unanticipated event—commonly leading to INJURY or other harm—in traffic, the workplace, or a domestic, recreational, or other setting. The primary event in a sequence that leads ultimately to injury if that event is genuinely not predictable. Epidemiological studies have demonstrated that the risk of accidents is often predictable and that many accidents and DISASTERS are preventable.

ACCUMULATION OF RISK The extent of cumulative damage to biological systems as the number, duration, or severity of exposures increase, and as body systems age and become less able to repair damage. The notion that LIFE COURSE exposures or insults gradually accumulate through episodes of illness and injury, adverse environmental and social conditions, and health damaging BEHAVIORS. Exposures increasing risk of disease may be independent or clustered.[13,23,24] See also DEVELOPMENTAL AND LIFE COURSE EPIDEMIOLOGY; THRIFTY PHENOTYPE HYPOTHESIS.

ACCURACY

1. The degree to which a measurement or an estimate based on measurements represents the true value of the attribute that is being measured. Relative lack of ERROR. In statistics, accuracy is sometimes measured as the MEAN SQUARED ERROR.[1,6,25,26] See also DISCRIMINATORY ACCURACY; MEASUREMENT, TERMINOLOGY OF; PRECISION; VALIDITY, MEASUREMENT.

2. The ability of a DIAGNOSTIC test to correctly classify the presence or absence of the target disorder. The diagnostic accuracy of a test is usually expressed by its SENSITIVITY and SPECIFICITY.

ACQUAINTANCE NETWORK The internal and external connections, relationships, and dynamics of a group of persons in regular or sporadic contact or communication, among whom transmission of knowledge, infectious agents, healthy and toxic habits, BEHAVIOR, and VALUES is common and whose social interaction often has as well individual and public health implications.[27,28] See also CONTEXT; NETWORK; TRANSMISSION OF INFECTION.

ACQUIRED IMMUNODEFICIENCY SYNDROME (AIDS) (Syn: acquired immune deficiency syndrome) The late clinical stage of infection with HUMAN IMMUNODEFICIENCY VIRUS (HIV), recognized as a distinct syndrome in 1981. The opportunistic or indicator diseases associated with AIDS include certain protozoan and helminth infections, fungal infections, bacterial infections, viral infections, and some types of cancer. The role of AIDS as an indicator in SURVEILLANCE has diminished since the advent of HIGHLY ACTIVE ANTIRETROVIRAL THERAPY (HAART).

ACTIVE LIFE EXPECTANCY See DISABILITY-FREE LIFE EXPECTANCY.

ACTIVITIES OF DAILY LIVING (ADL) SCALE A scale devised to score physical ability/disability, used to measure outcomes of interventions for various chronic, disabling conditions, such as arthritis.[29] It is based on scores for responses to questions about mobility, self-care, grooming, etc. Refinements or variations of the ADL scale have been developed.[30]

ACTIVITY SETTING The places, events, routines, and patterns that structure the experience of everyday life; e.g., a classroom, a neighborhood resident meeting, a commuter train, family meals, a waiting room in a hospital. A unit through which culture and community are propagated across time.[31] See also BEHAVIOR SETTING; CONTEXT.

ACTUARIAL RATE See FORCE OF MORTALITY.

ACTUARIAL TABLE See LIFE TABLE.

ACUTE

1. Referring to a health effect: of sudden onset, often brief; not necessarily clinically severe.

2. Referring to an exposure: brief, intense, or short-term; sometimes specifically referring to a brief exposure of high intensity. Contrast with CHRONIC.

ADAPTATION

1. The process by which organisms surmount environmental challenges.[13,32,33] See also RESILIENCE.

2. A heritable component of the phenotype that confers an advantage in survival and reproductive success.

ADDITIVE MODEL A model in which the combined effect of several factors on an outcome measure (such as a RISK or RATE) is the sum of the effects that would be produced by each of the factors in the absence of the others. For example, if factor X adds x to risk in the absence of Y, and factor Y adds y to risk in the absence of X, an additive model states that the two factors together will add $(x + y)$ to risk.[1,7,8,34] See also INTERACTION; LINEAR MODEL; MATHEMATICAL MODEL; MULTIPLICATIVE MODEL.

ADHERENCE Health-related behavior that adheres to the recommendations of a physician, other health care provider, or investigator in a research project. The word *adherence* aims to avoid the authoritarian connotations of COMPLIANCE, formerly used to describe this BEHAVIOR. *Concordance* is another alternative.[1,6,9,35]

ADJUSTMENT A summarizing procedure for a statistical measure in which the effects of differences in composition of the populations being compared have been minimized by statistical methods.[5,24,36-38] Examples are adjustment by STANDARDIZATION, by STRATIFICATION, by REGRESSION ANALYSIS, by INVERSE-PROBABILITY WEIGHTING, by G-ESTIMATION, by PROPENSITY SCORES, or by some combination of these techniques.[1,2] Adjustment is often performed on an EFFECT MEASURE, commonly because of differing distributions of age, sex, education or other known risk factors in the populations being compared.[39-42,797] See also STANDARDIZATION.

ADULT LITERACY RATE The percentage of persons 15 years of age and over who can read and write.[4,43]

ADVERSE HEALTH EVENT Any unfavorable and unintended sign, symptom, disease, or other relevant health event associated with the use of a medical product or procedure, or that occurred during a research study, regardless of the causal relationship.[6,26,44,45] See also ASSOCIATION.

ADVERSE REACTION An undesirable or unwanted consequence of a preventive, DIAGNOSTIC TEST, or therapeutic procedure. See also SIDE EFFECT.

ADVERSE SELECTION A phenomenon of major theoretical concern in health insurance markets, which occurs when people with health-related characteristics different from those of the average person can choose the amount of health insurance they purchase. Individuals who expect high health care costs and utilization differentially tend to prefer more generous and expensive insurance plans, whereas individuals who expect low costs and utilization choose more moderate plans.[46] Insurers may end up with clients who are costlier than expected; they may thus raise the premium above what the low- and average-risk people are willing to pay.[7] See also ASYMMETRY OF INFORMATION.

AETIOLOGY, AETIOLOGICAL See ETIOLOGY.

AGE The duration of time that a person has lived, conventionally measured in completed years of life. The WHO recommends that age should be defined by completed units of time, counting the day of birth as zero. In epidemiology age is a common independent variable, as well as a CONFOUNDER. It may be important to distinguish "BIOLOGICAL AGE" from chronological age; for example, milestones of human growth and development such as onset of puberty or closure of epiphyses are delayed by malnutrition.[24] See also COHORT ANALYSIS.

AGE DEPENDENCY RATIO See DEPENDENCY RATIO.

AGENCY RELATIONSHIP A conceptual approach to describe the doctor-patient relationship, in which the physician acts as agent for the patient (or other client). Such relationship arises because of the ASYMMETRY OF INFORMATION between the doctor, who possesses superior medical information, and the patient, who possesses superior information on her preferences (e.g., on treatment options). A doctor working as a perfect agent would make the same decision as the patient would were the patient to be party to the same clinical expertise as the doctor. In many systems doctors are expected to act not only for the "patient," but also for "society" (e.g., for other patients, an organization, taxpayers).[47] See also SUPPLIER INDUCED DEMAND.

AGENT (OF DISEASE) A factor (e.g., microorganism, chemical substance, form of radiation, mechanical, behavioral, social agent or process) whose presence, excessive presence, or (in deficiency diseases) relative absence is essential for the occurrence of a disease. A disease may have a single agent, a number of independent alternative agents (at least one of which must be present), or a complex of two or more factors whose combined presence is essential for or contributes to the development of the disease or other outcome. See also CAUSALITY; NECESSARY CAUSE.

AGE–PERIOD–COHORT ANALYSIS See COHORT ANALYSIS.

AGE–SEX PYRAMID See POPULATION PYRAMID.

AGE–SEX REGISTER A list of all clients or patients of a medical practice or service, classified by age (birthdate) and sex; it provides denominators for calculating age- and sex-specific rates.

AGE-SPECIFIC FERTILITY RATE The number of live births occurring during a specified period to women of a specified age group divided by the number of person-years lived during that period by women of that age group. When an age-specific fertility rate is calculated for a calendar year, the number of live births to women of the specified age is usually divided by the midyear population of women of that age.

AGE-SPECIFIC RATE A RATE for a specified age group. The numerator and denominator refer to the same age group. Example:

$$\text{Age-specific death rate [age } (25-34)] = \frac{\text{number of deaths among residents age } 25-34 \text{ in an area in a year}}{\text{average (for midyear) population age } 25-34 \text{ in the area in that year}} \times 100,000$$

The multiplier (usually 100,000 or 1 million) is chosen to produce a rate that can be expressed as a convenient number.

AGE STANDARDIZATION A procedure for adjusting rates (e.g., death rates) designed to minimize the effects of differences in age composition in comparing rates for different populations.[1,3,26] See also ADJUSTMENT; STANDARDIZATION.

AGGREGATION BIAS (Syn: ecological bias) See AGGREGATIVE FALLACY; ECOLOGICAL FALLACY.

AGGREGATE SURVEILLANCE The surveillance of a disease or health event by collecting summary data on groups of cases (e.g., general practitioners taking part in SURVEILLANCE schemes are asked to report the number of cases of specified diseases seen over a specified period of time).[48,49]

AGGREGATIVE FALLACY An erroneous application to individuals of a causal relationship observed at the group level. A type of ECOLOGICAL FALLACY (sometimes just a synonym) and an antonym of the ATOMISTIC FALLACY.[3,5,50]

AGING OF THE POPULATION An increase over time in the proportion of older persons in a defined population. It does not necessarily imply an increase in life expectancy or that people are living longer than they used to. In the past, the principal cause of aging of populations has been a decline in the birthrate: in the absence of a rise in the death rate at higher ages, when fewer children are born than in prior years, the proportion of older persons in the population increases. Nowadays, in developed societies, little further mortality reduction can occur in the first parts of life; thus, reductions in mortality that occur in the third and fourth quarters of life are leading to a rise in the proportion of older persons. See also DEMOGRAPHIC TRANSITION.

"AGNOSTIC" ANALYSIS In GENOME-WIDE ASSOCIATION STUDIES (GWAS), massive testing of multiple genetic markers without necessarily considering available knowledge on gene function, clinical or BIOLOGICAL PLAUSIBILITY, COHERENCE, or other prior evidence that some of such variants may be clinically more important than others, or more likely to have some ASSOCIATION with the clinical or physiological outcomes of interest.[51-55] See also ASSOCIATION STUDY; CANDIDATE GENE; DATA MINING; EXPLORATORY STUDY.

AGREEMENT See KAPPA INDEX.

AIDS See ACQUIRED IMMUNODEFICIENCY SYNDROME.

AIRBORNE INFECTION An infection whose agent is transmitted by particles, dust, or DROPLET NUCLEI suspended in the air. The infective agent may be transmitted by a patient or CARRIER in airborne droplets expelled during coughing and sneezing.[56] See also TRANSMISSION OF INFECTION.

ALGORITHM Any systematic process that consists of an ordered sequence of steps with each step depending on the outcome of the previous one. The term is commonly used to describe a structured process—for instance, relating to computer programming or health planning.[38] See also DECISION TREE.

ALGORITHM, CLINICAL An explicit description of steps to be taken in patient care in specified circumstances. This approach makes use of branching logic and of all pertinent data, both about the patient and from epidemiological and other sources, to arrive at decisions that yield maximum benefit and minimum risk.

ALLELE Alternative forms of a gene occupying the same locus on a CHROMOSOME. Each of the different states found at a polymorphic site.[54,57]

ALLOCATION BIAS An error in the estimate of an effect caused by failure to implement valid procedures for RANDOM ALLOCATION of subjects to intervention and control groups in a CLINICAL TRIAL or in another type of randomized study (randomized FIELD TRIALS, randomized COMMUNITY TRIALS).[58]

ALLOCATION CONCEALMENT Concealing the result of the RANDOM ALLOCATION between two or more arms of a study.[1,6] See also ALLOCATION BIAS; BLINDED STUDY.

ALLOSTASIS The adaptive processes that actively maintain homeostasis through physiological or behavioural changes.[59]

ALLOSTATIC LOAD The long-term cost of handling stress.[59] The cumulative biological burden or physiological consequences exacted on the body through repeated attempts to adapt to life's demands in the environment. When responses to these demands occur outside of normal ranges, "wear and tear" on the regulatory system is thought to occur, resulting in accumulation of allostatic load.[60]

ALMA-ATA DECLARATION See HEALTH CARE; HEALTH FOR ALL; PRIMARY HEALTH CARE.

ALPHA ERROR See ERROR, TYPE I.

ALPHA LEVEL (Syn: α-level) In statistical hypothesis testing, a prespecified cutoff point α used to judge whether a result is "statistically significant" or not. Typically, if the P value for the TEST HYPOTHESIS is below α ($P < \alpha$), the result will be declared "statistically significant" and the hypothesis will be rejected. An α of 0.05 is used routinely, but this usage is purely customary; in the original theory of hypothesis testing, α was supposed to be chosen based on the cost of errors, with α representing the maximum acceptable probability of Type I error (incorrect rejection).[1] See also ERROR, TYPE I.

AMBIENT Surrounding; pertaining to the environment in which events are observed.

ANALYSIS OF VARIANCE (ANOVA) A statistical technique that isolates and assesses the contribution of categorical independent variables to the variance of the mean of a continuous dependent variable. The observations are classified according to their categories for each of the independent variables, and the differences between the categories in their mean values on the dependent variable are estimated and tested.[1,3,7,34,37]

ANALYTICAL STUDY A study conceived to examine hypothesized causal relationships and to make CAUSAL INFERENCES. Hence, most such studies can be conceptualized as ETIOLOGICAL STUDIES. An analytical study is usually concerned with identifying or measuring the effects of RISK FACTORS or with the health effects of specific exposures or interventions. Contrast with DESCRIPTIVE STUDY, which does not test causal hypotheses. Some common types of analytical study are COHORT, and CASE-CONTROL. In an analytical study, individuals in the study population may be classified according to the absence or presence (or future development) of specific disease and according to "attributes" that may influence disease occurrence. Attributes may include age; race; sex; other diseases; genetic, biochemical, and physiological characteristics; social position; economic status; occupation; residence; and various aspects of the environment or personal behavior.[1,3,8,24,795] See also RESEARCH DESIGN.

ANAMORPHIC MAP A diagrammatic method of displaying administrative jurisdictions of a country or any other region in two-dimensional "maps" with areas proportional to any statistic related to the region. A popular variant is the ISODEMOGRAPHIC MAP.[61]

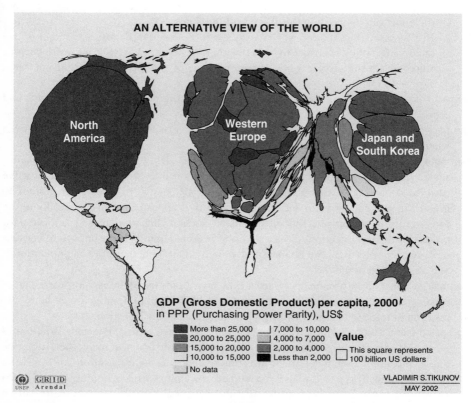

Anamorphic map. World economy cartogram. To highlight the distribution of wealth and power in the world, this cartogram sizes the countries according to their relative financial status, here presented through gross domestic product (GDP) per capita, offering an alternative world view to a regular map. Countries such as China and India become much smaller, next to giants in Western Europe, North America and Japan. Africa represents a minor speck, while South and Central America land somewhere in between. Source: GRID-Arendal.[62] With permission.

ANCILLARY STUDY (Syn: substudy, spin-off study, add-on study) A study that is secondary to another study. In a clinical trial, a medical test on a patient that is not a part of the original study design.[7,44]

ANECDOTAL EVIDENCE Evidence derived from descriptions of cases or events rather than systematically collected data that can be submitted to formal epidemiological and statistical analysis. Such evidence must be viewed with caution but sometimes is useful to raise a warning of danger or to generate hypotheses (e.g., as shown by voluntary reporting of adverse drug events).[5,63] See also CASE REPORTS.

ANIMAL MODEL A study in a group of laboratory animals that uses conditions of animals analogous to conditions of humans to model processes comparable to those that occur in humans.[64] See also EXPERIMENTAL EPIDEMIOLOGY; PATHOPHYSIOLOGY.

ANNUAL PARASITE INDEX (API) A measure of malaria morbidity for a given year at any given geographical level. It is calculated as the number of malaria-positive patients per 1,000 inhabitants (number of positive slides/total number of slides × 1000).[56,65]

ANTAGONISM (Opposite: SYNERGISM)
1. One of two main types of EFFECT MODIFICATION or INTERACTION: the EFFECT MODIFIER diminishes the effect of the putatively causal variable. The process in which the combined effect of two or more factors is smaller or weaker than that expected from the effect of one factor in the absence of the others.[1,3,66]
2. In a BIOASSAY, the situation when a response is produced by exposure to either of two factors but not by exposure to both together. Antagonism exists if there are persons who will get the disease when exposed to one of the factors alone but not when exposed to both.

ANTHROPOMETRY The technique dealing with the measurement of the size, weight, and proportions of the human body.

ANTHROPOPHILIC (adj.) Pertaining to an insect's preference for feeding on humans even when nonhuman hosts are available.

ANTIBODY Protein molecule produced in response to exposure to a "foreign" or extraneous substance (e.g., invading microorganisms responsible for infection) or active IMMUNIZATION. May also be present as a result of passive transfer from mother to infant, via immune globulin, etc. Antibody has the capacity to bind specifically to the foreign substance (antigen) that elicited its production, thus supplying a MECHANISM for protection against infectious diseases. Antibody is epidemiologically important because its concentration (titer) can be measured in individuals and, therefore, in populations[67] See also SEROEPIDEMIOLOGY.

ANTIGEN A substance (protein, polysaccharide, glycolipid, tissue transplant, etc.) that is capable of inducing specific immune response. Introduction of antigen may be by the invasion of infectious organisms, immunization, inhalation, ingestion, etc.

ANTIGENIC DRIFT The "evolutionary" changes that take place in the molecular structure of DNA/RNA in microorganisms during their passage from one host to another. It may be due to recombination, deletion, or insertion of genes, to point mutations, or to several of these events. This process has been studied in common viruses, notably the influenza virus.[68] It leads to alteration (usually slow and progressive) in the antigenic composition and thus in the immunological responses of individuals and populations to exposure to the microorganisms concerned.[67,69] See also ANTIGENIC SHIFT.

ANTIGENICITY (Syn: immunogenicity) The ability of agent(s) to produce a SYSTEMIC or a local immunological reaction in the host.[67]

ANTIGENIC SHIFT A mutation, or sudden change in molecular structure of DNA/RNA, in microorganisms, especially viruses, that produces new strains of the microorganism. Hosts previously exposed to other strains have little or no acquired immunity. Antigenic shift is believed to be the explanation for the occurrence of strains of the influenza A virus associated with large-scale EPIDEMIC and PANDEMIC spread.[67] See also ANTIGENIC DRIFT.

APACHE Acronym for Acute Physiology and Chronic Health Evaluation, a scoring system used to predict the outcome of critical illness or injury. This system and its variations (APACHE II, etc.) assign scores for state of consciousness, eye movements, reflexes, and physiological data such as blood pressure.[70]

APGAR SCORE A composite index used to evaluate neonatal status by assigning numerical scores (0–2) to heart rate, respiration, muscle tone, skin color, and response to stimulation. Developed by Virginia Apgar (1909–1974), a pediatrician/anesthetist. Low scores are associated with a poor prognosis. The 10-point Apgar scoring system has been used to assess the condition and prognosis of newborn infants throughout the world since 1952. Today it remains as relevant for the prediction of neonatal survival as it was over 60 years ago.[38,71]

APPLIED EPIDEMIOLOGY The application and evaluation of epidemiological knowledge and methods (e.g., in public health or in health care). It includes applications of etiological research, priority setting, and evaluation of health programs, policies, technologies, and services. It is epidemiological practice aimed at protecting and/or improving the health of a defined population. It usually involves identifying and investigating health problems, MONITORING changes in health status, and/or evaluating the outcomes of interventions. It is generally conducted in a time frame determined by the need to protect the health of an exposed population and an administrative context that results in PUBLIC HEALTH action.[28,72] See also FIELD EPIDEMIOLOGY; HOSPITAL EPIDEMIOLOGY.

ARBOVIRUS An *arthropod-borne virus*. Various RNA viruses transmitted principally by arthropods, including the causative agents of encephalitis, yellow fever and dengue. A group of taxonomically diverse animal viruses that are unified by an epidemiological concept, i.e., transmission between vertebrate host organisms by bloodfeeding (hematophagous) arthropod vectors such as mosquitoes, ticks, sand flies, and midges. The interaction of arbovirus, vertebrate host, and arthropod vector gives this class of infections unique epidemiological features. See VECTOR-BORNE INFECTION for terms that describe these features.[56,69]

AREA SAMPLING A method of sampling that can be used when the numbers in the population are unknown. The total area to be sampled is divided into subareas (e.g., by means of a grid that produces squares on a map); these subareas are then numbered and sampled using a table of random numbers. Depending upon circumstances, the population in the sampled areas may first be enumerated, and then a second stage of sampling may be conducted.

ARITHMETIC MEAN See MEAN, ARITHMETIC; AVERAGE.

ARM (of a trial) A group of persons whose outcome in a study is compared with that of another group or groups. When an active treatment is compared with a placebo or a standard of care, the arms of a CLINICAL TRIAL are commonly referred to as *experimental* and *control* groups.[73-77]

ARMITAGE-DOLL MODEL One of several models of CARCINOGENESIS,[78] in which time elapsed since exposure, not age, is a prime determinant of cancer.[79] The model postulates three phases: (1) A normal cell develops into a cancer cell after a small number of transition stages; (2) Initially the number of normal cells at risk is very large, and for each cell transition is a rare event; and (3) The transitions are independent of each other. There are no presumptions about precipitating causes of the transition from normal to cancerous cell. Named for Peter Armitage (1924–) and Richard Doll (1912–2005).[8,80-82] See also MULTISTAGE MODELS.

ARTIFICIAL INTELLIGENCE A branch of computer science in which attempts are made to duplicate human intellectual functions. One application is in clinical diagnosis, in which computer programs are based upon statistical analyses of data abstracted from clinical records.

ASCERTAINMENT The process of determining what are the characteristics, status, or events in a population or study group; e.g., household composition, exposure status (i.e., exposure ascertainment), occurrence of cases of specific diseases (the latter is also known as CASE FINDING).

ASCERTAINMENT BIAS Systematic failure to represent equally all classes of cases or persons supposed to be represented in a sample.[1,3,5,6,9,26,53,63] This bias may arise because of the nature of the sources from which persons come (e.g., a specialized clinic); from a diagnostic process influenced by culture, or idiosyncracy; or, in genetic studies, from the statistical CHANCE of selecting from large or small families. See also DETECTION BIAS; DISEASE PROGRESSION BIAS; REVERSE CAUSATION; SPECTRUM BIAS; VERIFICATION BIAS.

ASSAY The quantitative or qualitative evaluation of a (hazardous) substance in water food, soil, air, etc.; the results of such an evaluation. See also BIOASSAY.

ASSISTED REPRODUCTIVE TECHNOLOGY **(ART)** A term used to describe collectively a number of non-coital methods of conception that are used to treat infertility with donor or non-donor eggs and sperm. It comprises in vitro fertilization (IVF), gamete intrafallopian transfer (GIFT), and zygote intrafallopian transfer (ZIFT).

ASSOCIATION
1. Statistical dependence between two or more events, characteristics, or other variables. An association is present if the probability of occurrence of an event or characteristic, or the quantity of a variable, varies with the occurrence of one or more other events, the presence of one or more other characteristics, or the quantity of one or more other variables. The association between two variables is described as positive or direct when higher values of a variable are associated with higher values of another variable, and as negative or inverse when higher values of one variable are associated with lower values of the other variable. An association may be fortuitous or may be produced by various other circumstances; the presence of an association does not necessarily imply a CAUSAL relationship.[1-3,5,7,24,25,38,54,83] In epidemiological and clinical research the terms *association, relationship*, and *correlation* are sometimes loosely used interchangeably, but in statistics "correlation" is more often used to refer to the CORRELATION COEFFICIENT.
2. In his *Treatise of Human Nature* of 1739, one of three properties David Hume deemed necessary (but insufficient standing alone) for assigning cause; the other two properties of a cause are CONNECTION and TIME ORDER.[42,84,85]

ASSOCIATION, FORTUITOUS A relationship between two variables that occurs by CHANCE and is thought to need no further explanation. See also RANDOM; CORRELATION, NONSENSE.

ASSOCIATION, SPURIOUS An ambiguous term used with different meanings, which may refer to artifactual, fortuitous, false, or other noncausal associations owing to CHANCE or BIAS, including CONFOUNDING.[83]

ASSOCIATION STUDY (Syn: genetic association study) An approach commonly used in genetics and in genetic epidemiology to explore novel genetic markers associated with a particular TRAIT or the risk of developing a particular condition. The frequency of alleles or genotypes is compared between cases with the disease or trait under investigation and a group of individuals without that disease or trait (controls). A difference between the two groups in the frequency of the genetic marker, variant, or polymorphism under test suggests that such marker may increase the likelihood of the condition or trait, or be in LINKAGE DESIQUILIBRIUM with a genetic characteristic which does. One problem with the case-control design of association studies is that the genotype frequencies vary between ethnic or geographic regions. If cases and controls are not properly matched on these characteristics FALSE POSITIVE associations may occur due to the CONFOUNDING effects of POPULATION STRATIFICATION. Another common problem is the "flight to quantity" of samples (study size is maximized by including all possible case series regardless of quality or the source of controls), with inadequate and biased control groups (which are often not temporally or geographically matched to cases).[53,86-91] See also GENOME-WIDE ASSOCIATION STUDY (GWAS).

ASSORTATIVE MATING Selection of a mate with preference (or aversion) for a particular genotype (i.e., nonrandom mating).

ASYMMETRY OF INFORMATION Differences ("asymmetry") between a patient, or member of the public, and a health care professional, or insurer, in the information and knowledge available about illness and health. The belief that such informational advantages are all on one side (the professional's), is a too narrow view of what the relevant information is. While the professional generally possesses superior medical information, the patient possesses the best information on her preferences over the options, and she will usually be more competent in judging the value (utility) assigned to alternative clinical possibilities. The insurer will typically set premia according to broad averages of probability and expense to cover the expected liability, while the insured person may possess information (e.g., about private lifestyle) that is not available to the former.[92] See also ADVERSE SELECTION; AGENCY RELATIONSHIP; CARRIER.

ASYMPTOTIC Pertaining to a limiting value or property, for example, of a dependent variable, when the independent variable approaches zero or infinity. Most commonly in statistics, it refers to an approximation that becomes better as the sample size increases.[1,7] See LARGE SAMPLE METHOD.

ASYMPTOTIC CURVE A curve that approaches but never reaches zero or infinity (e.g., an exponential or reciprocal exponential curve).

ASYMPTOTIC METHOD See LARGE SAMPLE METHOD.

ATOMISTIC FALLACY An erroneous inference about causal relationships in groups of people made on the basis of relationships observed in individuals.[50] The opposite of the ECOLOGICAL FALLACY. A direct or mechanical translation of CAUSAL INFERENCES made in individuals to population groups may be wrong because different causal processes may operate when the individual is the unit of interest than when the unit is a population. The atomistic fallacy may occur when studies based on individuals (individual-level studies) are assumed to be valid and sufficient to make causal inferences at an upper level of aggregation (e.g., on the relationship between exposures and diseases at the group level). Relevant in particular when individual-level factors (e.g., income, gun ownership) and group-level factors (e.g., average income in the neighborhood, prevalence of gun holders in a city) capture or mediate different aspects of health risks.[38,93] See also AGGREGATIVE FALLACY; ECOLOGICAL FALLACY; INDIVIDUAL THINKING; MULTIPLE CAUSATION; POPULATION THINKING.

ATTACK "RATE" A type of RISK. Synonym for INCIDENCE PROPORTION used traditionally in outbreak investigations. The proportion of a group that experiences the outcome under study over a given period (e.g., the period of an epidemic). It can be determined empirically by identifying clinical cases or by seroepidemiology. It also applies in noninfectious problems and settings (e.g., mass poisonings). Because its time dimension is uncertain or arbitrarily decided, it should probably not be described as a rate.[1,5,69] See also INFECTION RATE; MASS ACTION PRINCIPLE; REED-FROST MODEL; SECONDARY ATTACK RATE.

ATTENUATION Weakening (dilution) of the concentration, as of an antigen in a vaccine; also of an effect, e.g., relative risk.

ATTRIBUTABLE BENEFIT Synonym for PREVENTED FRACTION.

ATTRIBUTABLE FRACTION (Syn: attributable proportion) The proportion of the caseload that can be attributed to a particular exposure. It is the causal RISK DIFFERENCE divided by the INCIDENCE PROPORTION in the group. It is the proportion by which the RISK would be reduced if the exposure were eliminated.[1,2,7,94,95] It may be estimated for the individuals exposed (ATTRIBUTABLE FRACTION AMONG THE EXPOSED) or for the whole population (ATTRIBUTABLE FRACTION FOR THE POPULATION).

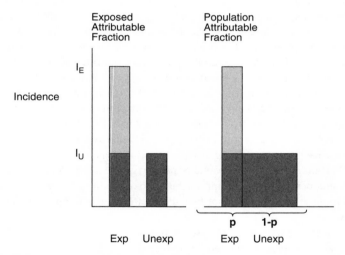

Attributable fractions. I_E and I_U are the incidence in the exposed and unexposed groups, p is the proportion of the population that is exposed, and 1-p the proportion not exposed. The lighter area represents cases that are attributable to the exposure (attributable risk, AR) and that would not have occurred in the absence of the exposure. It is assumed that in the absence of this hazardous exposure, the incidence would be I_U in the whole population. Source: Spasoff R.[96] With permission.

ATTRIBUTABLE FRACTION AMONG THE EXPOSED (Syn: attributable proportion among the exposed, attributable risk (exposed), relative attributable risk). With a given outcome, exposure factor, and population, the attributable fraction among the exposed is the proportion by which the INCIDENCE PROPORTION or the INCIDENCE RATE of the outcome among those exposed would be reduced if the exposure were eliminated. If there is no BIAS or CONFOUNDING, it may be estimated by the formula

$$AF_e = \frac{I_e - I_u}{I_e}$$

where I_e is the incidence proportion or the incidence rate among the exposed, and I_u is the incidence proportion or incidence rate among the unexposed; or by the formula

$$AF_e = \frac{RR-1}{RR}$$

where RR is the rate ratio, I_e/I_u. It should not be confused with the ETIOLOGICAL FRACTION AMONG THE EXPOSED or the PROBABILITY OF CAUSATION.[1]

ATTRIBUTABLE FRACTION FOR THE POPULATION (Syn: attributable proportion for the population, population attributable proportion, Levin's attributable risk) With a given outcome, exposure factor, and population, the attributable fraction for the population incidence proportion or incidence rate is the proportion by which the incidence proportion or incidence rate of the outcome in the entire population would be reduced if the exposure was eliminated. If there is no BIAS or CONFOUNDING, it may be estimated by the formula

$$AF_p = \frac{I_p - I_u}{I_p}$$

where I_p is the incidence proportion or the incidence rate in the total population and I_u is the incidence proportion or incidence rate among the unexposed. It should not be confused with the ETIOLOGICAL FRACTION FOR THE POPULATION.
The formula

$$AF_p = \frac{P_e(RR-1)}{1+P_e(RR-1)}$$

(where RR is the risk ratio or the rate ratio, I_e/I_u and P_e is the proportion exposed in the entire population) is often cited, but it is biased if the RR is adjusted for confounders, as is normally the case.[1]
A formula that does not suffer from this problem is

$$AF_p = \frac{P_c(RR-1)}{RR}$$

(where P_c is the exposure prevalence among cases).
Attributable fractions may also be calculated for other measures of disease frequency; e.g., the attributable fraction for the caseload over a defined time period is

$$(A_p - A_u)/A_p$$

where A_p is the caseload in the population and A_u is what the caseload would be if everyone were not exposed. This fraction equals the attributable fraction calculated from the incidence proportion, but is not the same as the quantity computed from the rates because the rate fraction does not account for the effect of exposure on PERSON-TIME.[1]

ATTRIBUTABLE NUMBER The excess caseload of a specific outcome attributable to an exposure over a defined time period. If there is no bias or confounding and the exposure has negligible effect on the PERSON-TIME at risk, it may be estimated using the formula

$$AN = T_e \left(I_e - I_u \right)$$

where I_e is the INCIDENCE RATE among the exposed, I_u is the incidence rate among the unexposed, and T_e is the person-time in the exposed population during the period in question.

ATTRIBUTABLE PROPORTION See ATTRIBUTABLE FRACTION

ATTRIBUTABLE RATE (Syn: causal rate difference) The rate of the outcome had everybody in the population been exposed minus the rate of the outcome had everybody in the population remained unexposed. It measures the proportion of the rate in exposed individuals that can be attributed to the exposure.

ATTRIBUTABLE RISK (Syn: causal risk difference) The risk of the outcome had everybody in the population been exposed minus the risk of the outcome had everybody in the population remained unexposed. The attributable risk measures the proportion of the risk in exposed individuals that can be attributed to the exposure.[1,3,5,7] Unfortunately, this term and ATTRIBUTABLE RATE have been used to denote a number of different concepts, including the ATTRIBUTABLE FRACTION FOR THE POPULATION, the ATTRIBUTABLE FRACTION AMONG THE EXPOSED, and the RATE DIFFERENCE. See also IMPACT NUMBERS.

ATTRIBUTABLE RISK (EXPOSED) This term has been used to denote the ATTRIBUTABLE FRACTION AMONG THE EXPOSED and the excess risk among the exposed. See also RATE DIFFERENCE.

ATTRIBUTABLE RISK PERCENT ATTRIBUTABLE FRACTION expressed as a percentage of the total rate or risk rather than as a proportion.

ATTRIBUTABLE RISK PERCENT (EXPOSED) The ATTRIBUTABLE FRACTION AMONG THE EXPOSED, expressed as a percentage of the total rate or risk among the exposed.

ATTRIBUTABLE RISK PERCENT (POPULATION) The ATTRIBUTABLE FRACTION FOR THE POPULATION, expressed as a percentage of the total rate or risk in the population.

ATTRIBUTABLE RISK (POPULATION) This term has been used to denote the ATTRIBUTABLE FRACTION FOR THE POPULATION and the population excess risk.

ATTRIBUTE A qualitative characteristic of an individual or an item.

ATTRITION Reduction in the number of participants in a study as it progresses (i.e., during FOLLOW-UP of a COHORT STUDY or a RANDOMIZED CONTROLLED TRIAL). Losses may be due to withdrawals, DROPOUTS, or protocol deviations.[1,3] See also CENSORING.

ATTRITION BIAS A type of SELECTION BIAS due to systematic differences between the study groups in the quantitative and qualitative characteristics of the processes of loss of their members during study conduct; i.e., due to ATTRITION among subjects in the study. Different rates of losses to follow-up in the exposure groups may change the characteristics of these groups irrespective of the studied exposure or intervention, or losses may be influenced by the positive or adverse effects of the exposures.[3,97,98]

AUDIT

1. An examination or review that establishes the extent to which a condition, process, or performance conforms to predetermined standards or criteria. Assessment or review of any aspect of HEALTH CARE to determine its quality; audits may be carried out on the provision of care, compliance with regulations, community response, completeness of records, etc.[17]

2. An evaluation of the quality of health care, the use of resources, and outcomes. See also HEALTH SERVICES RESEARCH.

3. The process of checking whether the accounts of an institution, company, or association are complete, accurate, and consistent; whether they agree with other records of activity; and whether they comply with legal requirements and professional standards.

AUSTRALIA ANTIGEN Hepatitis B surface antigen (HBsAg). So called because it was first identified in an Australian aborigine. HBsAg is a BIOMARKER for the prevalence of infection with the virus of hepatitis B.

AUTONOMY, RESPECT FOR

1. In ETHICS, the principle of respect for human dignity and the right of individuals to decide things for themselves.

2. In epidemiological practice and research, this principle is central to the concept of INFORMED CONSENT. It can conflict with the need to protect the population from identified risks (e.g., risks related to contagious disease) and with the need for access to personally identifiable health-related data and information. See also CONFIDENTIALITY; CONSENT BIAS; PRIVACY.

AUTOPSY DATA Data derived from autopsied deaths; used, for instance, to study aspects of the NATURAL HISTORY OF DISEASE or TRENDS in frequency of disease. Autopsies are done on nonrandomly selected persons; findings should therefore be generalized only with great caution. See also BIAS IN AUTOPSY SERIES.

AUXILIARY HYPOTHESIS BIAS A form of RESCUE BIAS and thus of INTERPRETIVE BIAS, which occurs in introducing ad hoc modifications to imply that an unanticipated finding would have occurred otherwise had the experimental conditions been different. Because experimental conditions can easily be altered in many ways, adjusting a hypothesis is a versatile tool for saving a cherished theory.[1,38,99]

AVERAGE

1. Most often, the ARITHMETIC MEAN. The arithmetic average of a set of n numbers is the sum of the numbers divided by n.

2. A measure of location, either the MODE or, in the case of numerical data, the MEDIAN or the MEAN.[1] See also MEASURE OF CENTRAL TENDENCY.

3. In everyday speech, ordinary, usual, or NORMAL; the normal or typical amount.

AVERAGE LIFE EXPECTANCY See EXPECTATION OF LIFE.

AXIS

1. One of the dimensions of a graph. A two-dimensional graph has two axes, the horizontal or x axis and the vertical or y axis. Mathematically, there may be more than two axes, and graphs are sometimes drawn with a third dimension. See also ABSCISSA; ORDINATE.

2. In NOSOLOGY, an axis of classification is the conceptual framework (e.g., etiological, topographical, psychological, sociological). The INTERNATIONAL CLASSIFICATION OF DISEASES (ICD), for example, is multiaxial: the primary axis is topographical (i.e., body systems), while secondary axes relate to etiology, manifestations of disease, detail of sites affected, severity, etc.

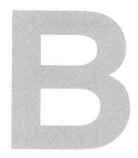

BACKDOOR (BIASING PATH) A path on a CAUSAL DIAGRAM from the exposure to the outcome that begins with an arrow pointing into the exposure. If control is not made for a variable on the path CONFOUNDING will be introduced.[1,2,34,100,101]

BACKDOOR FORMULA See G-FORMULA.

BACKGROUND LEVEL, RATE The concentration, often low, at which some substance, agent, or event is present or occurs at a particular time and place in the absence of a specific HAZARD or set of hazards under investigation. An example is the background level of the naturally occurring forms of ionizing radiation, to which everyone in an area would be exposed.

BACTERIA (singular: bacterium) Single-celled prokaryotic MICROORGANISMS found throughout nature, which can be beneficial or cause disease. One of two major types of prokaryotic (lacking a nucleus) single-celled organisms. Large numbers of bacteria and bacterial species are found in the human digestive system or on the skin. Epidemiology and medical microbiology through the 19th and 20th centuries focused on bacterially caused diseases as tuberculosis, typhoid, and cholera. More recently, there has been interest on issues such as the ecology of bacterial communities in normal individuals, on how disruption of that ecology may contribute to disease, or on antimicrobial resistance.

BAR CHART (Syn: bar diagram) A type of GRAPH for presenting DISCRETE DATA organized in such a way that each observation can fall into one and only one category of the variable. Frequencies are listed along one axis and categories of the variable along the other axis. The frequencies of each group of observations are represented by the lengths of the corresponding bars. An apparently simple way to visually display quantitative information.[102-108] See also HISTOGRAM.

BAR DIAGRAM See BAR CHART.

BARKER HYPOTHESIS See DEVELOPMENTAL ORIGINS OF HEALTH AND DISEASE.

BARRIER METHOD Contraceptive method that interposes a physical barrier between sperm and ovum (e.g., condom, cervical cap, diaphragm).

BARRIER NURSING (Syn: bedside isolation) Nursing care of hospital patients that minimizes the risks of cross-infection by use of antisepsis, gowns, gloves, masks for nursing staff, and ISOLATION of the patient, preferably alone in a single room. See also UNIVERSAL PRECAUTIONS.

BASELINE DATA A set of data collected at the beginning of a study.[1,6]

BASE POPULATION See POPULATION, SOURCE.

BASE, STUDY See STUDY BASE.

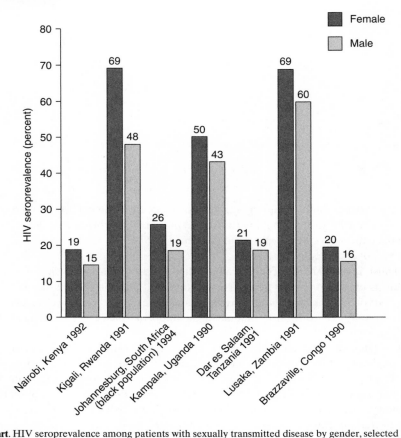

Bar chart. HIV seroprevalence among patients with sexually transmitted disease by gender, selected African countries, 1990–1993. Source: Mann JM, et al.[109]

BASIC REPRODUCTIVE RATE (R_0) A measure of the number of infections produced, on average, by an infected individual in the early stages of an epidemic, when virtually all contacts are susceptible. (Some authors use the symbol Z_0 for basic reproductive rate.).[67,110]

BAYESIAN STATISTICS A method of statistical inference that begins with formulation of probabilities of hypotheses (called *prior probabilities*) before the data under analysis are taken into account. It then uses the data and a model for the data probability (usually the same model used by other methods, such as a LOGISTIC MODEL) to update the probabilities of the hypotheses. The resulting updated probabilities are called *posterior probabilities*. Central to this updating is BAYES' THEOREM,[1,7,34,37,101,111] although not all Bayesian methods require explicit use of the theorem and not all uses of the theorem are Bayesian methods. Bayesian statistics can be used alongside or in place of other methods for many purposes (e.g., evaluation of diagnostic tests, studies of disease progression, and analyses of geographic studies, clinical trials, cohort studies, and case-control studies). Many types of Bayesian estimators have excellent FREQUENTIST (repeated-sampling) properties, and are identical in form to SHRINKAGE ESTIMATES.

BAYES' THEOREM A theorem of probability named for Thomas Bayes (1702–1761), a clergyman and mathematician; his *Essay Towards Solving a Problem in the Doctrine* *of Chances* (1763, published posthumously) contained this theorem. In epidemiology, it is often used to obtain the probability of disease in a group of people with some characteristic on the basis of the overall rate of that disease (the prior probability of disease) and of the likelihoods of that characteristic in healthy and diseased individuals. The most familiar application is in CLINICAL DECISION ANALYSIS, where it is used for estimating the probability of a particular diagnosis given the appearance of some symptoms or test result. A simplified version of the theorem is

$$P(D|S) = \frac{P(S|D)P(D)}{P(S|D)P(D) + P(S|\bar{D})P(\bar{D})}$$

where D = disease, S = symptom, $\bar{D}$ = no disease, $P(D)$ is the overall probability of disease (also called the crude, unconditional, or PRIOR PROBABILITY), $P(S|D)$ is the probability of the symptom given the disease, $P(S|\bar{D})$ is the probability of the symptom given no disease, and $P(D|S)$ is the probability of disease given the symptom (also called the conditional or POSTERIOR PROBABILITY). The formula emphasizes what clinical intuition often overlooks, namely, that the probability of disease given the symptom depends not only on how characteristic of the disease that symptom is but also on how frequent the disease is among the population being served.[1,7,34,37,38,101]

The theorem is sometimes presented in terms of the odds of disease before knowing the symptom (PRIOR ODDS) and after knowing the symptom (POSTERIOR ODDS). The theorem can also be used for estimating exposure-specific risks from case-control studies if there is information about the overall risk of disease $P(D)$ in that population. See also DENOMINATOR.

BEDSIDE ISOLATION See BARRIER NURSING; ISOLATION.

BEHAVIOR Anything a person does in response to internal or external events. Actions may be overt (motor or verbal) and directly measurable or, covert (activities not viewable but involving voluntary muscles) and indirectly measurable; behaviors are physical events that occur in the body and are controlled by the brain.[112] See also BEHAVIOR CHANGE INTERVENTION; BEHAVIOR CHANGE TECHNIQUE; HEALTHY LIFESTYLE.

BEHAVIORAL EPIDEMIC An epidemic attributable to the power of suggestion or to culturally influenced behavioral patterns. Examples include episodes of mass fainting or convulsions, crowd panic, and waves of fashion or enthusiasm. The communicable nature of the behavior is dependent not only on person-to-person transmission of the behavioral pattern but also on group reinforcement. Behavioral epidemics may be difficult to differentiate from outbreaks of organic disease (e.g., due to CONTAMINATION by a toxic substance) or may complicate them.

BEHAVIORAL RISK FACTOR A BEHAVIOR that is causally related to an increased (or decreased, if it is beneficial) probability of an outcome.[24,113] See also RISK FACTOR.

BEHAVIOR SETTING The place where a pattern or sequence of behavior regularly occurs; it includes the ordinary events and settings of daily life.[31] A forerunner of the concept of ACTIVITY SETTING.

BEHAVIOR CHANGE INTERVENTION A coordinated set of activities designed to modify a BEHAVIOR to produce a desired outcome. Such interventions include one or more BEHAVIOR CHANGE TECHNIQUES. Interventions are used to promote healthy lifestyles, self-management of health conditions (e.g., adherence to medication, monitoring symptoms), and optimal delivery and uptake of health care services (e.g., doctors implementing evidence based guidance, patient attendance for breast screening).[9,114] See also LIFESTYLE MODIFICATION.

BEHAVIOR CHANGE TECHNIQUE A systematic procedure delivered as an active component of an intervention designed to change behavior. Such techniques are observable, replicable, and irreducible components that are postulated to be active ingredients within interventions. They should be well specified so that their EFFECTIVENESS can be evaluated.[114,115]

BENCHMARK A slang or jargon term, usually meaning a measurement or point of reference taken at the beginning of a survey or project, used for comparison with subsequent measurements of the same variable; sometimes it means the best or most desirable value of the variable. Alternatively, an acceptable standard in evaluation (e.g., of air quality, of performance).[17,116]

BENCHMARKING The process of comparing the processes and performance of one organization to the best practices of other organizations to improve one's performance.

BENEFICENCE Literally, doing good. In bioethics, a principle underlying utilitarian approaches. It implies a certain obligation to promote benefits of things judged to be good, typically balancing potential or produced goods against risks. In PUBLIC HEALTH, it implies acting in the best interest of the population at stake.[13,117,118]

BENEFIT Positive effect, advantage, or improvement resulting from an exposure, intervention, or action or its avoidance. In epidemiology, public health, and medicine benefits of programs and policies may remain relatively invisible unless they are monitored.[13,28,32,119-122] This is also the case for the positive effects of educational, social, or environmental policies.[33,123] See also HEALTHY PUBLIC POLICIES; MINIMALLY IMPORTANT DIFFERENCE; PREVENTION.

BENEFIT-COST RATIO See COST-BENEFIT ANALYSIS.

BERKSONIAN BIAS A general term to indicate all types of bias that have the structure of SELECTION BIAS, based on the assumption that Berkson originally described a bias with that structure.

BERKSON'S BIAS (Syn: Berkson's fallacy) A form of SELECTION BIAS that arises when the variables whose association is under study affect selection of subjects into the study. It is a particular concern in hospital-based studies, especially when prevalent or previously diagnosed cases are not excluded. Joseph Berkson (1899-1982) described an imaginary hospital-based case-control study wherein the controls are patients with other diseases, and the "exposure" is also a disease; he noted that in such a study the association between the disease prevalences is expected to differ from the corresponding association in the general population.[124] This difference in the association has historically been referred to as Berkson's bias. Some authors restricted the use of the term to (prevalent) disease-disease associations, as in the original Berkson paper;[124] others extended it to exposure-disease associations (including situations in which two diseases affect the selection but the exposure is associated with one of the diseases). In Berkson's original example, hospitalization is a COLLIDER for two or more diseases whose prevalences are independent in the population, but for which different fractions of the population are hospitalized. The selection process into the hospital is such that a hospital-based case-control study inevitably yields an association between prevalent diseases. "Indirect Berkson's bias" refers to exposure-disease associations that arise because another disease is associated with the exposure under study;[125] this bias is largely attenuated by using incident cases, and prevented completely by excluding cases hospitalized because of another disease.[125,126] The causal structure of Berkson's bias is the same of all biases due to conditioning on a collider. See also M-BIAS.

BERNOULLI DISTRIBUTION The probability distribution associated with two mutually exclusive and exhaustive outcomes. The distribution of a Bernoulli (binary) variable. A variable that has only two possible values; e.g., death or survival.[7] See also BINOMIAL DISTRIBUTION.

BERTILLON CLASSIFICATION The International List of Causes of Death of 1893, progenitor of the INTERNATIONAL CLASSIFICATION OF DISEASES (ICD). The first numerically based NOSOLOGY in which disease entities were arranged in chapters, developed by Jacques Bertillon (1851–1922).[127] It descended from a nosology proposed in 1853 by Marc d'Espigne and William Farr.

BETA ERROR See ERROR, TYPE II.

BIAS Systematic deviation of results or inferences from truth. Processes leading to such deviation. An error in the conception and design of a study—or in the collection, analysis, interpretation, reporting, publication, or review of data—leading to results or conclusions that are systematically (as opposed to randomly) different from truth.[1-3,5-9,25,39-42,85,97-99,128]
Ways in which deviation from the truth can occur include:
1. Systematic variation of measurements or estimates from the true values.
2. Variation of statistical estimates (means, rates, measures of association, etc.) from their true values as a result of statistical artifacts or flaws in study design, conduct, or analysis.
3. Deviation of inferences from truth as a result of conceptual or methodological flaws in study conception or design, data collection, or the analysis or interpretation of results.
4. A tendency of procedures (in study design, data collection, analysis, interpretation, review, or publication) to yield results or conclusions that depart from the truth.
5. Prejudice leading to the conscious or unconscious selection of research hypotheses or procedures that depart from the truth in a particular direction or to one-sidedness in the interpretation of results.

The term *bias* does not necessarily carry an imputation of prejudice or any other subjective factor, such as the experimenter's desire for a particular outcome. This differs from conventional usage, in which *bias* refers to a partisan point of view—to prejudice or unfairness.[38] See also INTERPRETIVE BIAS.

BIAS ANALYSIS The analysis of systematic variation in estimates due to flaws in study design, conduct, analysis, or interpretation of results. Bias analysis is complementary to analysis of purely random variation in estimates, as in ANALYSIS OF VARIANCE.[1]

BIAS, ASCERTAINMENT See ASCERTAINMENT BIAS.

BIAS, BERKSON'S See BERKSON'S BIAS.

BIAS, COLLIDER See COLLIDER.

BIAS, CONFIRMATION See CONFIRMATION BIAS.

BIAS, CONFOUNDING See CONFOUNDING BIAS.

BIAS, CONSENT See CONSENT BIAS.

BIAS, DETECTION See DETECTION BIAS.

BIAS, DIAGNOSTIC SUSPICION See DIAGNOSTIC SUSPICION BIAS.

BIAS, DISCONFIRMATION See CONFIRMATION BIAS.

BIAS, DISEASE PROGRESSION See DISEASE PROGRESSION BIAS.

BIAS DUE TO DIGIT PREFERENCE See DIGIT PREFERENCE.

BIAS DUE TO INSTRUMENT ERROR Systematic error due to faulty CALIBRATION, inaccurate measuring instruments, contaminated reagents, incorrect dilution or mixing of reagents, etc. See also CONTAMINATION, DATA; INFORMATION BIAS; MEASUREMENT BIAS.

BIAS DUE TO WITHDRAWALS A difference between the true effect and the association observed in a study due to characteristics of subjects who choose to withdraw. See also ATTRITION; CENSORING; DROPOUT.

BIAS FORMULA An analytic formula that expresses the relationship between the biased estimator (due to CONFOUNDING, selection error, or measurement error) and the true effect in terms of parameters, such that the biased estimate and specification of the correct parameter values together would give an unbiased effect estimate. See also BIAS PARAMETERS.[129,130]

BIAS IN ASSUMPTIONS (Syn: conceptual bias) Errors arising from faulty logic or premises or mistaken beliefs on the part of the investigators. False conclusions about the explanation for associations between variables. See also BIOLOGICAL PLAUSIBILITY; COHERENCE.

BIAS, INFORMATION See INFORMATION BIAS.

BIAS IN HANDLING OUTLIERS Error arising from biased discarding of unusual values or exclusion of unusual values that should be included.[37]

BIAS IN PUBLICATION See PUBLICATION BIAS.

BIAS, INTERPRETIVE See INTERPRETIVE BIAS.

BIAS, LEAD-TIME See LEAD-TIME BIAS.

BIAS, LENGTH See LENGTH BIAS.

BIAS, MEASUREMENT See MEASUREMENT BIAS.

BIAS, MECHANISTIC See MECHANISTIC BIAS.

BIAS OF AN ESTIMATOR The difference between the expected (mean) value of an estimator of a parameter and the true value of this parameter. See also UNBIASED ESTIMATOR.

BIAS, INVESTIGATOR See INVESTIGATOR BIAS.

BIAS OF INTERPRETATION See INTERPRETIVE BIAS.

BIAS PARAMETERS Parameters such that a biased estimate in conjunction with the correct specification of the parameters together can yield an unbiased effect estimate.[129-131]

BIAS, PERFORMANCE See PERFORMANCE BIAS.

BIAS, PUBLICATION See PUBLICATION BIAS.

BIAS, RECALL See RECALL BIAS.

BIAS, RESCUE See RESCUE BIAS.

BIAS, RESPONSE See RESPONSE BIAS.

BIAS, REVERSE CAUSATION See REVERSE CAUSATION.

BIAS, SELECTION See SELECTION BIAS.

BIAS, SPECTRUM See SPECTRUM BIAS.

BIAS, VERIFICATION See VERIFICATION BIAS.

BIAS, WORKUP See WORKUP BIAS.

BIBLIOGRAPHIC IMPACT FACTOR (BIF) In SCIENTOMETRICS, a measure of the "average" frequency with which articles in a scientific periodical are cited by articles in journals that are chosen by Thomson Reuters to be included in the Science Citation Index (SCI) and related databases.[132-134] Given the virtues and limitations of BIF, and the well-known fact that scientific articles have a wide and skewed spectrum of impacts (or none),[133,134] it is clear that the cultural impact of BIF in EPISTEMIC COMMUNITIES is related to the SOCIOLOGY OF SCIENTIFIC KNOWLEDGE (and human nature).[38,135-137] Attributing bibliometric indicators for *journals* to *articles* or to individual *authors* is an ECOLOGICAL FALLACY. Main reasons why BIF is often not a valid or relevant indicator include: it is highly influenced by the number of articles chosen by Thomson Reuters for each journal as the denominator of BIF; such articles are usually not disclosed; the consistency of the application across journals of such choice is unknown; remarkably, citations to articles excluded from

BIF's denominator are counted in the numerator; citation distributions within journals are highly skewed; the properties of BIF are field-specific (e.g., field size); BIF can be manipulated by editorial policy; and data used to calculate it are neither transparent nor openly available.[133,134,138] If the *journal* is the unit of analysis, the total number of citations received by all articles published by such journal may be a better indicator. If the *article* is of interest, the total number of citations received by the article may the best place to start.[133]

BILLS OF MORTALITY Weekly and annual abstracts of christenings and burials compiled from parish registers in England, especially London, that date from 1538. Beginning in 1629, the annual bills were published and included a tabulation of deaths from plague and other causes. These were the basis for the earliest English vital statistics, compiled, analyzed, and discussed by John Graunt (1620–1674) in *Natural and Political Observations…on the Bills of Mortality* (London, 1662).[69]

BIMODAL DISTRIBUTION A DISTRIBUTION with two regions of high frequency separated by a region of lower frequency of observations. A two-peak distribution.

BINARY VARIABLE (Syn: dichotomous variable) A variable having only two possible values (e.g., *on* or *off*, 0 or 1).[1,3,34,37] See also BERNOULLI DISTRIBUTION; MEASUREMENT SCALE.

BINOMIAL DISTRIBUTION A probability DISTRIBUTION for the relative frequencies of two mutually exclusive outcomes (e.g., presence or absence of a clinical sign, death or survival) in a group of n independent units. The probability distribution of the number of occurrences of a binary event in a sample of n independent observations. The binomial distribution may be used to model the INCIDENCE PROPORTION and PREVALENCE of events when INDEPENDENCE is assumed. The BERNOULLI DISTRIBUTION is a special case of the binomial distribution with $n = 1$ (only 1 unit in the group or sample).[1,7,12,34,37,110]

BIOACCUMULATION Progressive increase in the concentration of a chemical compound in an organism, organ, or tissue when the rate of uptake exceeds the rate of excretion or metabolism. In humans exposure to and bioaccumulation of persistent chemical agents occurs largely through the fatty components of animal foods, including recycled animal fats, which are used as components of food products and animal feed. Bioaccumulation occurs within a trophic (food chain) level.[13,139,140] See also BIOMAGNIFICATION.

BIOASSAY The quantitative evaluation of the potency of a substance by assessing its effects on tissues, cells, live experimental animals, or humans. Bioassay may be a direct method of estimating relative potency: groups of subjects are assigned to each of two (or more) preparations, the dose that is just sufficient to produce a specified response is measured, and the estimate is the ratio of the mean doses for the two (or more) groups. In this method, the death of the subject may be used as the "response." The indirect method (more commonly used) requires study of the relationship between the magnitude of a dose and the magnitude of a quantitative response produced by it. See also INTERACTION.

BIODIVERSITY (Syn: biological diversity) The variety of species of plants, animals, and microorganisms in a natural community, of communities within a particular environment, and of genetic variation within a species (GENETIC DIVERSITY). Biodiversity is important for the stability of ecosystems. To many it is also a cultural value.[13,33,139]

"BIOLOGICAL AGE"

1. An attribute of body tissue that is relevant in PATHOGENESIS; e.g., "age" of breast tissue, which develops after puberty, in relation to breast cancer risk.[141] See also ARMITAGE-DOLL MODEL.

2. People age with different "speed" at equal "calendar age," and this is expressed in external appearance, body characteristics, or physical and social functioning. It can be calculated from a model based on measured aging-related characteristics.[142-144]

BIOLOGICAL MARKER See BIOMARKER.

BIOLOGICAL MONITORING See BIOMONITORING.

BIOLOGICAL PLAUSIBILITY The CAUSAL CONSIDERATION that an observed, potentially causal ASSOCIATION between an exposure and a health outcome may plausibly be attributed to causation on the basis of existing biomedical and epidemiological knowledge. On a schematic continuum including *possible, plausible, compatible*, and *coherent*, the term *plausible* is not a demanding or stringent requirement, given the many biological mechanisms that often can be hypothesized to underlie clinical and epidemiological observations; hence, in assessing CAUSALITY, it may be logically more appropriate to require COHERENCE (biological as well as clinical and epidemiological). *Plausibility* should hence be used cautiously, since it could impede development or acceptance of new knowledge that does not fit existing biological evidence, pathophysiological reasoning, or other evidence. Valid and relevant clinical and epidemiological discoveries may precede the acquisition of knowledge on the biological mechanisms of such events; i.e., biologically relevant epidemiological evidence may precede biological evidence derived from laboratory experiments. Biological associations often have small clinical or epidemiological effects (e.g., many genetic variants confer a slightly increased or decreased risk for DISEASES OF COMPLEX ETIOLOGY).[25,51-54,91,145] See also COHERENCE; HILL'S CONSIDERATIONS FOR CAUSATION.

BIOLOGICAL TRANSMISSION See VECTOR-BORNE INFECTION. See also PATHOGEN.

BIOMAGNIFICATION (Syn: biological magnification, bioamplification) Sequence of processes in an ecosystem by which higher concentrations (e.g., of a persistent toxic substance) are attained in organisms at higher levels in the food chain. The increase in concentration of an element or compound, such as a pesticide, that occurs in a food chain. Biomagnification occurs across trophic (food chain) levels.[13,139,140] See also BIOACCUMULATION.

BIOMARKER, BIOLOGICAL MARKER A substance, structure, or process that can be measured in biological specimens or media and may be associated with health outcomes or biological effects. A cellular, biochemical, or molecular indicator of exposure; of biological, subclinical, or clinical effects; or of possible SUSCEPTIBILITY. A biological indicator of internal dose, biologically effective dose, early biological response, altered structure, or altered function. Some uses of the term are ambiguous, suggesting insufficient understanding of the physico-chemical, pathophysiological, or mechanistic nature, properties, and role of the "marker."[1,5,12,146-149] See also DISEASE PROGRESSION BIAS; MOLECULAR EPIDEMIOLOGY; REVERSE CAUSATION.

BIOMEDICALIZATION See MEDICALIZATION.

BIOMETRY Literally, measurement of life. The application of statistical methods to the study of numerical data based on observation of biological phenomena. The term was made popular by Karl Pearson (1857–1936), who founded the journal *Biometrika*. Francis Galton (1822–1911) has been deemed the founder of biometry, but others—e.g., Pierre-Charles-Alexandre Louis (1787–1872)—preceded him in the study of phenomena now classified under that heading.[42]

BIOMONITORING (Syn: biological monitoring) Conception, performance, analysis, and interpretation of biological measurements aimed at MONITORING levels and changes in exposures (and health status, in human populations), in an environmental compartment (e.g., water, air, or soil), or in other health DETERMINANTS (e.g., food samples, animal feed).

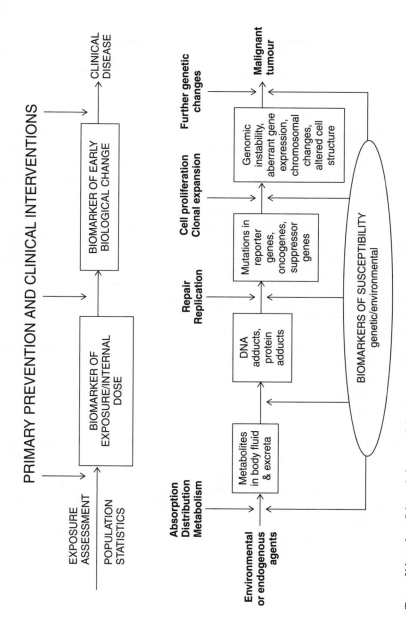

Types of biomarkers. Schematic framework for the use of biomarkers in molecular epidemiology studies of cancer. Source: Gallo V, et al.[146]

Monitoring of concentrations of suspected or known toxic or hazardous substances using biological means in well-defined populations (e.g., analyses of concentrations of environmental chemical agents in samples of urine, blood, or adipose tissue). Well-established biomonitoring programs in representative samples of the general population exist in countries as the United States and Germany.[12,147-151] See also SURVEILLANCE.

BIOSTATISTICS Application of STATISTICS to biological problems. The term should not be restricted to mean the application of statistics to medical problems (MEDICAL STATISTICS), since its real meaning is broader, subsuming agricultural statistics, forestry, and ecology, among other applications.[7]

BIPHASIC See NONMONOTONIC.

BIRTH CERTIFICATE Official, legal document recording details of a live birth, usually comprising name, date, place, identity of parents, and sometimes additional information such as birth weight. It provides the basis for vital statistics of birth and birthrates in a political or administrative jurisdiction and for the DENOMINATOR for infant mortality and certain other vital rates.

BIRTH COHORT The location of a person in historical time as indexed by his or her year of birth. Birth cohorts are often differentially affected by social events. Numerous COHORT variations in factors that have long-term effects on health (e.g., childbearing, smoking, physical activity) have been documented. Cohort effects are easiest to distinguish when disease TRENDS have accelerated, decelerated, or changed direction; where they are steady and linear, they can hardly be distinguished reliably from period effects.[1,3,7,23,24] See also COHORT ANALYSIS; DEVELOPMENTAL AND LIFE COURSE EPIDEMIOLOGY; LIFE COURSE.

BIRTH COHORT ANALYSIS See COHORT ANALYSIS.

BIRTH INTERVAL Time interval between termination of one completed pregnancy and the termination of the next. Time interval between the birth of one offspring and the birth of the next offspring of the same mother.

BIRTH INTERVAL, CLOSED This applies to the population of women who gave birth to two or more living children: it counts only birth intervals between two completed pregnancies (i.e., the interval is closed by next pregnancy).

BIRTH INTERVAL, OPEN This applies also to the population of women who gave birth to two or more living children, but it counts only birth intervals after completed pregnancies.

BIRTH ORDER The ordinal number of a given live birth in relation to all previous live births of the same woman. Thus, 4 is the birth order of the fourth live birth occurring to the same woman. This strict demographic definition may be loosened to include all births, i.e., STILLBIRTHS as well as live births. More loosely, the ranking of siblings according to age, starting with the eldest in a family.

BIRTHRATE A summary rate based on the number of live births in a population over a given period, usually 1 year.

$$\text{Birthrate} = \frac{\begin{array}{c}\text{Number of live births to residents} \\ \text{in an area in a calendar year}\end{array}}{\begin{array}{c}\text{Average or midyear population} \\ \text{in the area in that year}\end{array}} \times 1000$$

Demographers refer to this as the *crude birthrate*. See also PERINATAL MORTALITY.

BIRTH WEIGHT Infant's weight recorded at the time of birth and, in some countries, entered on the birth certificate. Certain variants of birth weight are precisely defined. Low birth weight (LBW) is below 2500 g. Very low birth weight (VLBW) is below 1500 g. Ultra-low birth weight (ULBW) is below 1000 g. Large for gestational age (LGA) is birth weight above the 90th percentile. Average weight for gestational age (AGA) (syn: appropriate or adequate) is birth weight between the 10th and 90th percentiles. Small for gestational age (SGA) (syn: small for dates) is birth weight below the 10th percentile.

"BLACK BOX"

1. A method of reasoning or studying a problem in which the methods and procedures are not described, explained, or perhaps even understood. Nothing is stated or inferred about the method; discussion and conclusions relate solely to the empirical relationships observed.

2. A method of formally relating an input (e.g., quantity of a drug administered, exposure to a putative causal factor) to an output or an observed effect (e.g., amount of the drug eliminated, disease), without making detailed assumptions about the MECHANISMS that have contributed to the transformation of input to output within the organism (the "black box").

"BLACK-BOX EPIDEMIOLOGY" A common epidemiological approach, used both in research and in public health practice, in which the focus is on assessing putative causes and clinical effects (beneficial or adverse) rather than the underlying biological MECHANISMS. It is not a formal branch or specialty of epidemiology, nor is it an epidemiological method or philosophy. Loosely speaking, it is an opposite of MECHANISTIC EPIDEMIOLOGY.

BLINDED STUDY (Syn: masked study) A study in which one or more of the involved groups (participant subjects, investigators, data collectors, outcome assessors, laboratory personnel, data analysts) are kept unaware of the exposure or treatment group to which the subjects are assigned, as in a blinded EXPERIMENT, or of the population from which the subjects come, as in a blinded nonexperimental study. A DOUBLE-BLIND study usually refers to a situation in which the data collectors and subjects do not know the treatments assignment. If the data analysts are also unaware of the group to which subjects belong, the study is sometimes described as TRIPLE-BLIND. The intent of blinding is to minimize differences among study groups in the effects that knowledge of treatment or exposure status might have for the subjects (e.g., reporting of beneficial and adverse effects, PLACEBO EFFECTS), data collectors (measurement bias), or data analysts. Those describing a a study should provide a specific description of who among those involved in the study were blinded. To avoid confusion about the meaning of *blind*, some authors prefer to use *masked*.[1,6,24,26,58,73-77] See also ALLOCATION CONCEALMENT; PERFORMANCE BIAS.

BLINDING See BLINDED STUDY; DOUBLE-BLIND TRIAL; TRIPLE BLIND STUDY.

BLOCKED RANDOMIZATION (Syn: restricted randomization) A procedure used in a RANDOMIZED CONTROLLED TRIAL that helps achieve a similar number of subjects allocated to each group, often within defined baseline categories.[1,26,73-77] For example, for allocation in two groups (A and B) in blocks of four, there are six variants: (1) A A B B; (2) A B A B; (3) A B B A; (4) B B A A; (5) B A B A; (6) B A A B. To create the allocation sequence, such blocks are used at random. As a result of this procedure, the number of subjects in two groups at any time differs by no more than half the block length. Block size is usually a multiple of the number of groups in the trial. Small blocks are used at the beginning of the trial to balance subjects in small participating clinics or centers. Large blocks control balance less well but mask the allocation sequence better. It may be seen as an analogue in a RANDOMIZED

CONTROLLED TRIAL of individual matching in an observational study. See also RANDOM ALLOCATION; STRATIFIED RANDOMIZATION.

BODY BURDEN The concentration (e.g., in specific tissues, blood, urine) or the total amount of an agent, element or substance present in the body (e.g., a virus, a radioactive element, a synthetic chemical). A term commonly used in analytical chemistry, BIOMONITORING programs, or ENVIRONMENTAL EPIDEMIOLOGY to refer to the internal dose of a BIOMARKER used to measure an environmental chemical compound temporarily present or more permanently stored in the body.[12,13,146-153]

BODY MASS INDEX (BMI) (Syn: Quetelet's index) Anthropometric measure, defined as weight in kilograms divided by the square of height in meters. The measure was suggested by Lambert Adolphe Jacques Quetelet (1796–1857) and known as Quetelet's index II. It correlates closely with body density and skinfold thickness; in this respect it is superior to the PONDERAL INDEX. It is a standard measure to detect overweight (BMI among 25 and 29.9), and obesity (BMI over 30).[154-158]

BONFERRONI CORRECTION See MULTIPLE COMPARISON TECHNIQUES.

BOOSTER PHENOMENON In people who have a TUBERCULOSIS infection, an initial false-negative result of a TUBERCULIN SKIN TEST due to a diminished response, becoming positive on subsequent testing. This boosted reaction may be misinterpreted as a test conversion from a newly acquired infection and, thus, two-step testing is recommended.

BOOTSTRAP (Syn: resampling) A technique for estimating the VARIANCE and BIAS of an estimator by repeatedly drawing random samples with replacement from the observations at hand, with the resamples having the same size as the original sample. One applies the estimator to each sample drawn, thus obtaining a set of resample estimates. The empirical variance of this set is the naïve bootstrap estimate of variance

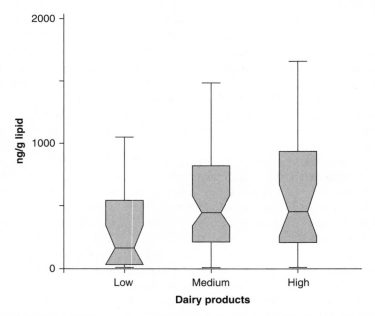

Box-and-whiskers plot. Serum concentration of p,p'-DDT in patients with exocrine pancreatic cancer by reported intake of dairy products. Source: Gasull M, et al.[160] With permission.

("naïve" because better estimates can be created from the resamples by using more complex formulas). The difference between the mean of the set of resample estimates and the original estimate is the bootstrap estimate of bias. Many more sophisticated uses of the repeated samples have been developed.[1,34,37]

BOX-AND-WHISKERS PLOT (Syn: box plot, cat-and-whiskers plot) A type of graph used to present the DISTRIBUTION of a variable measured on a numerical scale. The midpoint (or sometimes, the median) of the distribution is often represented by a horizontal line; the values above and below this line divided into quartiles by horizontal lines (the "hinges" of the box) are the two quartiles nearer the midpoint; values beyond the hinges are represented by lines (the "whiskers") extending to the extreme value in each direction. The box-and-whiskers plot and the STEM-AND-LEAF DISPLAY were developed by the statistician John Tukey (1915–2000).[37,159]

"BRAIN SPARING" A human baby receiving an inadequate supply of nutrients or oxygen may protect its brain. One way in which it does is by diverting more blood to the brain at the expense of the blood supply to the trunk. The growth of organs such as the liver is therefore "traded off" to protect growth of the brain. Brain sparing may also be effected through metabolic processes as insulin resistance.[161] See also DEVELOPMENTAL ORIGINS OF HEALTH AND DISEASE; PLASTICITY; THRIFTY PHENOTYPE HYPOTHESIS.

BREAKPOINT

1. A point where a plotted quantity shifts or jumps abruptly. A point of discontinuity in a plot or function.
2. The critical mean wormload in a community below which the helminth mating frequency is too low to maintain reproduction. A value exceeding the breakpoint of a wormload means that the wormload will increase until equilibrium is reached;

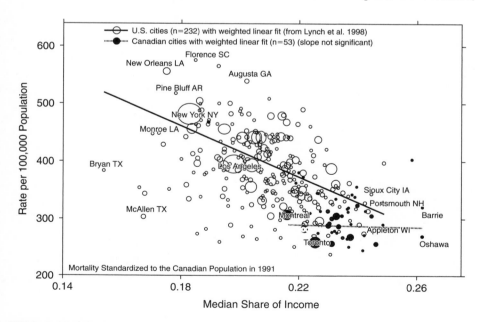

Bubble plot. Standardized mortality rates of working-age people by proportion of income of the less-well-off half of households, U.S. and Canadian cities, 1990–1991. U.S. cities open circles, Canadian cities solid circles. Source: Ross NA, et al.[162] With permission.

a value less than or equal to the breakpoint means that the wormload will decrease progressively.

BUBBLE PLOT A type of graph that displays three sets of variables, two of which form a scatter diagram while the third is represented by circles of varying diameter.

BURDEN OF DISEASE The impact of disease in a population. An approach to the analysis of health problems, including loss of healthy years of life. It is an important concept for PUBLIC HEALTH and for other professions interested in the societal impact of ill-health, including injuries and disabilities. It may be expressed as lost HEALTHY LIFE YEARS (HEALYS), DISABILITY-ADJUSTED LIFE YEARS (DALYs), or QUALITY-ADJUSTED LIFE YEARS (QALYS). Methodologies used in GLOBAL BURDEN OF DISEASE studies enable the combined measurement of mortality and non-fatal health outcomes, and provide comparable and comprehensive measures of population health across countries. They are also relevant to investigate the costs, efficacy, effectiveness, and other impacts of major health interventions applied in diverse settings.[17,28,95,163-166] The World Health Organization offers guidance for the estimation of disease burden at national or local levels for selected environmental and occupational risk factors.[167-169] Since many diseases cannot be completely eradicated with most known interventions, policies should also be based on the likely impact of interventions, available resources, and values. See also ATTRIBUTABLE FRACTION.

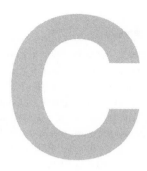

CALIBRATION

1. Adjustment of an instrument or its measurements so the distribution of measurements matches a standard. In multicenter studies, calibration ensures a common standard and therefore comparability of measurements.

2. In statistics, a situation in which an asserted frequency property of a statistical procedure is in fact true. Suppose, for example, that a procedure produces interval estimates that are asserted to be 95% confidence intervals; if those intervals would indeed contain the true parameter in at least 95% of repeated samplings or trials, the procedure is said to be calibrated (or frequency valid).[1,6,7,26,796] See also FREQUENTIST STATISTICS.

CALIPER MATCHING See MATCHING.

CAMPBELL COLLABORATION An independent international nonprofit organization that aims to improve decisions about the effects of interventions in the social, behavioral, and educational arenas. An international network of social scientists that produces and disseminates SYSTEMATIC REVIEWS of research evidence on the effectiveness of social interventions. Also known as "C2" because of its relationship with the COCHRANE COLLABORATION.[170]

CANCER EPIDEMIOLOGY A branch or subspecialty of epidemiology that studies factors influencing the occurrence (e.g., incidence, population distribution) of neoplastic and preneoplastic diseases and related disorders. Primary outcomes include incidence, prevalence, survival, and mortality from all types of cancers.[81,82,149,171]

CANCER MORTALITY: INCIDENCE RATIO (Syn: cancer MIR, cancer mortality-to-incidence ratio) The ratio of mortality to incidence for each of several cancer sites being considered in a study. It is one diagnostic technique among several that can be used to gain some sense of cancer data quality; its main use is in studies of the natural history and survival rates of malignancies. Because not all patients with cancer die of cancer, the number of new cases in any one year should exceed cancer deaths in that same year, and—if cancer mortality and incidence are reported accurately—the ratio between the two should be proportional to the known survival for each specific site. For example, cancers with poor survival, such as pancreatic cancer, would be expected to have an MIR closer to unity than cancers with better survival, such as testicular cancer. If MIR exceeds unity, concern should arise about the quality of the data.[172,173]

$$\text{Cancer MIR} = \frac{\text{no. of cancer-specific deaths over a specified length of time}}{\text{no. of cancer-specific new cases in the same time period}}$$

CANCER REGISTRY See REGISTER.

CANDIDATE GENE One or more genes thought of being implicated in the PATHOPHYSIOLOGY of a disease or another phenotype that are selected for study based on a priori knowledge (e.g., of the gene's biological and physiological function, of its clinical RELEVANCE).[54] See also "AGNOSTIC" ANALYSIS.

CANDIDATE GENE-ENVIRONMENT INTERACTION A GENE-ENVIRONMENT INTERACTION that is selected for study based on available knowledge on its potential role in influencing disease risk, severity, or prognosis.[174,175]

CANDIDATE GENE APPROACH An approach used in GENETIC ASSOCIATION STUDIES which focuses on associations between genetic variation within CANDIDATE GENES and phenotypes such as a disease. Both a strength and a limitation are its reliance on existing empirical or theoretical knowledge about the biology and pathophysiology of the clinical phenotype.[53,86] It thus contrasts with GENOME-WIDE ASSOCIATION STUDIES (GWAS).

CAPITAL See SOCIAL CAPITAL.

CAPTURE-RECAPTURE METHOD A method of estimating the size of a target population or a subset of this population that uses overlapping and presumably incomplete but intersecting sets of data about that population.[7,24,176,177] The method originated in wildlife biology, where it relied on tagging and releasing captured animals and then recapturing them. The method was adopted in veterinary epidemiology and later in vital statistics (census taking) and epidemiology. If two independent sources or population estimates are available, with (a) cases found by both, (b) cases found only by the first source, or (c) cases found only by the second source, the maximum likelihood population estimate is the product of the total in each source divided by the total found in both sources, i.e., $(a + b) \times (a + c) / a$. If the two sources are positively (negatively) dependent, the result will be biased toward an underestimate (overestimate). If three or more sources are available, log-linear methods can sometimes be used to model the degrees of dependency among the sources. Although the capture-recapture methods have some limitations, they are useful to estimate numbers of cases and numbers at risk in elusive populations, such as homeless people and sex workers. See also SNOWBALL SAMPLING.

CARCINOGEN A substance or agent that can cause cancer. A physical, chemical, or biological agent that may induce or otherwise participate in the causation of cancer. A carcinogen may or may not be MUTAGENIC. Some compounds do not bind to DNA and are not mutagenic, yet they are carcinogenic in animal models and in humans. Carcinogens act through GENOTOXIC and NONGENOTOXIC mechanisms. "Complete carcinogens" (e.g., some polycyclic aromatic hydrocarbons [PAHs]) can induce both somatic (acquired) mutations in genes through DNA binding (tumor "initiation" phase) and subsequent outgrowth of irreversibly transformed cells (tumor "promotion" phase). In the early 1980s, carcinogenic PAHs were shown to induce activating mutations in *ras* genes. Today, about 200 different chemical compounds and mixtures are officially recognized as "known" or "anticipated to be" human carcinogens.[13,14,78,80-82,178-182]

The International Agency for Research on Cancer (IARC) classifies CARCINOGENS as follows: *Sufficient evidence.* A positive causal relationship has been established between exposure and occurrence of cancer. *Limited evidence.* A positive association has been observed between exposure to the agent and cancer for which a causal interpretation is credible, but chance, bias, or confounding cannot be ruled out. *Inadequate evidence.* Available studies are of insufficient quality, consistency, or statistical power to permit a conclusion regarding the presence or absence of a causal relationship. *Evidence suggesting lack of carcinogenicity.* Several adequate studies covering the full range of doses to which humans are known to be exposed are mutually consistent in not showing a positive association between exposure to the agent and any studied cancer at any level of exposure. Overall evaluation: Taking all the evidence into account, the agent is assigned to one of the following categories: *Group 1*: The agent is carcinogenic to humans. *Group 2*: At one extreme, the evidence for human carcinogenicity is almost sufficient (group 2A, probably carcinogenic); at the other, there are no human data but there is experimental evidence of carcinogenicity (group 2B, possibly carcinogenic). *Group 3*: The agent is not classifiable as to its human carcinogenicity. *Group 4*: The agent is probably not carcinogenic to humans.

CARCINOGENESIS The process by which cancer is produced. Carcinogenesis is a multistage process driven by carcinogen-induced accumulation of genetic and EPIGENETIC damage in susceptible cells, which gain a selective growth advantage and undergo clonal expansion as the result of activation of (proto)oncogenes and inactivation of tumor suppressor genes. Accumulation of genetic and epigenetic alterations is hence a key causal process linking environment exposure and the occurrence of DISEASES OF COMPLEX ETIOLOGY.[14,78,80-82,178,183-187] The traditional stages of carcinogenesis are as follows: *Initiation.* The primary step of tumor INDUCTION; the irreversible transformation of a cell's growth-regulatory processes whereby the potential for unregulated growth is established, usually through genetic damage by a chemical or physical CARCINOGEN. *Promotion.* The second stage, in which a promoting agent induces an initiated cell to divide abnormally. *Progression.* Transition of initiated promoted cells to a phase of unregulated growth and invasiveness, frequently with metastases and morphological changes in the cancer cells. Research in EPIGENETICS and MOLECULAR EPIDEMIOLOGY often clarifies carcinogenic mechanisms.

CARDIOVASCULAR EPIDEMIOLOGY A branch or subspecialty of epidemiology that studies factors influencing the occurrence of diseases that affect the cardiovascular system, like coronary heart disease and stroke. Established and putative RISK FACTORS include individual-level behavioral factors (e.g., diet, smoking, physical activity) and psychosocial risk factors, as well as macro-, aggregate-, or higher-level socioeconomic factors and processes (e.g., environmental and economic characteristics of neighbourhoods or cities).

CARRIER

1. A person or animal harboring a specific INFECTIOUS AGENT in the absence of discernible clinical disease and which serves as a potential source of infection. The carrier state may occur in an individual with an infection that is inapparent throughout its course (known as a healthy or asymptomatic carrier) or the carrier state may exist only during the incubation period, convalescence, and postconvalescence of an individual with a clinically recognizable disease (known as an incubatory carrier or convalescent carrier). The carrier state may be of short or long duration (temporary or transient carrier or chronic carrier).[20-22,56,188]

2. An insurance carrier provides reimbursement of part or all of medical expenses for health insurance policy holders.[116] See also ADVERSE SELECTION; ASYMMETRY OF INFORMATION.

3. When the INHERITANCE of a disorder is recessive, each parent contributes one abnormal copy of the gene to the child who has the disorder, and the two abnormal copies must be present for the individual to be affected. While heterozygous individuals (such as the parents of the affected child) do not show the abnormal

phenotype, they are called *carriers* because they have one normal and one abnormal copy of the gene.[57] An individual who is heterozygous for a specified recessive allele and who thus does not normally display the characteristics associated with that allele but who may, with appropriate mating, produce homozygous offspring that exhibit the recessive characteristic.[189]

4. A component of a biological membrane that effects the transfer of a substance from one side of the membrane to the other. Still other biological meanings of *carrier* may be relevant in some epidemiological contexts.[59,189,190]

CARRIER, CHRONIC An individual remaining in a carrier state for a long period of time after convalescence.[20-22,56,188]

CARRIER FREQUENCY (Syn: carrier rate) The proportion of individuals in a population who have a single copy of a recessive allele. Also sometimes applied to the prevalence of variants in dominantly acting genes such as BRCA1 and BRCA2.

CARRYING CAPACITY FOR HUMANS In a community of subsistence farmers, the carrying capacity denotes the maximum number of people that a hectare of land can support sustainably in an average year at a practicable level of technology and at a specified standard of living—commonly mere survival. For example, if a hectare of land grows 1 ton of maize and 250 kg will feed one person for a year, the carrying capacity of that land is four people to the hectare. There is uncertainty about the earth's carrying capacity: some experts argue that there is abundant unused capacity, while others believe that the earth is already exceeding its carrying capacity.

CARRYING CAPACITY FOR OTHER SPECIES The maximum sustainable size of a resident population in a given ecosystem.

CARRYOVER EFFECT

1. A BIAS that may occur when the effects of an exposure persist into a subsequent period when a second exposure of interest is acting.
2. In a CROSSOVER CLINICAL TRIAL the effect of the treatment given in the first period may continue ("carryover") into the second treatment period.
3. Treatments may be randomly allocated to paired organs (eyes, arms, hips, kidneys) if treatments act only locally. However, CONTAMINATION may occur if there is a carryover effect of the experimental treatment to the control organ of the pair.[9]

CARTOGRAM A type of map in which the size of areas (e.g., countries, counties, electoral regions) varies in proportion to the value of the statistical variable displayed on the map. An example is the ISODEMOGRAPHIC MAP.

CASE A particular disease, health disorder, or condition under investigation found in an individual or within a population or study group. A person having a particular disease, disorder or condition (e.g., a case of cancer, a case in a case-control study). A variety of criteria may be used to identify cases; e.g., individual physicians' diagnoses, registries and notifications, abstracts of clinical records, surveys of the GENERAL POPULATION, SURVEILLANCE systems, screening programs. An epidemiological definition of a case may not be the same as the clinical definition.[1,6,9,24,58,69,160,191]

CASE, AUTOCHTHONOUS In infectious disease epidemiology, a case of local origin. Literally, "native where it arises." See also CASE, IMPORTED; CASE, INDIGENOUS.

CASE-BASE STUDY A variant of the case-control study in which the controls are drawn from the same STUDY BASE as the cases, regardless of their disease status.[1,192] Cases of the disease of interest are identified, and a sample of the entire base population (cases and noncases) forms the controls. This design provides for estimation of the RISK RATIO or rate ratio without any RARE DISEASE ASSUMPTION. Specific examples include the CASE-COHORT STUDY and the DENSITY CASE-CONTROL STUDY.

CASE-CASE STUDY A type of CASE-ONLY STUDY in which cases of a given disease with a specific characteristic are compared with other cases with the same disease but without the characteristic; the latter may be, for instance, an acquired (somatic) genetic alteration or an inherited genetic variant. The aim is to identify etiological or susceptibility factors specific to the subset of cases with the characteristic.[193] The design is also used in infectious disease epidemiology to detect different transmission ways between subtypes of one disease.[194-197] To analyze infectious disease outbreaks, exposures of an outbreak cluster are compared with exposures among individuals infected by another subtype of the same disease.

CASE-COHORT STUDY A variant of the case-control study in which the controls are drawn from the same COHORT as the cases regardless of their disease status. Cases of the disease of interest are identified, and a sample of the entire starting cohort (regardless of their outcomes) forms the controls. This design provides an estimate of the RISK RATIO without any RARE DISEASE ASSUMPTION.[1,3,5,8,24] A type of CASE-BASE STUDY. See also DENSITY CASE-CONTROL STUDY; NESTED CASE-CONTROL STUDY.

CASE, COLLATERAL A case occurring in the immediate vicinity of a case that has been the subject of an epidemiological investigation; a term used mainly in malaria control programs, equivalent to the term *contact* as used in infectious disease epidemiology.[56]

CASE CLASSIFICATION In SURVEILLANCE epidemiology, gradations in the likelihood of being a case (e.g., suspected/probable/confirmed); a useful method when early reporting of cases is important, and where there are difficulties in making a definitive diagnosis (e.g., because specialized laboratory tests are required) or when the diagnosis is based on a scoring system.[160]

CASE-COMPARISON STUDY A term considered a synonym for CASE-CONTROL STUDY in the past.

CASE-CONTROL STUDY (Syn: case-referent study) The observational epidemiological study of persons with the disease (or another outcome variable) of interest and a suitable CONTROL GROUP of persons without the disease (comparison group, reference group). The potential relationship of a suspected RISK FACTOR or an attribute to the disease is examined by comparing the diseased and nondiseased subjects with regard to how frequently the factor or attribute is present (or, if quantitative, the levels of the attribute) in each of the groups (diseased and nondiseased).[1,3,6,7,24,26,58,149,197]

It is not correct to call "case-control study" any comparison of a group of people having a specific outcome with another group free of that outcome.[42] The case-control study used to be called "retrospective" because, conceptually, it goes from disease onset backward to the postulated causal factors. Yet cases and controls in a case-control study are often accumulated prospectively: the conduct of the study starts before cases have been diagnosed and, as each new case is diagnosed and identified, it enters the study. Subjects in a RANDOMIZED CONTROLLED TRIAL should not be described as *cases* and *controls*.

CASE-CROSSOVER STUDY A type of CASE-ONLY STUDY and an observational analogue of a CROSSOVER STUDY. It can be used when a brief exposure triggers an outcome or causes a transient rise in the risk of a disease with an acute onset.[1,3,5,24,198] In this design each case serves as its own matched control. The exposure status of each case is assessed during different time windows, and the exposure status at the time of case occurrence is compared to the status at other times. Conditions to be met include the following: (1) acute cases are needed, an abrupt outcome applies best; (2) crossover in exposure status (there must be a sufficient number of individuals who crossed from higher to lower exposure level and vice-versa); (3) brief and transient exposures (the exposure or its effects must be short-lived); and (4) selection of control time periods must be unrelated to any general TRENDS in exposure. Properly applied, the design allows estimation of the rate ratio without need for a RARE DISEASE ASSUMPTION. See also CASE-TIME CONTROL STUDY.

CASE DEFINITION A set of criteria (not necessarily diagnostic criteria) that must be fulfilled in order to identify a person as representing a case of a particular disease or condition. It is different from CASE diagnosis. Case definition can be based on geographic, clinical, laboratory, or combined clinical and laboratory criteria or on a scoring system with points for each criterion that matches the features of the disease. Where the diagnosis is based on a scoring system, it is important to abide by the system for SURVEILLANCE purposes and in deciding whether to include or exclude cases in an epidemiological study.[69,160,199]

CASE FATALITY RATE The proportion of cases of a specified condition that are fatal within a specified time.

$$\text{Case fatality rate (usually expressed as a percentage)} = \frac{\text{Number of deaths from a disease (in a given period)}}{\text{Number of diagnosed cases of that disease (in the same period)}} \times 100$$

This definition can lead to paradox when more persons die of the disease than develop it during a given period. For instance, chemical poisoning that is slowly but inexorably fatal may cause many persons to develop the disease over a relatively short period of time, but the deaths may not occur until some years later and may be spread over a period of years during which there are no new cases. Thus, in calculating the case fatality rate, it is necessary to acknowledge that the time dimension varies: it may be brief (e.g., covering only the period of stay in a hospital); of finite duration (e.g., 1 year); or of longer duration still. The term *case fatality rate* is then better replaced by a term such as *survival rate* or by the use of a survivorship table.[5,24] See also ATTACK RATE; SURVIVORSHIP STUDY.

CASE FINDING
1. (Syn: Contact tracing). A standard procedure in the control of certain CONTAGIOUS DISEASES (e.g., tuberculosis and sexually transmitted diseases) whereby diligent efforts are made to locate and treat persons who have had close or intimate contact with a known case. Also, seeking persons who have been exposed to risk of other potentially harmful factors, like toxic substances, epidemic conditions, or outbreaks such as food poisoning.[69]
2. SECONDARY PREVENTION through EARLY CLINICAL DETECTION of cases among persons using health services for other reasons (e.g., checking blood pressures of all patients who attend a physician's office).

CASE HISTORY STUDY
1. In clinical medicine, a CASE REPORT or a report on a CASE SERIES.
2. A term considered a synonym for CASE-CONTROL STUDY in the past.[197]

CASE IMPACT NUMBER See IMPACT NUMBERS.

CASE, IMPORTED In infectious disease epidemiology, a case that has entered a region by land, sea, or air transport, in contrast to one acquired locally. See also CASE, AUTOCHTONOUS.

CASE, INDIGENOUS In infectious disease epidemiology, a case in a person residing in the area.

CASE, INDUCED In malaria epidemiology, a case occurring in a person who has received a transfusion of blood containing malaria parasites; the term is generalizable to other conditions that can be transmitted by infected blood (e.g., HIV, hepatitis C).[56,188,196]

CASE INVESTIGATION In SURVEILLANCE epidemiology, examination to determine whether an individual is or is not involved in an epidemic, especially an INDEX CASE.[69,160]

CASE-MIX INDEX **(CMI)** A measure of the complexity of illness. Among hospital patients, it is based on the relative severity indexes assigned to a DIAGNOSIS-RELATED GROUP. A high CMI indicates a high proportion of complex cases and justifies higher rates of reimbursement in medical care insurance systems such as Medicare.

CASE-ONLY STUDY A type of study in which cases are the only subjects used to estimate or test hypotheses about effects (e.g., cases with the disease of interest); thus, it does not use an independent comparison group for reference.[1,9,24,57] Variants include the CASE-CASE STUDY, the CASE-CROSSOVER STUDY, CASE-SPECULAR designs and even CASE SERIES.[200] Under some assumptions, case-only designs may be used to assess gene-gene and GENE-ENVIRONMENT INTERACTIONS, and etiologic, diagnostic, and prognostic heterogeneity.

CASE REFERENT STUDY See CASE-CONTROL STUDY.

CASE REPORTS Detailed descriptions of a few patients or clinical cases (frequently, just one sick person) with an unsual disease or complication, uncommon combinations of diseases, an unusual or misleading SEMIOLOGY, CAUSE, or OUTCOME (maybe a surprising recovery). They often are preliminary observations that are later refuted. They cannot estimate disease frequency or risk (e.g., for lack of a valid DENOMINATOR). Alternatives are available for COMPLETING THE CLINICAL PICTURE. However, as Pierre Charles Alexandre Louis, Claude Bernard, Thomas Lewis, Austin Bradford Hill, and many others have shown (e.g., more recently, Jan P. Vandenbroucke or Gordon Guyatt, or organizations like the COCHRANE COLLABORATION), many problems worthy of investigation in medicine are first identified by observations at the bedside.[26,58,201,202] Indeed, case reports may thoughtfully integrate clinical, anatomopathological, genetic, pathophysiological, occupational, or biochemical information and reasoning; they may thus build a sound mechanistic or pragmatic hypothesis and set the foundation for (micro)biological studies and for larger clinical and epidemiological studies. They may also raise a thoughtful suspicion of a new adverse drug event and are an important means of SURVEILLANCE for rare clinical events. They help to reflect on and learn from medical error.[6,9,24,63,69,203]

CASE SERIES A collection of subjects (usually, patients) with common characteristics used to describe some clinical, pathophysiological, or operational aspect of a disease, treatment, exposure, or diagnostic procedure. Some are similar to the larger CASE REPORTS and share their virtues. The number of subjects does not attenuate the limitations of the design. A case series does not include a comparison group and is often based on prevalent cases and on a SAMPLE of convenience.[6,8,9,24,26,58,63] Common selection biases and CONFOUNDING severely limit their power to make CAUSAL INFERENCES. See also INCEPTION COHORT; VALIDITY.

CASE-SPECULAR STUDY A type of CASE-ONLY STUDY that obtains the actual distribution of exposure among the dwellings of the cases and a reflected or "specular" exposure distribution, which is what the exposure distribution would have been if the dwellings had been placed on the opposite side of the street. From these two distributions (i.e., the actual and the specular distribution) and some assumptions, including a RARE DISEASE ASSUMPTION, a relative risk estimate for the effect of exposure can be calculated, much as it can for a case-control study, albeit with different assumptions.[1] For example, the distance of each case's front door from an electrical wire is matched with the distance from the same wire of a hypothetical front door located exactly across the street.[204]

CASE STUDY A detailed analysis of the occurrence, development, and outcome of a particular problem or innovation, often over a period of time. A detailed description of a concrete situation requiring ethical analysis, judgment, and — sometimes — action.[13]

CASE-TIME-CONTROL STUDY A study in which exposure of cases and controls during one period is compared in matched-pair analyses to their own exposure during another period of similar length.[205] See also CASE-CROSSOVER STUDY.

CASUISTRY A method of reasoning and decision-making based on experience with and decisions about similar cases in the past; traditionally used in clinical medicine or in ETHICS. Medical *casuistics* is the study of cases of disease.

CAT-AND-WHISKERS PLOT See BOX-AND-WHISKERS PLOT.

CATASTROPHE THEORY A branch of mathematics dealing with large changes in the total system that may result from small changes in a critical variable in the system. An example is the sudden change in the physical state of water into steam or ice with rise or fall of temperature beyond a critical level. Certain epidemics, HERD IMMUNITY, gene frequencies, and behavioral phenomena in populations may abide by similar mathematical rules. See also CHAOS THEORY.

CATCHMENT AREA Region from which the clients of a particular health facility are drawn. Such a region may be well or ill defined.

CATEGORIZATION One way of organizing information on objects or ideas. The process of recognition, differentiation, and understanding of objects by grouping into categories, usually for statistical analysis or graphic representation.[1] Category is from late Latin *categoria*—a division within a system of CLASSIFICATION. See also CLUSTERING; DIRECTORY; ONTOLOGY; TAXONOMY.

CAUSAL CRITERIA or CAUSAL CONSIDERATIONS Considerations (often informally or misleadingly called "criteria") that help to guide judgments about causality and to make causal inferences.[1,5-9,25,39-42,58,85,101,206-208] Examples close to epidemiological and clinical research include John Stuart MILL'S CANONS, the "rules" of David Hume, EVANS'S POSTULATES, HENLE-KOCH POSTULATES, or HILL'S CONSIDERATIONS FOR CAUSATION.

CAUSAL DIAGRAM (Syn: causal graph, path diagram) A graphical display of causal relations among variables, in which each variable is assigned a fixed location on the graph (called a *node*), and in which each direct causal effect of one variable on another is represented by an arrow with its tail at the cause and its head at the effect.[100] Direct noncausal associations are usually represented by lines without arrowheads. Graphs with only directed arrows (in which all direct associations are causal) are called *directed graphs*. Graphs in which no variable can affect itself (no feedback loop) are called *acyclic*. Methods have been developed to determine from causal diagrams which sets of variables are sufficient to control CONFOUNDING and for when control of variables leads to BIAS.[1,2,34,84,101,209,210]

CAUSAL INFERENCE The quantification of the causal effect of an exposure or treatment on an outcome.[2] The thought processes and methods that assess whether a relation of cause to effect exists, or that estimate the size of a causal relationship using some EFFECT MEASURE. In epidemiology, causal inference is often conducted under the POTENTIAL OUTCOME or COUNTERFACTUAL models. See also ANALYTICAL STUDY; ASSOCIATION; GENERALIZABILITY; HILL'S CONSIDERATIONS FOR CAUSATION; PROBABILITY OF CAUSATION; PROPERTIES OF A CAUSE; RISK FACTOR; VERIFICATION.

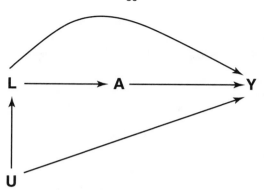

Causal diagram representing outcome Y, exposure A, their unmeasured common cause U, and risk factor L. Graph theory can be used to show that data on L are sufficient to eliminate the confounding, caused by the presence of U, for the effect of A on Y.

CAUSALITY The relation of causes to the effects they produce. The property of being causal. The presence of cause. Ideas about the nature of the relations of cause and effect. The potential for changing an outcome by changing the cause. Most of clinical, epidemiological, and public health research concerns forms of causality. In the health and life sciences, causality is often approached by INTEGRATION of biological, clinical, epidemiological, and social or environmental evidence, as appropriate to the hypothesis at stake. Several types of causes can be distinguished.[1-3,5,8,24,25,26,38,101,110,206,207,798] A cause is termed "necessary" when it must always precede an effect. This effect need not be the

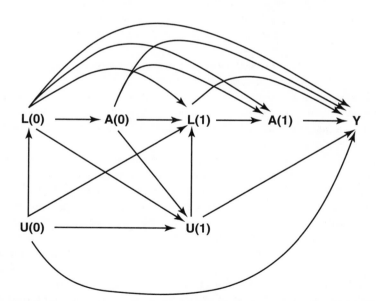

Causal diagram representing outcome Y and time-varying exposure A(t), their unmeasured common cause U(t), and risk factor L(t) at times t = 0 and t = 1. Graph theory can be used to show that data on L(0) and L(1) are sufficient to eliminate the confounding, caused by the presence of U(0) and U(1), for the joint effect of A(0) and A(1) on Y.

sole result of the one cause. A cause is termed "sufficient" when it inevitably initiates or produces an effect. Any given cause may be necessary, sufficient, neither, or both. Hence, there are four general conditions under which antecedent variable X may cause Y:

	X is necessary	X is sufficient	
1.	+	+	$X \rightarrow Y$
2.	+	−	X and $Z \rightarrow Y$
3.	−	+	$X \rightarrow Y; Z \rightarrow Y$
4.	−	−	X and $Z \rightarrow Y; W$ and $K \rightarrow Y$

1. X is necessary and sufficient to cause Y. Both X and Y are always present together, and nothing but X is needed to cause $Y; X \rightarrow Y$. For example, the measles virus is necessary to cause measles in an unimmunized individual or population.
2. X is necessary but not sufficient to cause Y. X must be present when Y is present, but Y is not always present when X is. Some additional factor(s) must also be present; X and $Z \rightarrow Y$. *Mycobacterium tuberculosis* is the necessary cause of tuberculosis but often is not a SUFFICIENT CAUSE: poverty, poor nutrition, or overcrowding must also operate.
3. X is not necessary but is sufficient to cause Y. Y is present when X is, but X may or may not be present when Y is present, because Y has other causes and can occur without X. For example, an enlarged spleen can have many separate causes that are unconnected with each other; $X \rightarrow Y; Z \rightarrow Y$. Lung cancer can be caused by cigarette smoking, asbestos fibers, or radon gas.
4. X is neither necessary nor sufficient to cause Y. Again, X may or may not be present when Y is present. Under these conditions, however, if X is present with Y, some additional factor must also be present. Here X is a contributory cause of Y in some causal sequences; X and $Z \rightarrow Y; W$ and $Z \rightarrow Y$.

See also ASSOCIATION; CAUSAL CRITERIA; DISEASES OF COMPLEX ETIOLOGY; HILL'S CONSIDERATIONS FOR CAUSATION; NECESSARY CAUSE.

CAUSAL NULL HYPOTHESIS The hypothesis or condition that there is no effect of one variable (e.g., the treatment or exposure) on another (e.g., the outcome or disease).[1]

CAUSATION OF DISEASE, FACTORS IN While they are not mutually exclusive, the following factors can be differentiated:

1. PREDISPOSING FACTORS are those that prepare, sensitize, condition, or otherwise create a situation such as a level of immunity or state of susceptibility so that the host tends to react in a specific fashion to a disease agent, personal interaction, environmental stimulus, or specific incentive. Examples include age, sex, marital status, family size, educational level, previous illness experience, presence of concurrent illness, dependency, working environment, and attitudes toward the use of health services. These factors may be "necessary" but are rarely "sufficient" to cause the phenomenon under study.
2. ENABLING FACTORS are those that facilitate the manifestation of disease, disability, ill-health, or the use of services or conversely those that facilitate recovery from illness, maintenance or enhancement of health status, or more appropriate use of health services. Examples include income, health insurance coverage, nutrition,

climate, housing, personal support systems, and availability of medical care. These factors may be "necessary" but are rarely "sufficient" to cause the phenomenon under study.

3. PRECIPITATING FACTORS are those associated with the definitive onset of a disease, illness, accident, behavioral response, or course of action. Usually one factor is more important or recognizable than others. Examples include exposure to specific disease, amount or level of an infectious organism, treatment, noxious agent, physical trauma, personal interaction, occupational stimulus, or new knowledge.

4. REINFORCING FACTORS are those tending to perpetuate or aggravate the presence of a DISEASE, DISABILITY, IMPAIRMENT, attitude, pattern of behavior, or course of action. They may tend to be repetitive, recurrent, or persistent and may or may not necessarily be the same or similar to those categorized as predisposing, enabling, or precipitating. Examples include repeated exposure to the same noxious stimulus (in the absence of an appropriate immune response) such as an infectious agent, work, household, or interpersonal environment, presence of financial incentive or disincentive, personal satisfaction or deprivation. See also PROBABILITY OF CAUSATION.

CAUSE-DELETED LIFE TABLE A life table constructed using death rates lowered by eliminating the risk of dying from a specified cause; its most common use is to calculate the gain in life expectancy that would result from the elimination of one cause. See also COMPETING RISK.

CAUSE, PROPERTIES See PROPERTIES OF A CAUSE.

CAUSES, COMPONENTS See COMPONENT CAUSES.

CAUSES IN PUBLIC HEALTH SCIENCES In epidemiology and other population and social sciences (e.g., economy), causes include contextual factors, even if some such factors can seldom be manipulated experimentally to produce change, given the following facts: causal factors, causal processes, and causal systems operate at upper, aggregate, global, and distal levels as well as across macro- and micro-levels (e.g., climate, geographic location, food availability, trade in SYSTEMIC economies); some causes are fairly constant or immutable conditions (such as gender); others show large variations across time and space in the extent to which they change in an individual's LIFE COURSE (e.g., educational and occupational achievement, work conditions, income, social mobility and status, living arrangements).[1-3,5,8,13,19-26,28,33,38,83, 84,93,101,110,121,164,165,211-215,798] Hence, causes of individual and population health often change with global and local societal and geopolitical processes, and many act in specific periods of susceptibility, often with long latencies, or throughout life. None of these characteristics per se excludes or refutes CAUSALITY. Research on the causes of diseases is a "natural meeting place" for basic science (one of whose objectives is knowledge on biological mechanisms), clinical sciences, and epidemiology (one of whose aims is to generate knowledge for primary prevention).[208,216] See also ATTRIBUTABLE FRACTION; STRATEGY, "POPULATION."

CAUSES OF DEATH See DEATH CERTIFICATE.

CAUSE-SPECIFIC RATE A rate that specifies events, such as deaths, according to their cause.

CENSORING

1. Loss or ATTRITION of subjects from a follow-up study; the occurrence of the event of interest among such subjects is uncertain after a specified time when it was known that the event of interest had *not* occurred; it is not known, however, if or when the event of interest occurred subsequently. Such subjects are described as *censored*. For example, in a follow-up study with myocardial infarction as the outcome of interest, a

subject who has not had an infarct but is killed in a traffic crash in year 6 is described as censored as of year 6, since it cannot be known when, if ever, he might have had an infarct at a later time of follow-up. This is censoring by competing risk; other sources of censoring include loss to follow-up and termination of the study. Censoring can be an important influence on observed PERSON-TIME at risk. Analysis of data to account for censoring requires special analytical methods, such as LIFE-TABLE ANALYSIS.[1-3,7] See also ATTRITION; DROP-OUT; LOST TO FOLLOW-UP.

2. Observations with unknown values from one end or a particular interval of a frequency distribution. Left-censored data come from the left-hand portion, or low end, and right-censored data come from the right-hand portion, or high end, of the distribution. Data may also be censored within intervals between the extremes of the data; e.g., when someone drops out but later rejoins a study.

CENSUS An enumeration of a population, originally intended for purposes of taxation and military service. Ancient civilizations such as the Romans conducted censuses; Jesus of Nazareth was born in Bethlehem because Mary and Joseph had gone there to be counted in a Roman census. Census enumeration of a population usually records identities of all persons in every place of residence, with age or birth date, sex, occupation, national origin, language, marital status, income, and relationship to head of household in addition to information on the dwelling place. Many other items of information may be included, e.g., educational level (or literacy) and health-related data such as permanent disability. A de facto census allocates persons according to their location at the time of enumeration. A de jure census assigns persons according to their usual place of residence at the time of enumeration.

CENSUS TRACT An area for which details of population structure are separately tabulated at a periodic census; normally it is the smallest unit of analysis of census tabulations. Census tracts are chosen because they have well-defined boundaries, sometimes the same as local political jurisdictions, sometimes defined by conspicuous geographical features such as main roads or rivers. In urban areas census tracts may be further subdivided (e.g., into city blocks), but published tables do not contain details to this level. Census tracts are usually relatively homogeneous in demographic, socioeconomic, and ethnic composition.

CENTILE See QUANTILES.

CESSATION EXPERIMENT Controlled study in which an attempt is made to evaluate the termination of an exposure to a risk factor (e.g., a smoking cessation experiment).

CHAIN OF INFECTION (Syn: infectious disease cycle, chain of transmission) A set of parameters involved in the transmission of an infectious agent (e.g., the source of infection, the vectors, a susceptible host).[20,56,217-219]

CHAINS OF RISK A sequence of linked EXPOSURES and other RISK FACTORS that increase (or decrease) disease RISK because one negative (or positive) experience or exposure tends to lead to another. See also LIFE COURSE.

CHANCE

1. Frequency PROBABILITY.

2. Accidental, unanticipated, unplanned, fortuitous, serendipitous (e.g., a chance finding during DATA DREDGING).[1-3,5-9,37,38] See also ASSOCIATION, FORTUITOUS; SERENDIPITY.

CHAOS THEORY Branch of mathematics dealing with events and processes that cannot be predicted by conventional mathematical theorems or laws because small, localized perturbations have widespread general consequences. Examples include long-range weather changes and turbulence in fast-flowing water. The unpredictable course of some epidemics and metastases in many kinds of cancer accord with chaos theory.[7]

CHART The medical dossier of a patient. See also BAR CHART; INFORMATION SYSTEM; MEDICAL RECORD.

CHECK DIGIT A single digit, derived from a multidigit number such as a case identification number, that is used as a screening test for transcription errors.

CHEMOPROPHYLAXIS The administration of a chemical, including antibiotics, to prevent the development of an infection or to slow progression of the disease to a clinically manifest form. Applicable to infectious and noninfectious diseases.

CHEMOTHERAPY The use of a chemical to treat a clinically recognizable disease or to limit its further progress.

CHILD (1-4 YEARS) MORTALITY RATE The number of deaths of children age 1–4 years in a given year per 1000 children in this age group. This term was originally defined as "mortality from 1-4 years," but is more often used as a synonym for the UNDERFIVE MORTALITY RATE.

CHILD NUTRITION, MEASURES OF WHO and UNICEF define several aspects of infant and child nutrition:

Stunting A deficit in length (for children aged under two years) or in height (for children aged two years or more) relative to the child's age, according to a standard that reflects optimal growth. Most frequently, stunting is defined as two standard deviations or more below the median value of the WHO Growth Standards.[220] Stunting reflects long-term exposure to inadequate diets, infectious diseases, or inappropriate child care.

Underweight A deficit in weight relative to a child's age. Like stunting, it is usually defined as two standard deviations or more below the WHO standards for weight for age. Underweight can be a result of stunting, wasting or a combination of both.

Wasting A deficit in weight relative to a child's length or height, usually defined as two standard deviations or more below the WHO standards for weight for length or height. Wasting is most often an indicator of acute food shortage or severe infectious disease.

Overweight An excess in weight relative to a child's length or height, usually defined as more than two standard deviations above the WHO standards for weight for length or height. It is also defined in terms of a child's body mass index (BMI) for age.

CHI-SQUARE (χ^2) DISTRIBUTION (Syn: chi-squared distribution) A variable is said to have a chi-square distribution with K degrees of freedom if it is distributed like the sum of the squares of K independent random variables, each of which has a NORMAL DISTRIBUTION with mean zero and variance one.[12,34,37]

CHI-SQUARE (χ^2) TEST (Syn: chi-squared test) A statistical test based on comparison of a test statistic to a chi-square DISTRIBUTION.[7,34,37] The oldest and most common chi-square tests are for detecting whether two or more population distributions differ from one another; these tests usually involve counts of data and may involve comparison of samples from the distributions under study or the comparison of a sample to a theoretically expected distribution. The Pearson chi-square test is probably the best known; another is the MANTEL-HAENSZEL TEST. (Statisticians disagree about the terminal letter; most of those who contributed to the discussion of this entry prefer *chi-square* rather than *chi-squared*. Either usage is acceptable.)

CHOROPLETHIC MAP A type of map in which previously defined areas (e.g., countries, counties, electoral regions) are shaded or patterned in proportion to the value of the statistical variable displayed on the map.

CHROMOSOME Discrete physical structures inside a cell nucleus that contain DNA organized into genes. Different organisms have different numbers of chromosomes. Humans have 23 pairs of chromosomes: 22 pairs of AUTOSOMES and one pair of sex chromosomes, X and Y. Each parent contributes one chromosome to each pair.

CHRONIC

1. Referring to a health-related state: lasting a long time. A disease that lasts from several weeks to many years.[24,163-169] The U.S. National Center for Health Statistics defined a "chronic" condition as one of 3 months' duration or longer. Contrast with ACUTE.

2. Referring to exposure: prolonged or long-term; sometimes, throughout life; sometimes, with an additional specific reference to low intensity or at low concentrations. In some DISEASES OF COMPLEX ETIOLOGY it is likely that chronic exposure at relatively low doses is more causally relevant than brief exposure at high doses.

CHRONIC CARRIER See CARRIER, CHRONIC.

CHRONOBIOLOGY The study of biological processes that possess periodicity (e.g., circadian rhythms, the menstrual cycle).

CIRCULAR EPIDEMIOLOGY Needlessly repetitive epidemiological studies ("me too studies") that merely reiterate what has already been done and demonstrated unequivocally.[222]

CIRCULAR REASONING

1. Reasoning that requires that the conclusion be used to support one of the premises. Circularity may be a problem in definitions.[223]

2. An argument whose conclusion is implicitly assumed in one of the premises.

As with the assessment of a TEMPORAL RELATIONSHIP, detection of circular reasoning may need to be based on knowledge on substantive matter and methodology.

CLASS A term used in the theory of frequency distributions. The total number of observations made upon a particular variate may be grouped into classes according to convenient divisions of the variate range in order to make subsequent analyses less laborious or for other reasons. A group so determined is called a *class*. The variate values that determine the upper and lower limits of a class are called *class boundaries*, the interval between them is the *class interval*, and the frequency falling into the class is the *class frequency*. See also SET; SOCIAL CLASS.

CLASSIFICATION

1. Assignment to predesignated classes on the basis of perceived common characteristics.

2. A means of giving order to a group of disconnected facts.

Ideally, a classification should be characterized by naturalness—the classes correspond to the nature of the thing being classified, exhaustiveness—every member of the group will fit into one (and only one) class in the system, usefulness—the classification is practical, simplicity—the subclasses are not excessive, and constructability—the set of classes can be constructed by a demonstrably systematic procedure. See also CATEGORIZATION; TAXONOMY.

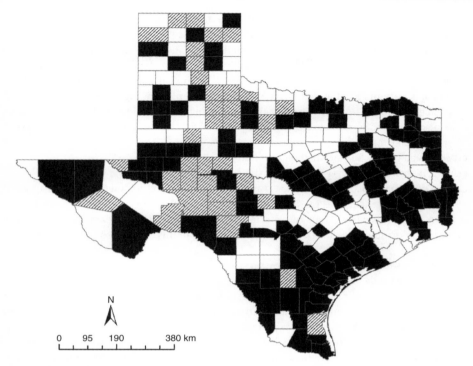

Choroplethic map. County-specific asthma incidence per 100 person-years among Medicaid-enrolled children in Texas, aged 1–17 years, 2005–2007. Counties shaded in black are those with incidence above the statewide incidence rate, while those shaded in white were below the state rate. Counties with hash marks had fewer than 16 cases, and therefore incidence rates were not calculated. Source: Wendt JK et al.[221]

CLASSIFICATION OF DISEASES Arrangement of diseases into groups having common characteristics. Useful in efforts to achieve STANDARDIZATION, and therefore comparability, in the methods of presentation of mortality and morbidity data from different sources. May include a systematic numerical notation for each disease entry.[24] Examples include the INTERNATIONAL CLASSIFICATION OF DISEASES (ICD) and the See INTERNATIONAL CLASSIFICATION OF PRIMARY CARE. See also FAMILY OF CLASSIFICATIONS.

CLASS INTERVAL The difference between the lower and upper limits of a class.

CLINICAL DECISION ANALYSIS Application of DECISION ANALYSIS in a clinical setting, often to assess probabilities of outcomes of alternative decisions (e.g., surgical procedures or drug treatment for myocardial ischemia). It considers three aspects of the decision: choices (options available to the patient), chances (probabilities of outcome for each choice), and values (quantitative expression of the desirability of different outcomes). It can be applied to small numbers of cases and even to a single patient. A method to systematically assess available treatment options, possible outcomes, and the desirability of each possible outcome. See also DECISION ANALYSIS; N-OF-ONE STUDY.

CLINICAL EPIDEMIOLOGY The application of epidemiological knowledge, reasoning, and methods to study clinical issues and improve clinical care. "Clinical" should not be restricted to "medical. "Medical epidemiology" is a complementary and commonly used term. Research often addresses etiological, mechanistic, diagnostic, therapeutic, and prognostic medical issues, is conducted in clinical settings, is led by clinicians, and has patients as study subjects. While clinical epidemiology uses epidemiological principles mostly to aid decision-making involving sick individuals, the wider CONTEXT is also commonly considered.[6,9,26,42,58,128,201,203,224,225] See also CLINICAL DECISION ANALYSIS; N-OF-ONE STUDY.

CLINICAL IMPORTANCE See SIGNIFICANCE, CLINICAL.

CLINICAL INFECTION See INFECTION, CLINICAL.

CLINICALLY MEANINGFUL See MINIMALLY IMPORTANT DIFFERENCE; NUMBER NEEDED TO TREAT; RELEVANCE; SIGNIFICANCE, CLINICAL.

CLINICAL PREDICTION RULE A set of criteria used to estimate the probability of a specific outcome or outcomes, particularly in a group of patients.[6,9] See also CLINICAL DECISION ANALYSIS.

CLINICAL RESEARCH ASSOCIATE See STUDY MONITOR.

CLINICAL SIGNIFICANCE See SIGNIFICANCE, CLINICAL.

CLINICAL STUDY (Syn: clinical investigation) An investigation involving persons and aiming to understand or control disease and other HEALTH states in persons. Often—but not exclusively—carried out on patients, by physicians, and in a health care setting. Problems found worthy of investigation in caring for patients are frequently taken to the laboratories; yet the nature and purpose of the investigation often remains clinical, and the laboratory results must be tested again on actual persons—eventually by integrating epidemiological and statistical reasoning with clinical, pathophysiological, and microbiological or preclinical (e.g., genetic) reasoning.[6,9,26,58,201,202] See also CASE REPORTS; CLINICAL EPIDEMIOLOGY; INDIVIDUAL THINKING; INTEGRATIVE RESEARCH.

CLINICAL TRIAL (Syn: therapeutic trial) A research activity that involves the administration of a test regimen to humans to evaluate its efficacy or its effectiveness and safety. The term is broadly polysemic: meanings include from the first test of a drug in humans without any control treatment to a rigorously designed RANDOMIZED CONTROLLED TRIAL.[1,6,9,26,58,73-77,110,226,227] Four phases of clinical trials or types of trials are distinguished:

Phase I trial It is the first test of a drug (or a candidate vaccine) in a small group of humans to determine its safety and mode of action. It usually involves a relatively small number of healthy volunteers. The focus is on safety and pharmacological profiles; it may also assess dose and route of administration.

Phase II trial Pilot efficacy studies. Initial trial to examine efficacy, usually in volunteers; with vaccines, the focus is on immunogenicity, and with drugs, on demonstration of safety and efficacy in comparison to existing regimens. Usually but not always, subjects are randomly allocated to the study and CONTROL groups.

Phase III trial Extensive clinical trial. This phase is intended for complete assessment of safety and efficacy. It commonly involves large numbers of patients with the disease or condition of interest, sometimes thousands; it uses random allocation to study and CONTROL groups.

Phase IV trial Postmarketing clinical trial. Conducted after the regulatory authority has approved registration and marketing begins. The common aim is to estimate the incidence of rare adverse reactions and other potential effects of long-term use in real life; it may also uncover potentially new uses and indications. It is part of POSTMARKETING SURVEILLANCE, which also includes OBSERVATIONAL STUDIES. See also COMMUNITY TRIAL.

CLINICAL TRIAL, NEGATIVE See NEGATIVE STUDY; NULL STUDY.

CLINICAL TRIAL, SPLIT-MOUTH A type of study used frequently in oral research: the mouth is divided into two or more subunits. Active and control (comparison) treatments are applied to the subunits (e.g., to the left and right sides). Treatments are compared within each patient. The design may reduce interpatient variability, much as in a CROSSOVER CLINICAL TRIAL. See also CARRYOVER EFFECT.

CLINIMETRICS The domain concerned with indexes, rating scales, and other expressions used to describe or measure symptoms, physical signs, and other distinctly clinical phenomena in clinical medicine.[225] Such measurements are an essential part of many preclinical, clinical, and epidemiological studies.[6,9,30,58] See also CLINICAL EPIDEMIOLOGY.

CLOSED COHORT A population in which membership begins at a defined time or with a defined event and ends only through occurrence of the study outcome or the end of eligibility for membership. An example is a population of women in labor being studied to determine the vital status of their offspring (i.e., whether live or stillborn).[1,3]

CLOSED POPULATION A population that gains no new members and loses members only to death.[24] Compare to CLOSED COHORT.

CLUSTER Aggregations of relatively uncommon events or diseases in space and/or time in amounts that are believed or perceived to be greater than could be expected by chance. Putative disease clusters are often perceived to exist on the basis of ANECDOTAL EVIDENCE, and much effort may be expended by epidemiologists and biostatisticians in assessing whether a true cluster of disease exists.[1,7,12,56]

CLUSTER ANALYSIS A set of statistical methods used to group variables or observations into interrelated subgroups (e.g., to detect clusters in routine SURVEILLANCE of disease).

CLUSTERING (Syn: disease cluster, time cluster, time-place cluster) A closely grouped series of events or cases of a disease or other health-related phenomena with well-defined distribution patterns in relation to time or place or both. The term is normally used to describe aggregation of relatively uncommon events or diseases (e.g., leukemia, multiple sclerosis).[1,7,8,12]

CLUSTER RANDOMIZED CONTROLLED TRIAL A form of RANDOMIZED CONTROLLED TRIAL in which entire groups of participants (i.e., clusters), instead of individual participants, are randomized. It is used to reduce the risk of CONTAMINATION between participants receiving the experimental and the control intervention.[73-77,110,228]

CLUSTER SAMPLING A sampling method in which each unit selected is a group of persons (all persons in a city block, a family, etc.) rather than an individual.[7] See also AREA SAMPLING; SAMPLING UNIT.

CNN APPROACH "Condoms, Needle exchange, Negotiation." A set of strategies aiming to combat the HIV/AIDS PANDEMIC, other sexually transmitted diseases, and other blood-borne infections. Harm reduction approaches to reducing the rate of HIV transmission through the adoption of safer sex and through risk reduction in intravenous drug users by provision of clean needles. See also ABC APPROACH.

COCHRANE COLLABORATION An international organization of clinicians, epidemiologists, other professionals, and patients that aims to help make well-informed decisions about HEALTH CARE by preparing, maintaining, disseminating, and promoting the accessibility of SYSTEMATIC REVIEWS of the effects of health care interventions.[229-231] *Cochrane Reviews* are prepared and updated by collaborating authors using explicitly defined methods to minimize the effects of bias; where appropriate and feasible, META-ANALYSIS is used. The collaboration honors Archibald L. Cochrane (1909–1988),[232,233] who advocated preference (including financial advantage) for interventions that have been assessed and found to be effective and efficient. See also EFFECTIVENESS.

COCHRAN-MANTEL-HAENSZEL TEST See MANTEL-HAENSZEL TEST.

CODE A numerical and/or alphabetical system for classifying information (e.g., about diagnostic categories).

CODING Translation of information (e.g., questionnaire responses) into numbered categories for entry in a data processing system.[1]

CODE OF CONDUCT A formal statement of desirable conduct that research workers and/or practitioners are expected to honor; there may be penalties for violation. Examples include the Hippocratic Oath, the Nürnberg (Nuremberg) Code, and the Helsinki Declaration, which govern requirements for research on human subjects. See also GUIDELINES.

CODOMINANCE The state in which both alleles of a gene are expressed to an equal extent. A relationship between two forms or versions of a gene. Individuals receive one version of a gene, an ALLELE, from each parent. If the alleles are different, the dominant allele usually will be expressed, while the effect of the other (recessive) allele is masked. In codominance, however, none of the alleles is recessive and the phenotypes of both of them are expressed.[189]

COEFFICIENT OF CONCORDANCE A measure of the agreement among several rankings or categories. See also CONCORDANCE.

COEFFICIENT OF VARIATION The ratio of the standard deviation to the mean. This is meaningful only if the variable is measured on a ratio scale. See MEASUREMENT SCALE.

COERCION Excessive pressure or influence to force or entice a person to act in a given way (e.g., to enroll in a research study or a public health program). May be exercised by offering excessive incentives, applying social pressure, using authority figures, or otherwise manipulating the vulnerable person or group.[118] See also INFORMED CONSENT.

COGNITIVE DISSONANCE The state of having inconsistent thoughts, beliefs, perceptions (i.e., cognitions), or attitudes, especially as relating to behavioral decisions and attitude change.[234] The drive to reduce *dissonance* in one's system of beliefs may lead to surprising strategies of belief formation and retention.[235] A theory that addresses competing or contradictory elements of cognition and behavior (e.g., why do people continue smoking when they know that smoking damages health?). Dissonance reduction may be attained through a change in behavior (e.g., quit smoking), in attitude, or in beliefs.[13,27,38,58,236]

COGNITIVE DISSONANCE BIAS A form of INTERPRETIVE BIAS that occurs when the belief in a given mechanism increases rather than decreases in the face of contradictory evidence.[38,58,237] See also CONFIRMATION BIAS.

COHERENCE The extent to which a hypothesized causal ASSOCIATION agrees with preexisting theory and knowledge.[25,38,206] Biological coherence requires more than just BIOLOGICAL PLAUSIBILITY or compatibility with biological knowledge derived from studies of nonhuman species or experimental systems.

COHERENCE, EPIDEMIOLOGICAL The extent to which a biological, clinical, or social observation is coherent with epidemiological evidence.[216] A consideration for causal inference in the

Cohort curves for years of birth, 1860–1950 *

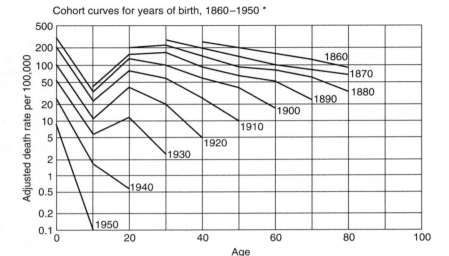

* The line associated with each year indicates death rates
by age-group for persons born in that year

Cohort slopes. Tuberculosis mortality rates of successive birth generations; death rates for tuberculosis by age, United States, 1900–1960, per 100,000 population, logarithmic scale. Source: Susser MW, et al.[238]

biological and clinical sciences, approximately but not fully reciprocal or symmetrical to the consideration of BIOLOGICAL PLAUSIBILITY in epidemiological causal inference.[208]

COHORT (From Latin *cohors*, warriors, the tenth part of a legion)

1. The component of the population born during a particular period and identified by period of birth so that its characteristics (e.g., causes of death and numbers still living) can be ascertained as it enters successive time and age periods.

2. The term "cohort" has broadened to describe any designated group of persons who are followed or traced over a period of time, as in COHORT STUDY (prospective study). See also BIRTH COHORT; HISTORICAL COHORT STUDY.

COHORT ANALYSIS The tabulation and analysis of morbidity or mortality rates in relation to the ages of a specific group of people (COHORT) identified at a particular period of time and followed as they pass through different ages during part or all of their life span. In certain circumstances (e.g., studies of migrant populations), cohort analysis may be performed according to duration of residence of migrants in a country, rather than year of birth, in order to relate the health or mortality experience to duration of exposure. The aim is to detect age, period, and BIRTH COHORT effects. Age-period-cohort models can be fitted to distinguish these effects; because of the dependency among the three factors, they require assumptions in order to estimate the parameters of the model.[1,3,5,8,24,37,149,153,800] See also ACCUMULATION OF RISK; BIRTH COHORT; DEVELOPMENTAL AND LIFE COURSE EPIDEMIOLOGY; REVERSE CAUSATION.

COHORT COMPONENT METHOD A method of population projection that takes the population distributed by age and sex at a base date and carries it forward in time on the basis of separate allowances for fertility, mortality, and migration.

COHORT EFFECT See GENERATION EFFECT.

COHORT INCIDENCE See INCIDENCE.

COHORT SLOPES (Syn: graphical cohort analysis) Arrangement of data so that when plotted graphically, lines connect points representing the age-specific rates for population segments from the same generation of birth (see diagram). These slopes represent changes in rates with age during the life experience of each cohort.

COHORT STUDY (Syn: concurrent, follow-up, incidence, longitudinal, panel, prospective study) The analytic epidemiological study in which subsets of a defined population can be identified who are, have been, or in the future may be exposed or not exposed—or exposed in different degrees—to a factor or factors hypothesized to influence the occurrence of a given outcome.[1-3,5-9,13,24,42,85,128,149,224,225,800] A common feature of a cohort study is comparison of incidences in groups that differ in exposure levels. The denominators used for analysis may be persons or PERSON-TIME.[239] See also BIAS; COHORT ANALYSIS; REVERSE CAUSATION; VALIDITY.

COHORT STUDY, HISTORICAL (Syn: historical prospective study, nonconcurrent prospective study, prospective study in retrospect) A COHORT STUDY conducted by reconstructing data about persons at a time or times in the past. This method uses existing records about the health or other relevant aspects of a population as it was at some time in the past and determines the current (or subsequent) status of members of this population with respect to the condition of interest. Different levels of past exposure to risk factor(s) of interest must be identifiable for subsets of the population. RECORD LINKAGE systems are often used in historical cohort studies. Growing public concern about protection of PRIVACY threatens such studies, which in the past have often made very valuable contributions to scientific understanding of disease causation. Ethical reviewers of research proposals for historical cohort studies increasingly require the investigators to obtain the informed consent of persons whose archived records are to be used in the study. If the study involves very large numbers and/or some or all of the persons are dead or cannot be traced, it is not feasible to obtain their INFORMED CONSENT.

COINTERVENTION In a RANDOMIZED CONTROLLED TRIAL, the application of additional diagnostic or therapeutic procedures to members of either or both the experimental and the control groups.

COLD CHAIN A system of protection against high environmental temperatures for heat-labile vaccines, sera, and other active biological preparations. Unless the cold chain is preserved, such preparations are inactivated and IMMUNIZATION procedures, etc., will be ineffective. Preservation of the cold chain is an integral part of the WHO expanded program on immunization in tropical countries.[67,240]

COLLAPSIBILITY Equality of stratum-specific measures of association or effect with the crude (collapsed), unstratified measure. Often, lack of collapsibility is equated with CONFOUNDING, but may instead signal inappropriate stratification (as in BERKSON'S BIAS and some forms of SELECTION BIAS), or the use of an outcome-frequency measure (such as an ODDS or INCIDENCE RATE) for which the stratifying factors affect the denominators as well as the numerators.[1,2,8,101,241] See also CONFOUNDING BIAS.

COLLIDER A variable directly affected by two or more other variables ("parents" of the variable) in the CAUSAL DIAGRAM;[1,2,34,100,101,209,242,243] e.g., a variable that is the common effect of an exposure and an outcome. In the following "inverted fork" $X \rightarrow C \leftarrow Y$ the arrow represents a direct effect of the tail variable on the head variable; C is then a collider on the X-C-Y pathway in the graph. Conditioning on a collider (i.e., controlling for the collider through stratification, restriction, or adjustment) will tend to induce a noncausal association (often referred to as *collider bias*) between the parent variables (i.e., the shared direct causes) of the collider.

COLLIDER BIAS See COLLIDER.

COLLINEARITY The presence of very strong linear relationship between two or more REGRESSOR variables in a REGRESSION MODEL. Collinearity is a concern when the correlation between the regressors nears −1 or 1; it can then can result in inflated variances for the estimated coefficients, and (in nonlinear models) bias in the estimated coefficients. A common solution in such situations is to remove one of the collinear variables from the model, although this can lead to CONFOUNDING BIAS if the removed variable is actually a confounder.[1,3,7,244]

COLONIZATION See INFECTION.

COMMENSAL Literally, eating together (sharing the same table). An organism or microorganism that lives on or in a host harmlessly. An organism in the HUMAN MICROBIOME that is not pathogenic to the host, and provides no apparent benefit. Examples include numerous bacteria that live in the mucosa or in the digestive tract.[20-22,56,188,217-219] See also METAGENOME; MUTUALISM; XENOBIOTIC. Contrast with PARASITE.

COMMON DISEASE GENETIC AND EPIGENETIC (CDGE) HYPOTHESIS The CDGE hypothesis argues that in addition to genetic variation, EPIGENETICS provides an added layer of variation that might mediate the relationship between GENOTYPE and internal and external environmental factors. This epigenetic component may help to explain the marked increase in common diseases with age as well as the frequent discordance of diseases between monozygotic twins.[245]

COMMON GOOD Shared values or benefits deemed to be good, either explicitly or tacitly, for individuals and for society. While the definition is important for PUBLIC HEALTH, in democratic societies it may be difficult to achieve consensus on certain "goods." For epidemiological and public health practice, elements of the larger public good include health itself as a social value, and the broader value of "assuring conditions under which people can be healthy."[28,118,246]

COMMON SOURCE EPIDEMIC (Syn: common vehicle epidemic) See EPIDEMIC, COMMON SOURCE.

COMMON VEHICLE SPREAD Transmission of a disease agent (infectious pathogen, toxic chemical, etc.) from a source that is common to those who acquire the disease. Common vehicles include air, water, food, and injected substances. Legionellosis is an example of common vehicle spread in air that has passed through air conditioning equipment contaminated by the causal organism. HIV disease and hepatitis B and C can be spread among intravenous drug users by the common vehicle of contaminated needles and syringes. Cholera and many other waterborne diseases are spread by the common vehicle of contaminated water.[56,69,188,196,217-219] The principal modes of foodborne common vehicle spread were sonorously summarized by an anonymous author (probably Sir Andrew Balfour) in *Memoranda on Medical Diseases in Tropical and Subtropical Areas*,[247] published by the British War Office in 1914–1918: "...careless carriers, contact cases, chiefly cooks, dirty drinking water, the dust of dried dejecta and the repulsive regurgitation, dangerous droppings, and filthy feet of faecal-feeding flies fouling food."

COMMUNICABLE DISEASE (Syn: transmissible disease) A disease whose causal agent can be transmitted from successive hosts to healthy subjects, from one individual to another. An illness due to a specific INFECTIOUS AGENT or its toxic products that arises through transmission of such agent or products from an infected person, animal, or reservoir to a susceptible host, either directly or indirectly through an intermediate plant or animal host, vector, or the inanimate environment. All INFECTIONS and INFESTATIONS are communicable diseases; thus, not all communicable diseases are infectious diseases. A disease can be communicable (transmissible) but not CONTAGIOUS if it requires a VECTOR for its transmission (e.g., tetanus). Thus, communicable diseases include contagious and noncontagious diseases. The latter include diseases genetically inherited and diseases exclusively transmitted through vectors.[8,20-22,56,69,188,217-219] See also CONTAGION; NON-COMMUNICABLE DISEASE; TRANSMISSION OF INFECTION.

COMMUNICABLE PERIOD The time during which an INFECTIOUS AGENT may be transferred directly or indirectly from an infected person to another person, from an infected animal to humans, or from an infected person to an animal, including arthropods. See also TRANSMISSION OF INFECTION.

COMMUNITARIAN ETHICS An approach to ethics emphasizing communal values, the COMMON GOOD, or social goals. Closely aligned with the cooperative virtues and a community's shared understanding of life. Need not be pitted against individual rights.[117,118,248,249]

COMMUNITY A group of individuals organized into a unit or manifesting some unifying TRAIT or common interest; loosely, the locality or catchment area population for which a service is provided or, more broadly, the state, nation, or body politic.

COMMUNITY DIAGNOSIS The process of appraising the health status of a community, including analysis of health-related statistics and information on health DETERMINANTS. The term may also denote the findings of this diagnostic process. It may be comprehensive or restricted to specific health conditions, determinants, or subgroups. Jeremiah N. Morris (1910 - 2009) identified community diagnosis as one of the uses of epidemiology.[250]

COMMUNITY HEALTH See PUBLIC HEALTH.

COMMUNITY MEDICINE An interdisciplinary field that aims at dealing integrally with the preservation and restitution of HEALTH, as well to prevent disease, not only at an individual level but also in groups of defined communities, taking into consideration health and social DETERMINANTS. A main goal is to identify health problems and NEEDS, and to evaluate the extent to which clinical and public health services meet such needs.

COMMUNITY NEED ASSESSMENT A method of identifying the needs of the community so that corrective measures can be taken.

COMMUNITY-ORIENTED PRIMARY HEALTH CARE Integration of COMMUNITY MEDICINE with the primary health care of individuals. The PRIMARY HEALTH CARE practitioner or team is responsible for health care both at the individual and the community or population levels.[17,28] See also PUBLIC HEALTH; SOCIAL MEDICINE.

COMMUNITY TRIAL An EXPERIMENT in which the unit of allocation to receive a preventive, therapeutic or social intervention is an entire community or part of an organization.[73-77,110] See also CLINICAL TRIAL; FIELD TRIAL; RANDOMIZED CONTROLLED TRIAL.

COMORBIDITY Disease(s) that coexist(s) in a study participant in addition to the index condition that is the subject of study.

COMPARATIVE EFFECTIVENESS RESEARCH The generation and synthesis of evidence that compares the benefits and harms of alternative methods to prevent, diagnose, treat, and monitor a clinical condition or to improve the delivery of care. Its purpose is to assist consumers, clinicians, purchasers, and policy makers to make informed decisions that will improve health care at both the individual and population levels.[231,251,252] The results often are summarized in a SYSTEMATIC REVIEW. See also PATIENT-REPORTED OUTCOMES; SIGNIFICANCE, CLINICAL.

COMPARISON GROUP Any group to which the index group is compared.[6,26] Usually synonymous with CONTROL GROUP. See also CASE SERIES; CONTROL; GROUP COMPARISON; STANDARD POPULATION.

COMPETING RISK (Syn: competing cause, competing event) An event that removes a subject from being at risk for the outcome under investigation. For example, in a study of smoking and cancer of the lung, a subject who dies of coronary heart disease is no longer at risk of lung cancer; in this situation, coronary heart disease is a competing risk. In considering a particular cause of death (or other inevitable outcome), one must take account of other causes of death, which are commonly called competing risks. When the frequency of previously common causes of death is reduced, competing risks must become more prominent. For instance, among young adults, pneumonia and other infections were a common cause of death until about mid-twentieth century; their control has increased the incidence of some competing risks as myocardial infarction and various cancers.[1,7,8,794]

COMPLETED FERTILITY RATE The number of children born alive per woman in a COHORT of women by the end of their childbearing years. See also TOTAL FERTILITY RATE.

COMPLETING THE CLINICAL PICTURE The use of epidemiology to define all modes of presentation of a disease, its full spectrum, and outcomes in a defined population. One of the "uses of epidemiology" identified by J. N. Morris.[250]

COMPLETION RATE The proportion or percentage of persons in a SURVEY for whom complete data are available for analysis.[160] See also RESPONSE RATE.

COMPLEX TRAIT (Syn: polygenic trait, multifactorial TRAIT) Any PHENOTYPE that results from the effect of multiple genes at two or more loci, often from environmental influences as well.[57]

COMPLIANCE See adherence.

COMPONENT CAUSES Multiple factors that act jointly to cause a given effect. They do so in different combinations, each combination of component causes capable of giving rise to particular effects. No component cause is sufficient to produce the effect. In some processes (e.g., diseases), one of the component causes is necessary, but in other instances this is not so (i.e., none of the component causes may be necessary). The frequency of the components of a SUFFICIENT CAUSE influences their relative strength. This heuristic model is useful when it also integrates the analysis of antecedent causes, the sequence and TIME ORDER of causal events, and causal processes that operate at different levels.[1-3,5,39,84,101,206-210,253,798]

COMPOSITE INDEX An index, such as the APGAR SCORE, or the Tumor/Nodes/Metastases (TNM) system to stage cancer, that contains contributions from categories of several different variables.

COMPOSITIONAL EFFECTS Effects of individual-level factors (i.e., characteristics of individuals within a group or area, such as individual income) on individual-level outcomes after accounting for the effects of relevant group- or area-level factors (referred to as CONTEXTUAL EFFECTS). They are estimated using MULTILEVEL ANALYSIS.[158,254,255] See also CAUSES IN PUBLIC HEALTH SCIENCES.

COMPRESSION OF MORBIDITY A term describing abbreviation of the average period of life when chronic illness or disability affects physical, mental, or social function. In theory, as health promotion and disease prevention become more efficacious, this period of long-term morbidity is compressed into a smaller proportion of the total life span. Empirical observations in several countries have failed to demonstrate the phenomenon. Others envisage an EXPANSION OF MORBIDITY or a state of balance. See also RECTANGULARIZATION OF MORTALITY.

CONCENTRATION CURVE See CONCENTRATION INDEX.

CONCENTRATION INDEX A means of quantifying the degree of income-related inequality in health. A measure of how much a health attribute is concentrated toward the rich or the poor. If there is no income-related inequality, the concentration index is zero. The concentration curve shows the cumulative percentage of the population or sample on the horizontal, x axis, ranked by income, beginning with the poorest; it shows the cumulative percentage of ill-health on the vertical, y axis. The concentration index is calculated as twice the area between the concentration curve and the "line of equality" (the latter defined as the 45° line running upward from origin, $y = x$). By convention the index takes a negative value when the curve lies above the "line of equality," indicating disproportionate concentration of ill health among the poor, and a positive value when it lies below the "line of equality."[256,257] See also GINI COEFFICIENT; LORENZ CURVE; SLOPE INDEX OF INEQUALITY; RELATIVE INDEX OF INEQUALITY.

CONCORDANCE In MATCHED STUDIES, concordance is present when subjects that are matched have the same value for the variable under investigation; such subjects are said to be concordant.[5] See also ADHERENCE; KAPPA INDEX.

CONCORDANT In TWIN STUDIES, a twin pair in which both twins exhibit or fail to exhibit a TRAIT under investigation.[5]

CONCURRENT STUDY See COHORT STUDY.

CONCURRENT VALIDITY See VALIDITY, MEASUREMENT.

CONDITIONAL LOGISTIC REGRESSION A statistical technique that fits a LOGISTIC MODEL using conditional maximum likelihood. See also LOGISTIC MODEL; MAXIMUM LIKELIHOOD ESTIMATE.

CONDITIONAL PROBABILITY The probability of an event given that another event has occurred. If D and E are two events and P (...) is "the probability of (...)," the conditional probability of D given that E occurs is denoted $P(D|E)$, where the vertical slash is read "given" and is equal to $P(D$ and $E)/P(E)$. The event E is the "conditioning event." Conditional probabilities obey all the axioms of probability theory.[1,7,34,37] See also BAYES' THEOREM; PROBABILITY THEORY.

CONFIDENCE INTERVAL (CI) The conventional form of an INTERVAL ESTIMATE in FREQUENTIST STATISTICS. If the underlying statistical model is correct and there is no BIAS, a confidence interval derived from a valid analysis will, over unlimited repetitions of the study, contain the true parameter with a frequency no less than its confidence level (often 95% is the stated level, but other levels are also used).[1,7,37,258]

CONFIDENCE LIMITS The upper and lower boundaries of the confidence interval.

CONFIDENTIALITY The obligation not to disclose information; the right of a person to withhold information from others. Information in medical records, case registries, and other data files and bases is generally confidential, and epidemiologists are required to obtain permission before being given access to it. This may be the INFORMED CONSENT of the person to whom the records relate or the permission of an INSTITUTIONAL REVIEW BOARD. Epidemiologists have an obligation to preserve confidentiality of information they obtain during their studies.[8,117,118,259-265] See also INFORMED CONSENT; PRIVACY.

CONFIRMATION BIAS A form of bias that may occur when evidence that supports one's preconceptions is evaluated more favorably than evidence that challenges these convictions.[99] The tendency to test one's beliefs or conjectures by seeking evidence that might confirm or verify them and to ignore or discount evidence that might disconfirm or refute them. The latter discounting is sometimes called *disconfirmation bias*.[38,117,237] See also CONSISTENCY; INTERPRETIVE BIAS.

CONFLICT OF INTEREST   Compromise of a person's objectivity when that person has a vested interest (e.g., in PEER REVIEW, in the outcome of a study). It occurs when the person could benefit financially or in other ways (e.g., promotion, prestige) from some aspect of a study, report, or other professional activity. Conflicts of interest are not limited to research settings, nor to the health sciences.[13,83,138,266,267] See also DISCLOSURE OF INTERESTS; INVESTIGATOR BIAS.

CONFOUNDER   (Syn: confounding variable) A variable that can be used to decrease CONFOUNDING BIAS when properly adjusted for. The identification of confounders requires expert or substantive knowledge about the causal NETWORK of which exposure and outcome are part (e.g., pathophysiological and clinical knowledge). Attempts to select confounders solely based on observed statistical associations may lead to bias.[1-3,8,24,101,209,268]

CONFOUNDING   (From the Latin *confundere*, to mix together)

1. Loosely, the distortion of a measure of the effect of an exposure on an outcome due to the association of the exposure with other factors that influence the occurrence of the outcome. Confounding occurs when all or part of the apparent association between the exposure and the outcome is in fact accounted for by other variables that affect the outcome and are not themselves affected by exposure.[1-3,24,25,39-42,268-270]

2. An association between the POTENTIAL OUTCOMES under alternative exposure or treatment possibilities and the actual exposures or treatments received by the persons under study. This condition is equivalent to a violation of IGNORABILITY.[1,2]

CONFOUNDING BIAS

1. Bias of the estimated effect of an exposure on an outcome due to the presence of common causes of the exposure and the outcome. Example: The effect of aspirin use on the risk of stroke will be confounded if aspirin is more likely to be prescribed to individuals with heart disease, which is hence both an indication for treatment and a RISK FACTOR for the disease. Heart disease may be a risk factor for stroke if it has a direct causal effect on stroke (heart disease is then the common cause of aspirin use and stroke) or if atherosclerosis causes both heart disease and stroke (atherosclerosis is then the common cause).[1-3,5-9,24,25,39-42,101,269,270,272,800]

2. Bias of the estimated effect of an exposure on an outcome due to either presence of common causes of the exposure and the outcome, or due to selection that occurred prior to the exposure of interest (e.g., M-BIAS).[242,271] Some authors include M-BIAS as an example of SELECTION BIAS and restrict CONFOUNDING to definition 1. Confounding bias has also been mistakenly defined as lack of COLLAPSIBILITY, but the latter concept is purely numerical, not causal.[1,2]

CONFOUNDING BY INDICATION   A type of CONFOUNDING BIAS that occurs when a symptom or sign of disease is judged as an indication (or a contraindication) for a given therapy, and is therefore associated both with the use of a drug or medical procedure (or its avoidance) and with a higher probability of an outcome related to the disease for which the agent is indicated (or contraindicated). The reason to initiate treatment can be assessed by a health professional, a patient (self-medication), or a relative. As a result, crude comparisons of risks for such outcomes between exposed and unexposed subjects would be biased toward a higher risk among the exposed. Confounding by indication generally arises in a common clinical situation and in full coherence with clinical logic: before beginning to receive a given therapy or procedure patients who are prescribed the drug have a poorer prognosis (or a higher risk of a disease-related adverse outcome) than patients who do not receive the agent. The confounding stems from this initial difference in the prognostic expectations of treated and nontreated subjects.[272] It shares some features with "susceptibility bias", "procedure selection bias", and PROTOPATHIC BIAS. Some biostatisticians call it "selection by indication." referring to the physician (or self-) selection of high-risk patients to receive the treatment. OBSERVATIONAL STUDIES on health care are prone to this BIAS.

CONFOUNDING, NEGATIVE Confounding that produces a downward bias in the effect estimate. Alternatively, confounding that dilutes, underestimates, obscures, or attenuates (rather than overestimates) the estimated effect of an exposure on an outcome. These alternative definitions coincide for adverse causal factors but are opposites for preventive factors.[3]

CONFOUNDING, POSITIVE Confounding that produces an upward bias in the effect estimate. Alternatively, confounding that creates, overestimates, or exaggerates (rather than underestimates) the estimated effect of an exposure on an outcome. These alternative definitions coincide for adverse factors but are opposites for preventive factors.[3]

CONFOUNDING, UNMEASURED See RESIDUAL CONFOUNDING.

CONGENITAL A condition or TRAIT present or recognized at (or before) birth and developed during intrauterine life. It may arise as a result of infections (e.g., the rubella virus), genetic factors, environmental conditions (e.g., in utero exposure to a pollutant), or a combination of them. Congenital malformations include all disorders present at birth, whether they are inherited or caused by an environmental factor.[116,190]

CONNECTION Something that can be shown to make a difference: an observed change in state (the effect) is consequent on change in an independent antecedent state (the cause) and not vice versa. One of the three essential PROPERTIES OF A CAUSE specified by David Hume, along with ASSOCIATION and TIME ORDER. It requires the elimination of alternative explanations (e.g., CONFOUNDING).[84,85,101] See also DIRECTION.

CONSANGUINE Related by a common ancestor within the previous few generations.

CONSENT BIAS Lack of GENERALIZABILITY that occurs when the sample of subjects, records, or specimens included in the study is systematically different from the original sample because of asking for INFORMED CONSENT (e.g., to be interviewed for the study, to access medical records, to store biological specimens).[1,2]

CONSILIENCE Agreement or harmony among two or more disparate scholarly disciplines regarding concepts or underlying principles. Consilience occurs when inductive explanations of two or more different kinds of phenomena are discovered separately, but unexpectedly lead scientists to the same underlying causes.[223]

CONSISTENCY

1. Close conformity between the findings in different samples, strata, or populations, or at different times or in different circumstances, or in studies conducted by different methods or investigators. Consistency may be examined in order to study an EFFECT MODIFIER. Consistency of results on replication of studies is an important consideration in judgments of CAUSALITY.[1,2,52,55,270,273] See also CONFIRMATION BIAS; HILL'S CONSIDERATIONS FOR CAUSATION.

2. *Internal consistency* is a measurement property of a measurement instrument: the degree of the interrelatedness among the items of the instrument.[274]

3. In statistics, an estimator is said to be consistent if the probability of its yielding estimates close to the true value approaches 1 as the sample size grows larger.

4. A POTENTIAL or COUNTERFACTUAL OUTCOME under exposure level *a* is said to be consistent when, for each individual actually exposed to level *a*, its value equals that of the observed outcome.

CONSORT Consolidated Standards of Reporting Trials. An evidence-based and structured approach to reporting CLINICAL TRIALS. Its central features include a checklist and a flow diagram spelling out the important features of the trial (i.e., protocol, methods, participant [subject] assignment, masking procedures, details of analysis, participant flow, results, and follow-up). The aim is to improve the quality of reporting of randomized trials.[275-277] See also EQUATOR; PRISMA; QUADAS-2; QUOROM; STARD; STROBE.

CONSTRUCT VALIDITY See VALIDITY, MEASUREMENT.

CONTACT, DIRECT A mode of TRANSMISSION OF INFECTION between an infected host and a susceptible host. Direct contact occurs when skin or mucous surfaces touch, as in shaking hands, kissing, and sexual intercourse. See also CONTAGION.

CONTACT, INDIRECT A mode of TRANSMISSION OF INFECTION involving FOMITES or VECTORS. Vectors may be mechanical (e.g., filth flies) or biological (when the disease agent undergoes part of its life cycle in the vector species).[20,22,56,69,188,217-219]

CONTACT, PRIMARY Person(s) in direct contact or associated with a COMMUNICABLE DISEASE case.

CONTACT, SECONDARY Person(s) in contact or associated with a primary contact.

CONTACT (OF AN INFECTION) A person or animal that has been in such association with an infected person or animal or a contaminated environment as to have had opportunity to acquire the infection.[56,69]

CONTACT TRACING See CASE FINDING.

CONTAGION The TRANSMISSION OF INFECTION by direct contact, droplet spread, or contaminated FOMITES. These are the modes of transmission specified by Fracastorius (1484–1553) in *De Contagione* (1546). Contemporary usage is sometimes looser, but use of this term is best restricted to description of INFECTION transmitted by direct contact.[56,69]

CONTAGIOUS DISEASE (From Latin *contagium*, contact). A disease transmitted by direct or indirect contact with a host that is the source of the pathogenic agent. The same disease can be contagious in some species and not in others.[20-22,56,69,188,217-219] See also COMMUNICABLE DISEASE.

CONTAINMENT The concept of regional eradication of a communicable disease, first proposed by Soper in 1949 for the elimination of smallpox.[278] Containment of a worldwide COMMUNICABLE DISEASE demands a globally coordinated effort, so that countries that have effected an interruption of transmission do not become reinfected following importation from neighboring endemic areas.[56,69]

CONTAMINATION

1. The presence of an INFECTIOUS AGENT, a toxic, or an otherwise harmful agent (radioactive material, other biological or chemical compounds) on or in the body—or in clothes, bedding, toys, medical devices, surgical instruments or dressings, other objects; in air, water, and food; or on buildings or land. Contamination of a body surface does not imply a CARRIER state.[56,69] The agent causing POLLUTION or present in the polluted environment is noxious but not infectious.[33] See also INFECTION; NETWORK; SOURCE OF INFECTION; TRANSMISSION OF INFECTION.

2. The situation that exists when a population being studied for one condition or factor also possesses other conditions or factors that modify results of the study. In

a RANDOMIZED CONTROLLED TRIAL, the application of the experimental procedure to members of the control group or failure to apply the procedure to members of the experimental group.

CONTAMINATION, DATA In computing, the intentional or accidental alteration of data (e.g., in a computer system).

CONTENT VALIDITY See VALIDITY, MEASUREMENT.

CONTEXTUAL ANALYSIS Analysis of CONTEXTUAL EFFECTS.

CONTEXT The location of a person by time and place; the latter refers to both geographical location and to group membership (e.g., in terms of family, friends, age, class, ethnicity, residence, gender). Context may affect exposure to risk and the response strategies.[23,38,158,255,279]

CONTEXTUAL EFFECTS Effects of group- or area-level factors (e.g., neighborhood poverty) on individual-level outcomes after accounting for the effects of relevant individual-level confounders (referred to as COMPOSITIONAL EFFECTS). They are estimated using MULTILEVEL ANALYSIS.[158,254,255] See also INTEGRATIVE RESEARCH.

CONTINGENCY TABLE A tabular cross-classification of data such that subcategories of one characteristic are indicated horizontally (in rows) and subcategories of another characteristic are indicated vertically (in columns). Tests of association between the characteristics in the columns and rows can be readily applied. The simplest contingency table is the fourfold or 2×2, table. Contingency tables may be extended to include several dimensions of classification.[7,37] See also DENOMINATOR.

CONTINGENT VARIABLE See INTERMEDIATE VARIABLE.

CONTINUING SOURCE EPIDEMIC (OUTBREAK) An epidemic in which new cases of disease occur over a long period, indicating persistence of the disease source.

CONTINUOUS DATA, CONTINUOUS VARIABLE Data (variable) with a potentially infinite number of possible values along a continuum (e.g., height, weight, enzyme output).[3]

CONTOUR PLOT Diagrammatic presentation, usually computer generated, of data involving three variables, one each on the horizontal and vertical axes and a third represented by lines of constant value. See also PERSPECTIVE PLOT.

CONTRACT RESEARCH ORGANIZATION (CRO) An organization that provides support to the pharmaceutical and biotechnology industries in the form of research services outsourced to the CRO on a contract basis. It may provide services such as biopharmaceutical development, biologic assay development, preclinical and clinical research, and pharmacovigilance.

CONTROL

1. (v.) To regulate, restrain, correct, restore to normal, to prevent DYSREGULATION.
2. (v.) To take into account or to adjust for extraneous factors, influences, or observations, whether by design or analysis.
3. (n. or adj.) Applied to many communicable and some non-communicable conditions, it refers to the ongoing operations, programs, or policies aimed at eliminating or reducing the occurrence of such conditions.
4. (n.) As used in the context of a COHORT STUDY and a RANDOMIZED CONTROLLED TRIAL, *control* refers to persons in a group that is used for reference in the comparison to an exposed group or a treated group, respectively.[1-3,5,7,24,25,38] See also CONTROL GROUP; GROUP COMPARISON.
5. (n.) As used in the expression CASE-CONTROL STUDY, it refers to persons in a group that is used for reference in the comparison to a case group.[197] See also CASE SERIES, CONTROL GROUP.

6. (adj.) The expression *control variable* refers to an independent variable other than the hypothetical causal variable that has a potential effect on the dependent variable and is subject to control by analysis.[1,3,5,270] See also INSTRUMENTAL VARIABLE.

CONTROL GROUP, CONTROLS Subjects with whom a comparison is made in a CASE-CONTROL STUDY, a RANDOMIZED CONTROLLED TRIAL, or other types of studies. Some uses of the noun *control* to describe the reference group may be confusing. Controls in a randomized controlled trial may be asked to undergo a regimen or procedure that may affect their health; their informed consent is therefore essential. By contrast—this is an essential ethical distinction—there is no intervention on the part of the researchers in the lives of the controls (and of the cases) in a case-control study. In a case-control study, controls are often defined as noncases or by other postexposure events, making them especially susceptible to SELECTION BIAS. Selection of appropriate controls is crucial to the VALIDITY of epidemiological and clinical studies.[6-8,197]

CONTROLS, HISTORICAL Persons or patients used for comparison who had the condition or treatment under study at a different time, generally at an earlier period than the study group or cases. Historical controls are often unsatisfactory because other factors affecting the condition under study may have changed to an unknown extent in the time elapsed.

CONTROLS, HOSPITAL Persons used for comparison who are drawn from the population of patients in a hospital. If wrongly chosen, hospital controls may be a source of SELECTION BIAS.

CONTROLS, MATCHED Controls who are selected so that they are similar to cases in specific characteristics. Some commonly used matching variables are age, sex, race, and socioeconomic status.[1-3,269,270,280] See also MATCHING.

CONTROLS, NEGATIVE Precautionary procedures taken to detect possible sources of spurious associations. A study thus includes conditions under which it is expected to produce a null result, and researchers verify whether it does. In experiments, procedures include leaving out an essential agent, inactivating the hypothesized active agent or using an inert substance; in observational and experimental studies, checking for an effect impossible by the hypothesized mechanism (based on subject matter knowledge). Associations can be assessed among subjects exposed to doses clearly too low to produce the effect: if such association is present, the validity of the design, information, or analytic strategy should be questioned. Another example is the inclusion in questionnaires of irrelevant variables ("probe variables") to assess if recall bias might be responsible for the observed magnitude of the associations between self-reported exposures and an outcome. A negative control outcome is one that cannot be affected by the exposure; e.g., mortality prior to influenza season for influenza vaccination. Similar to the INSTRUMENTAL VARIABLE design, a carefully selected negative control outcome variable may potentially be used to correct for unobserved confounding. The purpose of a negative control is to reproduce a condition that cannot involve the hypothesized causal mechanism but is likely to involve the same sources of bias that may have been present in the original association. The potential benefits of employing negative controls must be weighed against their cost and the possibility that their assumptions are wrong.[281,282]

CONTROLS, NEIGHBORHOOD Persons used for comparison who live in the same locality as cases and therefore may resemble cases in environmental and socioeconomic experience. Such use may lead to OVERMATCHING.

CONTROLS, SIBLING Persons used for comparison who are the siblings of cases and therefore share genetic makeup.

CONVENIENCE SAMPLE See SAMPLE.

COORDINATES In a two-dimensional graph, the values of ordinate and abscissa that define the locus or position of a point.

COPY NUMBER VARIANTS (CNV) Variation in the number of copies of a particular gene from one individual to another. They comprise insertions, deletions, and duplications of segments of DNA. CNV account for a significant proportion of the genetic variation between individuals, but the extent to which they contribute to human disease is not yet known.

CORDON SANITAIRE The barrier erected around a focus of infection. Used mainly in the ISOLATION procedures applied to exclude cases and contacts of life-threatening COMMUNICABLE DISEASES from society. Mainly of historical interest.

CORRELATION
1. In ordinary English, the degree to which variables change together. How closely two (or more) variables are related. Sometimes used as a synonym for ASSOCIATION.[1,3]
2. In statistics, a synonym for CORRELATION COEFFICIENT.[37]

CORRELATION COEFFICIENT A measure of association that indicates the degree to which two variables have a linear relationship. This coefficient, represented by the letter r, can vary between +1 and –1; when $r = +1$, there is a perfect positive linear relationship in which one variable varies directly with the other; when $r = -1$, there is a perfect negative linear relationship between the variables. The measure can be generalized to quantify the degree of linear relationship between one variable and several others, in which case it is known as the multiple correlation coefficient. Kendall's Tau, Spearman's Rank Correlation, and Pearson's Product Moment Correlation are special varieties with applications in clinical and epidemiological research.[3,7,8,26,37,283,284] Lack of correlation does not imply lack of relation, only lack of linear relation on the scale used to assess the correlation; therefore the use of correlation as a synonym for relation or association can be misleading. There are also several problems associated with attempting to interpret correlation coefficients as MEASURES OF EFFECT, among them that the correlation coefficient depends on the standard deviations of the causal and outcome variable. It can therefore vary greatly across populations and subgroups, even if the increase in the mean outcome, risk, or rate produced by exposure is identical across populations and subgroups.

CORRELATION, INTRACLASS A measure of the degree of relationship between two variables that presents the proportion of intersubject variance with respect to total variance (e.g., it compares the variance between patients to the total variance, including both between- and within-patient variance). It is used, for example, to assess interater RELIABILITY or the REPRODUCIBILITY of a diagnostic test.[24]

CORRELATION, NONSENSE A meaningless correlation between two variables. Nonsense correlations sometimes occur when social, environmental, or technological changes have the same TREND as incidence or mortality rates. An example is the correlation between the birthrate and the density of storks in parts of Holland. See also ASSOCIATION, FORTUITOUS; CONFOUNDING BIAS; ECOLOGICAL FALLACY.

COST The value of resources engaged in a service.[17,285]

COST, AVERAGE The average cost per unit; equals the total costs divided by the units of production.

COST, AVOIDED Costs caused by a health problem that are avoided by a health care intervention. Estimating avoided costs is one way to assess the value of benefits of health care interventions; sometimes known as benefits.

COST-BENEFIT ANALYSIS An analysis of the economic and social costs of medical care and the benefits of reduced loss of net earnings owing to the prevention of premature death or disability. The general rule for the allocation of funds in a cost-benefit analysis is that the ratio of marginal benefit (the benefit of preventing an additional case) to marginal cost (the cost of preventing an additional case) should be equal to or greater than 1. The benefit-cost ratio is the ratio of net present value of measurable benefits to costs. Calculation of a benefit-cost ratio is used to assess the economic feasibility or success of a public health program.[17,28,38,47,58]

COST, DIRECT Those costs borne by the health care system, the community, and patients' families (e.g., costs of diagnosis and treatment).

COST-EFFECTIVENESS ANALYSIS This form of analysis seeks to determine the costs and effectiveness of an activity or to compare similar alternative activities to determine the relative degree to which they will obtain the desired objectives or outcomes. The preferred action or alternative is one that requires the least cost to produce a given level of effectiveness or that provides the greatest effectiveness for a given level of cost. In the health care field, outcomes are measured in terms of health status.[17,58,231,232]

COST, FIXED Costs that, within a defined period, do not vary with the quantity produced (e.g., overhead costs of maintaining a building).

COST, INACTION See COSTS OF INACTION.

COST, INCREMENTAL The difference between marginal costs of alternative interventions.

COST, INDIRECT Lost productivity caused by disease and borne by the individual, the family, society, or the employer.

COST, INTANGIBLE Costs of pain, grief, suffering, loss of leisure time; the cost of a life is usually included in case of death.

COST, OPPORTUNITY See OPPORTUNITY COST.

COST, TOTAL All costs incurred in producing a set quantity of service.

COSTS, MARGINAL The additional costs from an increase in an activity. The additional cost incurred as a result of the production of one extra unit of output; the increase is equal to the cost of the next unit produced.

COSTS OF INACTION An expression in monetary terms of the damage that will be caused if no or limited intervention is taken. Inaction is the lack of development of policies, lack of development of policies beyond those which currently exist, or failure to enforce existing policies. Under an economics perspective the costs of inaction can be analogous to the benefits that it is feasible to obtain with proper regulation. In political decision-making processes, the burden of proof is often distributed such that policy makers only respond to early warning signals from hazards once the costs of inaction have been estimated. Such signals may provide a basis for a precautionary approach to the costs of inaction. The costs of PREVENTION are usually tangible, clearly allocated, and often short term, whereas the BENEFITS—and the costs of failing to act—are less tangible, less clearly distributed and usually longer term, posing particular problems of governance.[13,17,38,83,252,267,286,287]

COST-UTILITY ANALYSIS A form of economic evaluation in which the outcomes of alternative procedures or programs are expressed in terms of a single "utility-based" unit of measurement. A widely used utility-based measure is the QUALITY-ADJUSTED LIFE YEAR (QALY).[6,58] See also UTILITY.

COUNTERFACTUAL An event or condition (e.g., a treatment) that did not happen (i.e., is contrary to fact) but at one point was a logical possibility.[1,2,34,101]

COUNTERFACTUAL OUTCOME The outcome that an individual would have experienced if he had received a particular treatment or exposure value. There are as many counterfactual outcomes as possible treatment values. For each individual, the value of the counterfactual outcome under the treatment value that the individual actually received equals the observed outcome (a property of counterfactual outcomes known as consistency). Individual causal effects are defined by a contrast between an individual's counterfactual outcomes. Average causal effects are defined by a contrast between the average counterfactual outcomes in a group of individuals.[1,2,101] See also POTENTIAL OUTCOME.

COUNTERFACTUAL LOGIC Deductive reasoning that involves counterfactual premises or conditions; i.e., premises or conditions that are known to be contrary to fact. For example, in a thought experiment, an entity imagining that it had been exposed to the change agent is compared with the same entity had there been no exposure; or an entity that had no exposure to the change agent is compared with the same entity imagining that it had been exposed.[2,34,101,288] See also POTENTIAL OUTCOME.

COUNTERMATCHING A matching procedure for case-control studies nested within a COHORT when exposure status is known for all cohort members and information about confounders is acquired only on a matched sample of cases and controls, with controls selected to have the opposite exposure of their matched cases; this countermatching may improve the statistical efficiency of the study.[1,270,280,289]

COVARIATE A variable that is possibly predictive of the outcome under study. A covariate may be of direct interest to the study or may be a confounding variable or effect modifier.[1,36,37,101,797]

COVERAGE A measure of the extent to which the services rendered cover the potential need for these services in a community. It is expressed as a proportion in which the numerator is the number of services rendered and the denominator is the number of instances in which the service should have been rendered.[17] Example:

$$\text{Annual obstetric coverage in a community} = \frac{\text{Number of deliveries attended by a qualified midwife or obstetrician}}{\text{Expected number of deliveries during the year in a given community}}$$

COX MODEL See PROPORTIONAL HAZARDS MODEL.

CREATIVITY

1. The ability to produce ideas, knowledge, policies, and objects (including scientific knowledge and "knowledge objects") that are both novel or original and worthwhile or appropriate (i.e., useful, attractive, meaningful, relevant, and valid).[237]

2. In EPIDEMIOLOGICAL RESEARCH, the capacity of a set of studies to harmonize relevance, validity, meaning, innovation, feasibility, and precision—ideally, beauty and simplicity as well. An epidemiological study reflects creativity to the extent that it generates knowledge that is relevant, new, valid, practical, and precise. Complexity may be a plus; it need not clash with simplicity and elegance. Relevance may be social, environmental, sanitary, clinical, biological, methodological, ethical,

technological, intellectual.... Studies may blend, weave, knit, or weld such qualities in extraordinarily different ways.

3. A public health policy or program shows creativity when it is relevant, meaningful, useful, and attractive for populations, persons, companies, and institutions... when it is innovative, imaginative, simple... if effective and efficient in abating harmful determinants of health and significantly improving important health indicators. It may be morally and socially relevant if it increases freedom, justice, education, equity, or social cohesion. It needs to be culturally, environmentally, and economically sustainable. Creativity is an important value for epidemiology and the other health, life, and social sciences.[26,38,58,202,290,482]

CRITERION A principle or standard by which something is judged. See also STANDARD.

CRITERION VALIDITY See VALIDITY, MEASUREMENT.

CRITICAL APPRAISAL Application of rules of evidence to a study to assess the VALIDITY of the data, completeness of reporting, methods and procedures, SIGNIFICANCE of results, conclusions, compliance with ethical standards, etc.[1,5,6,24-26,30,34,37,38,42,58,202] See also HIERARCHY OF EVIDENCE.

CRITICAL PERIOD See SENSITIVE PERIOD.

CRITICAL REGION In tests of a statistical hypothesis, it is the set of values for the TEST STATISTIC that, if observed, would lead to rejection of the TEST HYPOTHESIS.[291]

CRITICAL TIME WINDOW (Syn: etiologically relevant exposure period) The period during which exposure to a causal factor is relevant to causation of a disease.

CRITICAL POPULATION SIZE The theoretical minimum host population size required to maintain an INFECTIOUS AGENT. This size varies depending on the agent and demographic, social, and environmental conditions (hygiene, ambient temperature, etc.) and, in the case of vector-borne diseases, the conditions required for survival and propagation of the vector species.

CRONBACH'S ALPHA (Syn: internal consistency reliability) An estimate of the correlation between the total score across a series of items from a rating scale and the total score that would have been obtained had a comparable series of items been employed.[7]

CROSS-CULTURAL STUDY A study in which populations from different cultural backgrounds are compared.[112,248,292]

CROSS-CULTURAL VALIDITY In clinical research, the degree to which the performance of the items on a translated or culturally adapted health related–patient reported outcomes (HR-PRO) instrument are an adequate reflection of the performance of the items of the original version of the HR-PRO instrument.[274] See also CULTURE; DISEASE.

CROSS-DESIGN SYNTHESIS A method for evaluating outcomes of medical interventions developed by the U.S. General Accounting Office (GAO).[293] It is conducted by pooling databases such as the results of a RANDOMIZED CONTROLLED TRIAL (RCT) and of routinely treated patients; the latter databases may come from hospital discharge statistics and other sources, and their validity should be carefully assessed. It may be seen as a variation of META-ANALYSIS.[9,25,294]

CROSS-INFECTION Infection of one person with pathogenic organisms from another and vice versa. Different from NOSOCOMIAL INFECTION, which occurs in a health care setting; cross-infection can occur anywhere (e.g., in military barracks, schools, workplaces).[20,22,56,69,188,217-219]

CROSS-LEVEL BIAS Biases occurring in ecological studies owing to aggregation at the population level of causes and/or effects that do not aggregate, operate, or interact at the individual level.[295] See also ECOLOGICAL FALLACY, AGGREGATIVE FALLACY, ATOMISTIC FALLACY.

CROSSOVER CLINICAL TRIAL, CROSSOVER EXPERIMENT A method of comparing two (or more) treatments or interventions in which subjects, upon completion of one treatment, are switched to the other. In the case of two treatments, A and B, half the patients are randomly allocated to receive these in the order "A first, then B," and half to receive them in the order "B first, then A." The outcomes cannot be permanent changes (e.g., they can be symptoms, functional capacity). A "washout" phase is often needed before beginning the second treatment. The analysis will have to check whether a CARRYOVER EFFECT was present. If the biological and clinical bases of the trial are coherent, the results will be unbiased and the design will help reduce "noise" and sample size requirements.[1,37] See also CASE-CROSSOVER STUDY; N-OF-ONE STUDY.

CROSS-PRODUCT RATIO See ODDS RATIO.

CROSS-SECTIONAL STUDY (Syn: disease frequency survey, prevalence study) A study that examines the relationship between diseases (or other health outcomes) and other variables of interest as they exist in a defined population at one particular time. The presence or absence of disease and the presence or absence of the other variables (or, if they are quantitative, their level) are determined in each member of the study population or in a representative sample at one particular time. The relationship between a variable and the outcome can be examined (1) in terms of the prevalence of the outcome in different population subgroups defined according to the presence or absence (or level) of the variables and (2) in terms of the presence or absence (or level) of the variables in the individuals with and without the outcome. Note that disease PREVALENCE rather than incidence is normally recorded in a cross-sectional study.[1,3,5,8,24,153,160,167,270] The TIME ORDER of cause and effect cannot necessarily be determined in a cross-sectional study. See also BIAS; COHORT STUDY; MORBIDITY SURVEY; REVERSE CAUSATION; VALIDITY.

CROSS-VALIDATION A statistical method for model development and testing based on splitting the data set into a *training sample* to which a model is fit, and *test sample* on which the model is tested. In modern applications, this process is repeated many times using different (possibly random) splits of the data, and the final model is derived by synthesizing over the results from each split. Cross-validated models tend to exhibit far better generalizability (out-of-sample performance) than conventionally fitted models. See also JACKKNIFE; MACHINE LEARNING; OVERFITTING.

CRUDE DEATH RATE See DEATH RATE.

CULTURE
1. In microbiology, the growth of an organism in or on a nutrient medium.
2. A set of beliefs; values; intellectual, artistic, and religious characteristics; customs, etc., common to and characteristic of a community, group, or nation. Health-related characteristics influenced by culture include diet, physical activity, violence, acceptable gender roles and occupations, and much health-related behavior.[26,112,292] See also INHERITANCE, CULTURAL.

CUMULATIVE DEATH RATE The proportion of a group that dies over a specified time interval. It is the incidence proportion of death. This may refer to all deaths or to deaths from a specific cause or causes. If follow-up is not complete on all persons, the proper estimation of this rate requires the use of methods that take account of CENSORING. Distinct from FORCE OF MORTALITY.

CUMULATIVE INCIDENCE (Syn: incidence proportion) See also RISK.

CUMULATIVE INCIDENCE RATIO (Syn: incidence proportion ratio, RISK RATIO).

CUMULATIVE SAMPLING In CASE-CONTROL STUDIES, the selection of controls restricted to those who never experience the study disease during the entire study period. Contrast with DENSITY SAMPLING, in which persons selected as controls may subsequently become cases before the study ends.[1-3,197,795]

CUSUM Acronym for cumulative sum (of a series of measurements). A way to demonstrate a change in TREND or direction of a series of measurements. Calculation begins with a reference figure (e.g., the expected average measurement). As each new measurement is observed, the reference figure is subtracted, and a cumulative total is produced by adding each successive difference; this cumulative total is the CUSUM.

CUT POINT (Syn: cutoff point) An arbitrarily chosen point or value in an ordered sequence of values used to separate the whole into parts. Commonly the cut point divides a DISTRIBUTION of values into parts that are arbitrarily designated as within or beyond the range considered normal. For example, a cut point of 85, 90, or 95 mm Hg differentiates normal from high blood pressure.[37]

CYCLICITY, SEASONAL The annual cycling of incidence on a seasonal basis. Certain acute infectious diseases, if of greater than rare occurrence, peak in one season of the year and reach the low point 6 months later (or in the opposite season). The onset of some symptoms of some chronic diseases also may show this amplitudinal cyclicity. Demographic phenomena, such as marriages, births, and mortality from all causes and certain specific causes may also exhibit seasonal cyclicity. See also CHRONOBIOLOGY.

CYCLICITY, SECULAR Fluctuation in disease incidence over a period longer than a year. For instance, in large, unimmunized populations, measles tends to have a 2-year cycle of high and low incidence. Empirical observations of secular and seasonal cycles of infectious diseases were the basis for epidemic theory (e.g., the MASS ACTION PRINCIPLE). Mass immunization programs, by raising HERD IMMUNITY levels, have eliminated many such cycles.[56,67,188,196,217-219,240]

CYST COUNT See WORM COUNT.

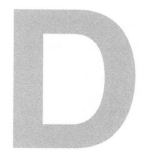

DAG (DIRECTED ACYCLIC GRAPH) See CAUSAL DIAGRAM.

DALY See DISABILITY-ADJUSTED LIFE YEARS.

DATA A collection of items of information. The singular of *data* is *datum*: the plural noun should not be accompanied by a singular verb.[5,7,37]

DATA COLLECTION The process of gathering information in a meaningful and reliable manner. Examples include reviewing medical records or personnel files, conducting interviews, or performing environmental measurements.[3,5,6,26]

DATA CONTAMINATION See CONTAMINATION, DATA.

DATABASE An organized set of data or collection of files that can be used for a specified purpose.[26]

DATA CLEANING The process of excluding the information in incomplete, inconsistent records or irrelevant information collected in a survey or other form of epidemiological study before analysis begins. This may mean excluding information that would distort the results if an attempt were made to edit and include it in the analysis, but it can also introduce biases. The fact that this step has been taken should be reported, along with the results of the study of analyzed data.[1,26] See also RAW DATA.

DATA DREDGING A jargon term meaning analyses done on a post hoc basis without benefit of prestated hypotheses. Such analyses are sometimes done when data have been collected on a large number of variables and unanticipated hypotheses are suggested by hypothesis-free analyses. The scientific validity of data dredging is dubious, usually unacceptable. An even less ethical practice is denoted by the expression "cherry-picking," usually referring to biased selection of patients, analysis of subsets of data, or reporting of results favorable to the interests of a researcher, organization, or sponsor.[6,26,87] See also AGNOSTIC ANALYSIS; CHANCE; CROSS-VALIDATION; EXPLORATORY STUDY; FISHING EXPEDITION; OVERFITTING; PUBLICATION BIAS; RANDOM.

DATA MINING The extraction of information from large databases or files, often with the use of ARTIFICIAL INTELLIGENCE technology and advanced statistical and bioinformatics methods.[7] An exploratory approach in "-omics" research (e.g., genomics, peptidomics, METABOLOMICS).[91] "The polite term for «DATA DREDGING»."[53] See also GENETIC EPIDEMIOLOGY; MOLECULAR EPIDEMIOLOGY.

DATA PROCESSING Conversion of items of information into a form that permits storage, retrieval, and analysis.

DATA REDUCTION The process of summarizing a set or sets of data in the form of an index, such as life expectancy or gross domestic product.

DATA SAFETY MONITORING BOARD (Syn: data monitoring committee) An independent group of experts who monitor patient safety and treatment efficacy data and advise the investigators at predetermined intervals during and at the end of the study.[7,26,58,73-77]

DEATH CERTIFICATE A vital record signed by a licensed physician or another designated health worker that includes cause of death, decedent's name, sex, birth date, places of residence and of death, and whether the deceased had been medically attended before death. Occupation, birthplace, and other information may be included. Immediate cause of death is recorded on the first line, followed by conditions giving rise to the immediate cause; the underlying cause is entered last. The underlying cause is coded and tabulated in official publications of cause-specific mortality. Other significant conditions may also be recorded separately, as is the mode of death, whether accidental or violent, etc. The most important entries on a death certificate are underlying causes of death and cause of death. These are defined in the tenth (1990) revision of the INTERNATIONAL STATISTICAL CLASSIFICATION OF DISEASES AND RELATED HEALTH PROBLEMS (ICD-10) as follows:

"*Causes of death:* The causes of death to be entered on the medical certificate of cause of death are all those diseases, morbid conditions, or injuries that either resulted in or contributed to death and the circumstances of the accident or violence which produced any such injuries.

Underlying cause of death: The underlying cause of death is (1) the disease or injury that initiated the train of events leading to death or (2) the circumstances of the accident or violence that produced the fatal injury."

Personal identifying information such as birthplace, parents' names (last name at birth), birth date, and personal identifying numbers are included on death certificates in some

INTERNATIONAL FORM OF MEDICAL CERTIFICATE OF CAUSE OF DEATH

Cause of death		Approximate interval between onset and death
I Disease or condition directly leading to death*	(a)	....
	due to (or as a consequence of)	
Antecedent causes Morbid conditions, if any, giving rise to the above cause, stating the underlying condition last	(b)	....
	due to (or as a consequence of)	
	(c)	....
	due to (or as a consequence of)	
	(d)	....
II Other significant conditions contributing to the death, but not related to the disease or condition causing it	....	....
	....	....
* This does not mean the mode of dying, e.g., heart failure, respiratory failure. It means the disease, injury, or complication that caused death.		

Death certificate. The International Standard Form. Source: World Health Organization.[296] With permission.

jurisdictions; this extra information makes possible a range of RECORD LINKAGE studies.[8] See also INTERNATIONAL FORM OF MEDICAL CERTIFICATE OF CAUSES OF DEATH.

DEATH RATE An estimate of the portion of a population that dies during a specified period. The numerator is the number of persons dying during the period; the denominator is the number in the population, usually estimated as the midyear population.[1] The death rate in a population is generally calculated by the following formula:

$$\frac{\text{Number of deaths during a specified period}}{\text{Number of persons at risk of dying during the period}} \times 10^n$$

This rate is an estimate of the PERSON-TIME death rate, i.e., the death rate per 10^n person-years. If the rate is low, it is also a good estimate of the cumulative death rate. This rate is also called the crude death rate.

DEATH REGISTRATION AREA A geographic area for which mortality data are collected and often published.

DEBIASING The reduction of cognitive, affective, and other types of BIAS.[38,297-299]

DECISION ANALYSIS A derivative of OPERATIONS RESEARCH and GAME THEORY to identify all available choices, and POTENTIAL OUTCOMES of each, in a series of decisions that have to be made (e.g., about aspects of patient care as diagnostic procedures, preventive and therapeutic regimens, prognosis). Epidemiological data play a large part in analyzing the probabilities of outcomes following each potential choice. The range of choices can be plotted on a DECISION TREE; at each branch of the tree, or decision node, the probabilities of each outcome that can be predicted are displayed. The decision tree thus portrays the choices available to those responsible for patient care and the probabilities of each outcome that will follow the choice of a particular action or strategy. The relative worth of each outcome is preferably described as a UTILITY or quality-of-life measure (e.g., a probability of life expectancy or of freedom from disability, often expressed as quality-adjusted life years, or QALYs).[6-9,14,38,58] See also CLINICAL DECISION ANALYSIS.

DECISION TREE The alternative choices expressed, in quantitative terms, available at each stage in the process of thinking through a problem may be likened to branches and the hierarchical sequence of options to a tree. Hence, decision tree. It is a graphic device used in DECISION ANALYSIS in which a series of decision options are represented as branches and subsequent possible outcomes are represented as further branches. The decisions and the eventualities are presented in the order in which they are likely to occur. The junction where a decision must be taken is called a decision node.[9,58]

DECOMPOSITION METHOD Comparison of groups by analyzing mathematical functions of rates, incidence densities, and exposure prevalence. This simplifies identification of relevant contributing factors in risk analysis.[301]

DEDUCTION Reasoned argument proceeding from the general to the particular.

DEDUCTIVE LOGIC Logic that predicts specific outcomes from prior general hypotheses — that is, it proceeds from the general to the particular. Logic based on derivation of necessary conclusions implied by explicit assumptions (premises), as in mathematics. See also HYPOTHETICO-DEDUCTIVE METHOD; INDUCTIVE REASONING.

DEGREES OF FREEDOM (df) The number of independent comparisons that can be made between the members of a sample. Roughly, it refers to the number of independent

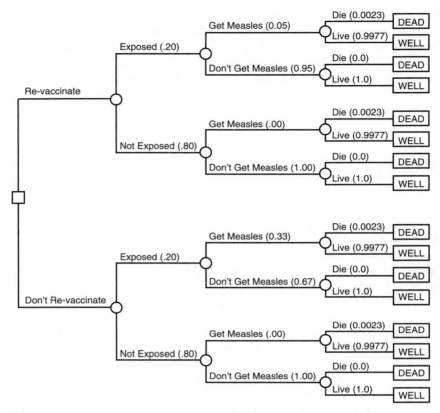

Decision tree. Probabilities of different outcomes with and without revaccination against measles. Source: Petitti DB.[300] With permission.

dimensions of variation in a sample under an assumed sampling model. More specifically, it is the number of independent contributions to a sampling DISTRIBUTION (such as χ^2, t, and F distribution) from the data-generating mechanism. For example, in a CONTINGENCY TABLE with fixed margins, the total degrees of freedom is one less than the number of row categories multiplied by one less than the number of column categories.[37] See also DIMENSIONALITY; DISTRIBUTION FUNCTION.

DELPHI METHOD Iterative circulation to a panel of experts of questions and responses that are progressively refined in light of responses to each round of questions; preferably participants' identities should not be revealed to each other. The aim is to reduce the number of viable options or solutions, perhaps to arrive at a consensus judgment on an issue or problem, or a set of issues or problems, without allowing any one participant to dominate the process. The method was developed at the RAND Corporation.

DEMAND (FOR HEALTH SERVICES) Willingness and/or ability to seek, use, and in some settings, pay for services. Sometimes further subdivided into *expressed demand* (equated with use) and *potential demand* or *need*. [17]

DEMOGRAPHIC TRANSITION The evolution from high to low fertility and mortality rates in a country. Formerly thought to be related to technological change and industrialization but probably more directly caused by improvements in female literacy and the status of women. It is accompanied by a change in the age composition of the population as birthrates and death rates decline; usually infant and child mortality rates decline as well. As a result there is a decrease in the proportion of children and young adults and an increase in the proportion of older persons in the population, i.e., an AGING OF THE POPULATION.[7,8] See also ECOLOGICAL TRANSITION; "EPIDEMIOLOGICAL TRANSITION" THEORY.

DEMOGRAPHIC ENTRAPMENT A community may be said to be demographically trapped if (1) it exceeds the CARRYING CAPACITY of its local ecosystem; (2) there is no other land to which it can migrate; and (3) it has too few exports to exchange for food and other essentials. Common outcomes include poverty, stunting, starvation, and violence. There may be a warning stage, during which starvation or violence can be expected (e.g., because population is increasing rapidly).

DEMOGRAPHY The study of populations, especially with reference to size and density, fertility, mortality, growth, age distribution, migration, and VITAL STATISTICS, and the interaction of all these with social and economic conditions.

DEMONSTRATION MODEL An experimental health care facility, program, or system with built-in provision for measuring aspects such as costs per unit of service, rates of use by patients or clients, and outcomes of encounters between providers and users. The aim usually is to determine the feasibility, efficacy, effectiveness, and/or efficiency of the model service.

DENOMINATOR The lower portion of a ratio.[1,7,28,34,37,106-108] Valid information on—as well as some psychological and cultural appreciation for—denominators and NUMERATORS is essential in clinical and EPIDEMIOLOGICAL RESEARCH, in many clinical and public health activities, DECISION ANALYSIS, HEALTH RISK APPRAISAL, HEALTH TECHNOLOGY ASSESSMENT, RISK ASSESSMENT, RISK MANAGEMENT, or policymaking. Along with other natural characteristics, mechanisms, biases, and influences of and on the common cognitive machinery (e.g., neglect of base rates and probabilities, duration neglect, availability cascades, substitution, insensitivity to the quality of information, intuitive judgments under uncertainty, risk aversion, framing, priming, anchoring, imagination, fear, other emotions),[38] *denominator neglect* is an important cause of differences in reasoning and decisions between some types of individuals and groups (e.g., patients, clinicians, counselors, politicians, other citizens) and others (e.g., statisticians, epidemiologists, risk assessors, other experts). See also CONTROL GROUP; POPULATION THINKING; RISK FACTOR.

DENSITY CASE-CONTROL STUDY A variant of the case-control study in which the controls are drawn in such a way that they represent the PERSON-TIME experience that generated the cases, usually by DENSITY SAMPLING.[1-3,197,795] This design provides an estimate of the rate ratio with no RARE DISEASE ASSUMPTION. A type of CASE-BASE STUDY. See also CASE-COHORT STUDY; RISK SET.

DENSITY-EQUALIZING MAP See ISODEMOGRAPHIC MAP.

DENSITY OF POPULATION Demographic term meaning numbers of persons in relation to available space.

DENSITY SAMPLING A method of selecting controls in a CASE-CONTROL STUDY in which cases are sampled only from incident cases over a specific time period and controls are sampled and interviewed throughout that period (rather than simply at one point in time, such as the end of the period). This method can reduce bias due to changing exposure patterns in the source population and allows estimation of the rate ratio without any rare-disease assumption. A density-sampled control may subsequently become a case, before the study ends, in contrast to CUMULATIVE SAMPLING.[1-3,7,8,197,270]

DEONTOLOGICAL A duty-based theoretical approach to ETHICS. Right actions stem from freely embraced obligations to universal moral imperatives, such as the obligation to respect persons as ends and not as means.[28,117,118,248-250,259-265]

DEPENDENCY RATIO Ratio of children and old people in a population in comparison to all others (i.e., the proportion of economically inactive to economically active); "children" are usually defined those below 15 years of age and "old people" as those 65 years of age and above.

DEPENDENT VARIABLE

1. A variable the value of which is dependent on the effect of other variable(s)—independent variable(s)—in the relationship under study. A manifestation or outcome whose variation we seek to explain or account for by the influence of independent variables.
2. In REGRESSION ANALYSIS, the variable whose average value is being studied in relation to regressors (covariates or "independent" variables).[36,244] See also INDEPENDENT VARIABLE; REGRESSAND; REGRESSOR.

DESCRIPTIVE EPIDEMIOLOGY Epidemiological studies and activities (e.g., SURVEILLANCE) whose descriptive components (e.g., aims, methods) are much stronger than their analytic components, or that fall within the descriptive area of the descriptive-analytic spectrum; e.g., studies more concerned with describing associations than with analyzing and explaining causal effects. Descriptive study of the occurrence of disease and other health-related characteristics in human populations. General descriptions concerning the relationship of disease to basic characteristics such as age, gender, ethnicity, occupation, social class, and geographic location; even such general descriptions may have analytic dimensions. Major categories in descriptive epidemiology are persons, place, and time. Descriptive epidemiology is always observational, never experimental; observational epidemiological studies may be descriptive or analytic.[3,7,8,48,160] See also ANALYTIC STUDY; CASE REPORTS; ETIOLOGICAL STUDY; OBSERVATIONAL STUDY; RISK FACTOR.

DESCRIPTIVE STUDY A study concerned with and designed only to describe the existing distribution of variables without much regard to causal relationships or other hypotheses. An example is a community health survey used to determine the health status of the people in a community. In a descriptive study, a parameter of disease occurrence is related to a determinant without concern for a causal interpretation of the relation.[28,270] Descriptive studies (e.g., analyses of population registries) can be used to measure RISKS and TRENDS in health indicators, generate hypotheses, or monitor health policies. Contrast with ANALYTIC STUDY; ETIOLOGICAL STUDY.

DESIGN See RESEARCH DESIGN.

DESIGN BIAS The difference between a true value and that obtained as a result of faulty study design. A BIAS in study findings attributable to the study design. Examples include uncontrolled studies where the effects of two or more processes cannot be separated for lack of measurement of key causes of the exposure or outcome (CONFOUNDING); and studies done on poorly defined populations or with unsuitable control groups.[1-3,795]

DESIGN EFFECT An effect of a study design feature on the performance or outcome of a statistical procedure. A specific form is bias attributable to intraclass correlation in CLUSTER SAMPLING. The design effect for a cluster design is the ratio of the variance for that design to the variance calculated from a simple random sample of the same size. If the latter incorrect variance is used in procedures instead of the correct cluster variance, the result will be a bias in the variance estimate.[7]

DESIGN VARIABLE
1. A study variable whose distribution in the subjects is determined by the investigator.
2. In statistics, a variable taking on the value 1 to indicate membership in a particular category and 0 or –1 to indicate nonmembership in the category. Used primarily in ANALYSIS OF VARIANCE. See also INDICATOR VARIABLE.

DESMOTERIC MEDICINE The practice of medicine in a prison. Derived from the Greek *desmoterion*, prison.

DETECTABLE PRECLINICAL PERIOD The period between the time when a disease is capable of yielding a positive screening test and the appearance of clinical symptoms and/or signs.[5,6,9,58] See also LEAD TIME.

DETECTION BIAS BIAS due to systematic differences between the study groups in ASCERTAINMENT, assessment, diagnosis, or verification of outcomes. As other biases, it has numerous mechanisms and forms.[1,3,6-9,42,53,63,270] An example is verification of diagnosis by laboratory tests in hospital cases but failure to apply the same tests to cases outside the hospital. See also SPECTRUM BIAS; VERIFICATION BIAS.

DETERMINANT(S) (Syn: risk factor) A collective or individual RISK FACTOR (or set of factors) that is causally related to a health condition, outcome, or other defined characteristic. The concept is probabilistic, and thus the term does not imply a DETERMINISTIC philosophy of health; e.g., it does not embody genetic, environmental, or social determinisms. In human health —and, specifically, in DISEASES OF COMPLEX ETIOLOGY— sets of determinants often act jointly in relatively complex and long-term processes. They commonly operate both at aggregate (e.g., social, regional, global) and distal levels, as well as at the individual, personal level; i.e., across macro- and micro-levels, SYSTEMICALLY.[14,17,28,158,213,215,279,302,306] See also CAUSALITY; CAUSES IN PUBLIC HEALTH SCIENCES.

DETERMINANT, DISTAL (DISTANT) (Syn: upstream determinant) A RISK FACTOR that is remote or far apart in scale, level, position, or time to the outcome of concern, making it more difficult to discern or trace within the causal pathway than other causal factors that are less far away from the outcome.[84,163-169,211,279,303-309] Examples include global climate warming and urban atmospheric pollution, which increase the risk of numerous acute and chronic diseases and disorders.[13,28,33,169,213,310] In infectious diseases, the microbial agent is more proximal to the disease than social factors such as poverty, which are more distant or upstream but no less influential on the individual risk of developing the disease and on its prevalence. See also STRATEGY, "POPULATION."

DETERMINANT, PROXIMAL (PROXIMATE) (Syn: downstream determinant) A RISK FACTOR that is near in scale, level, position, or time to the outcome of concern.[113] See also STRATEGY, "HIGH-RISK."

DETERMINISM, GENETIC A view of genetics according to which genetic INHERITANCE not only influences but strongly constrains human development, health, and behavior. It tends to disregard environmental influences on GENE EXPRESSION and social influences on health states. See also EPIGENETIC INHERITANCE; GENETIC PENETRANCE; HEREDITY; MONOGENIC DISEASES; POLYGENIC DISEASES.

DETERMINISTIC METHOD A method that predicts outcomes perfectly, without allowance for statistical (chance) variation.

DETERMINISTIC MODEL A representation of a system, process, or relationship in mathematical form in which relationships are fixed (i.e., they take no account of probability and CHANCE), so that any given input invariably yields the same result.[1,8,39,42,110,128] See also MATHEMATICAL MODEL.

DETERMINANT OF FERTILITY, PROXIMATE Factor having a direct influence on fertility, such as contraceptive use, age at marriage, age at first sexual intercourse, breast-feeding, or abortion.

DEVELOPMENTAL AND LIFE COURSE EPIDEMIOLOGY The study of long-term effects on later health or disease risk of physical or social exposures during gestation, childhood, adolescence, young adulthood, and later adult life. The premise or hypothesis is that various biological and social factors throughout life independently, cumulatively, or interactively influence health and disease in adult life. The aim is to elucidate biological, behavioral, and psychosocial processes that operate across an individual's LIFE COURSE or across generations to influence disease risk.[23,32,311,312]

DEVELOPMENTAL ORIGINS HYPOTHESIS See DEVELOPMENTAL ORIGINS OF HEALTH AND DISEASE.

DEVELOPMENTAL ORIGINS OF HEALTH AND DISEASE (DOHD) Originally, the hypothesis that cardiovascular disease and type 2 diabetes originate through developmental PLASTICITY in response to undernutrition. A hypothesis proposed in 1990 by the epidemiologist David Barker (1938 - 2013) that undernutrition and other insults during critical periods of fetal development not only reduce birth weight, but also have permanent effects on (or "program") the structure and metabolism of body tissues and systems, and cause hypertension, coronary heart disease, and non–insulin dependent diabetes in middle age.[161,313,314] Health during childhood is also influenced by in utero and neonatal exposures, and growth during infancy and early childhood is also linked to later disease; therefore, DOHD and *developmental origins hypothesis* are preferred to *fetal origins hypothesis*.[161] Evidence from human and animal studies suggests that early life programming contributes to other diseases, including cancer, chronic lung and kidney disease, osteoporosis, and mental illness.[315] The hypothesis is evolving to include evidence that exposure to environmental factors early in development involves EPIGENETIC modifications, which may increase the risk of adult disease;[32,80,153,186,187,316-319] e.g., protein restriction of pregnant rats leads to adult hypertension in the offspring, which is associated with altered methylation and expression of specific genes; these changes can be prevented by supplementing the protein-restricted dam with folic acid.[320] Also, in utero or neonatal exposure to bisphenol A (BPA) may be associated with higher body weight, increased risk of breast and prostate cancer, and altered reproductive function.[13,321]

DIAGNOSIS The process of determining the health status and the factors responsible for it; may be applied to an individual, family, group, society. The term is applied both to the process of determination and to its findings.[6,58] See also CASE; COMMUNITY DIAGNOSIS; DISEASE LABEL; SEMIOLOGY.

DIAGNOSIS-RELATED GROUP (DRG) Classification of hospital patients according to diagnosis and intensity of care required, used by insurance carriers to set reimbursement scales.

DIAGNOSTIC AND STATISTICAL MANUAL OF MENTAL DISORDERS (DSM) A manual that aims to systematize and standardize the definitions of mental disorders, developed by the American Psychiatric Association. It contains a listing of psychiatric disorders and their corresponding diagnostic codes; each disorder is accompanied by a set of diagnostic criteria and text containing information about the disorder. The first edition of DSM-5 was published in 2013.

DIAGNOSTIC INDEX A system for recording diagnoses, diseases, or problems of patients or clients in a medical practice or service, usually including identifying information (name, birthdate, sex) and dates of encounters.

DIAGNOSTIC SUSPICION BIAS A bias that may occur when knowledge of the subject's prior exposure to a putative cause (ethnicity, drug intake, a second disorder, an environmental exposure) influences both the intensity and the outcome of the diagnostic process.[6,9,26,203]

DIAGNOSTIC TEST A test to diagnose whether or not a person has a DISEASE or disorder. Not all biomedical (laboratory, imaging, genetic, other) tests have this aim. To protect individuals and groups from avoidable adverse effects of diagnostic activities, it is essential to distinguish related but different aims, such as diagnosing clinically overt disease; discovering occult disease (new process, recurrences); secondary and tertiary PREVENTION; determining the stage, characteristics, and activity of the disease; counseling; or monitoring the clinical course and effects of therapies.[6,8,9,24,26,58,322,323] See also ACCURACY; DETECTION BIAS; EARLY CLINICAL DETECTION; EARLY DETECTION OF DISEASE; QUADAS-2; SCREENING; SICKNESS "CAREER."

DICHOTOMOUS SCALE See MEASUREMENT SCALE.

DICHOTOMOUS VARIABLE See BINARY VARIABLE.

DIFFERENTIAL The difference(s) shown in tabulation of health and vital statistics according to age, sex, or some other factor; age differentials are the differences revealed in the tabulations of rates in age groups, sex differentials are the differences in rates between males and females, income differentials are differences between designated income categories, etc.

DIFFUSION THEORY
1. The concept that infectious pathogens and ideas diffuse through a population.[324]
2. Theories explaining the dissemination of ideas and customs to other populations.
3. The "innovation-diffusion theory" explains how innovative ideas spread through segments of society, including the role of opinion leaders and the media.

DIGITAL EPIDEMIOLOGY The use of epidemiologic knowledge and digital technologies to enable disease SURVEILLANCE and EPIDEMIOLOGICAL RESEARCH. For instance, in some outbreaks, digital disease surveillance has supplemented the critical laboratory studies and work in the trenches by public health officials and epidemiologists, by leveraging use of the Internet, mobile phones, and social media. Some of the added insights come from the general population. Both computational and EPIDEMIOLOGICAL INTELLIGENCE are required to extract meaningful information from data sets that are both extremely large and noisy.[48,160,325]

DIGIT PREFERENCE A preference for certain numbers that leads to rounding off measurements. Rounding off may be to the nearest whole number, even number, multiple of 5 or 10, or (when time units like a week are involved) 7, 14, etc. This can be a form of OBSERVER VARIATION or an attribute of respondent(s) in a survey.

DIMENSIONALITY The number of dimensions (i.e., scalar quantities) needed for accurate description of an element of a vector space. See also DEGREES OF FREEDOM.

DIRECT ADJUSTMENT, DIRECT STANDARDIZATION See STANDARDIZATION.

DIRECTED ACYCLIC GRAPH (DAG) See CAUSAL DIAGRAM.

DIRECTION Blalock's[326] synonym for David Hume's CONNECTION.[84] It indicates a linkage from cause to effect that is repeatedly demonstrable, hence predictable.

DIRECTIONALITY
1. The direction of inference of a study.[1-3,5-7,24,25,101,270] It may be retrospective (backward-looking, seeking causes of outcomes or effects) or prospective (forward-looking, seeking effects of treatments or exposures).
2. The sign of a relationship between variables. Correlation coefficients are directional measures of association because the sign changes if one of the variables is reversed.

DIRECTIVES See GUIDELINES.

DIRECT OBSTETRICAL DEATH See MATERNAL MORTALITY.

DISABILITY Temporary or long-term reduction of a person's capacity to function. See also DISABILITY; INTERNATIONAL CLASSIFICATION OF IMPAIRMENTS, DISABILITIES, AND HANDICAPS; HANDICAP.

DISABILITY-ADJUSTED LIFE YEARS (DALYs) A DALY lost is a measure of the BURDEN OF DISEASE on a defined population. It is hence an indicator of POPULATION HEALTH. DALYs are advocated as an alternative to QUALITY-ADJUSTED LIFE YEARS (QALYs). They are based on adjustment of LIFE EXPECTANCY to allow for long-term disability as estimated from official statistics; the necessary data to do so may not be available in some areas. The concept postulates a continuum from disease to disability to death that is not universally accepted, particularly by the community of persons with disabilities. DALYs are calculated using a "disability weight" (a proportion less than 1) multiplied by chronological age to reflect the burden of the disability. DALYs can thus produce estimates that accord greater value to fit than to disabled persons and to the middle years of life rather than to youth or old age.[248,327] See also DISABILITY-FREE LIFE EXPECTANCY.

DISABILITY-FREE LIFE EXPECTANCY (Syn: active life expectancy) The average number of years an individual is expected to live free of disability if current patterns of mortality and disability continue to apply.[328] A statistical abstraction based on existing age-specific death rates and either age-specific disability prevalences or age-specific disability transition rates.

DISASTER An ACCIDENT or other type of event that disrupts the normal conditions of existence and causes a level of suffering that exceeds the capacity of adjustment of the affected community.

DISASTER EPIDEMIOLOGY The application of epidemiological principles and tools to managing DISASTER and EMERGENCY public health programs (e.g., to reduce morbidity and mortality among displaced populations).

DISCLOSURE OF INTERESTS

1. In health sciences research and other professional activities (e.g., lecturing, consulting), the action of making researchers' interests on a given issue known. Widely used guidelines require that all participants in the PEER REVIEW and publication process must disclose all relationships that could present a potential conflict of interest.[6,13,26,83,138,266,267] Editors may use information disclosed in editorial decisions, and should publish it if they believe it is relevant in judging the manuscript. Editors should also publish regular disclosure statements of journal staff. A similar rationale is applied by governments and organizations that receive expert advice from health and other scientists. See also CONFLICT OF INTEREST.

2. In certain types of law, the obligation that each party has to the other parties to reveal or make known all facts relevant to the subject matter of the contract. The provision of financial and other types of information concerning a company to those with an interest in the economic activities of the company.

DISCONFIRMATION BIAS See CONFIRMATION BIAS.

DISCORDANT A term used in TWIN STUDIES to describe a twin pair in which one twin exhibits a certain TRAIT and the other does not. Also used in matched-pair case-control studies to describe a pair whose members had different exposures to the RISK FACTOR under study. Under conventional analytical methods, only the discordant pairs are informative about the association between exposure and disease.[1]

DISCOUNT RATE A measure of costs, benefits, and outcomes in relation to time that allows for the fact that money (and health) have greater value in the present than at some future time. A term used mainly in economics and in CLINICAL DECISION ANALYSIS.

DISCRETE DATA Data that can be arranged into naturally occurring or arbitrarily selected groups or sets of values as opposed to data in which there are no naturally occurring breaks in continuity (i.e., CONTINUOUS DATA).[1,37,110] An example is number of decayed, missing, and filled teeth (DMF).[5]

DISCRIMINANT FUNCTION ANALYSIS A statistical analytical technique used with discrete dependent variables; it is concerned with separating sets of observed values and allocating new values. Examples include normal linear discrimination and logistic discrimination (the latter being mathematically identical to LOGISTIC REGRESSION analysis). Kendall and Buckland[283] refer to this as "discriminatory analysis" and describe it as a rule for allocating individuals or values from two or more discrete populations to the correct population with minimal probability of misclassification under the assumed model.[7]

DISCRIMINATORY ACCURACY The power or capacity of a variable (e.g., a risk factor, a biomarker) to discriminate or predict cases and noncases with a given health outcome in the population. It is also known as *discriminatory power, predictive accuracy*, and *predictive capacity*. Measures of association alone are unsuitable for such discriminatory purpose; even a RISK FACTOR strongly associated with a disease (e.g., with an OR = 5) has a low capacity to discriminate cases and noncases in a population. To evaluate the discriminatory accuracy of a variable we may combine the true-positive fraction (TPF) (also known as SENSITIVITY or detection rate), and the false-positive fraction (FPF) (also known as 1- SPECIFICITY). We can also analyze: the *area under the* ROC CURVE (or "C-statistic"); a *risk assessment plot* (which represents the TPF and FPF against the predicted risk); the *explained variance*; the *incremental prognostic impact*; the *integrated discrimination improvement* (IDI); and the *net reclassification index* (NRI).[106-108,329-331,796] See also ATTRIBUTABLE FRACTION.

DISCRIMINATORY POWER See DISCRIMINATORY ACCURACY.

DISEASE
1. Literally, *dis-ease*, the opposite of *ease*, when something is wrong with a bodily function. A DISORDER that can be assigned to a diagnostic category.
2. *Disease, illness*, and *sickness* are better regarded as not synonymous:[24,50,332-334]
   i. DISEASE is the biological dimension of nonhealth, an essentially physiological dysfunction.
   ii. ILLNESS is a subjective or psychological state of the person who feels aware of not being well; the experience of a person with a disease; a social construct fashioned out of transactions between healers and patients in the context of their common culture.
   iii. SICKNESS is a state of social dysfunction of a person with a disease; the role that the individual assumes when ill; a result of being defined by others as "unhealthy."

In the real world, lay concepts of illness and medical concepts of disease interact and shape each other. Neither disease nor illness is infinitely malleable: both are constrained by biology and by culture.[211,248,335,336] See also DISORDER; EMBODIMENT; SEMIOLOGY; SICKNESS "CAREER."

DISEASE FREQUENCY SURVEY See CROSS-SECTIONAL STUDY; MORBIDITY SURVEY.

DISEASE INTENSITY See FORCE OF MORBIDITY.

DISEASE LABEL The identity of the condition from which a patient suffers. It may be the name of a precisely defined disorder identified by a battery of tests, a probability statement based on consideration of what is most likely among several possibilities, an opinion based on pattern recognition, or even a RISK FACTOR. See also CASE; DIAGNOSIS; "DISEASE MONGERING"; SEMIOLOGY; SICKNESS "CAREER".

DISEASE MAPPING A method for displaying spatial distribution of cases of disease, most often used in veterinary epidemiology. Disease maps may display raw numbers or rates (i.e., CHOROPLETHIC MAPS). See also GEOGRAPHICAL INFORMATION SYSTEM; GEOMATICS; MEDICAL GEOGRAPHY; SATELLITE EPIDEMIOLOGY.

DISEASE MODEL Quantitative simulation of the natural history of a disease (incidence, progression, prognosis, etc.) based on epidemiological data. A *public health model* is population based and is used in planning and evaluating health services, whereas a *clinical model* is used in individual patient care.[122]

"DISEASE MONGERING" The practice of breaking and widening evidence-based diagnostic and therapeutic boundaries of illnesses and disorders, of inflating frequencies and risks, and of publicly promoting such exaggerated visions in order to expand the markets for those who sell and deliver health-related services and products, which may include segments of some pharmaceutical and biotechnological companies, health professionals, media, and consumer and patient organizations. Part of the process of MEDICALIZATION and GENETIZATION of ordinary life, in which social construction of illness is strongly influenced by corporate interests and DYSREGULATION.[323,337-339] See also IATROGENESIS; PREVENTION, QUATERNARY.

DISEASE ODDS RATIO See ODDS RATIO.

DISEASE, PRECLINICAL Disease that has not yet developed signs or symptoms, or has not been diagnosed. See also EARLY CLINICAL DETECTION; INAPPARENT INFECTION.

DISEASE PROGRESSION BIAS

1. In studies on the clinical accuracy and validity of diagnostic tests, a BIAS that occurs if results of the diagnostic test under study and of the reference standard test are not collected on the same patients at the same time, and if spontaneous recovery or progression to a more advanced stage of disease takes place.[340] See also QUADAS-2.

2. In etiologic studies, biases that occur when disease progression entails metabolic or other pathophysiologic changes that alter the characteristics or concentrations (e.g., in blood, adipose tissue, target organs, peritumoral tissue) of the study exposure BIOMARKERS. Biomarkers of exposure collected during subclinical or overt disease will then not reflect exposures of true etiologic significance that took place in more distant time windows, and may hence cause REVERSE CAUSATION; e.g., lower blood concentrations of certain vitamins may not actually increase the risk of a disease, but be a consequence of the (subclinical) disease. Similarly, during the progression of some cancers, long before clinical diagnosis, blood concentrations of lipophilic substances of putative etiologic interest (e.g., lipophilic vitamins, organochlorine compounds) may be increased or decreased due to pathophysiologic changes associated with cancer-induced weight loss, cholestasis, or lipid mobilization.[146] See also PATHOPHYSIOLOGY.

DISEASE REGISTRY See REGISTER, REGISTRY.

DISEASE, SUBCLINICAL Disease that is detectable by specific tests but does not yet manifest signs or symptoms.

DISEASE TAXONOMY See TAXONOMY OF DISEASE.

DISEASE TRANSITION A measure of change in the individual disease status in two consecutive assessments independent of whether this was the first occurrence and/or whether prior data are missing.[341] Two types are distinguished:

1. *Positive transition:* the change from disease-free to diseased; defined as the number of subjects with a disease divided by the study population that was disease-free at the beginning of the transition period.
2. *Negative transition:* the change from diseased to disease-free; defined as the number of disease-free individuals divided by the study population that was diseased in the preceding assessment.

DISEASES OF COMPLEX ETIOLOGY Diseases that result from complex causal pathways (e.g., from interactions between sociocultural, environmental, clinical, genetic, and epigenetic processes), often developing over long periods of life. Common diseases with late-onset phenotypes often result from chronic interactions between the EPIGENOME, the GENOME, and environmental factors[86,145,316-321,799] See also PLEIOTROPY; POLYGENIC DISEASES; WEB OF CAUSATION.

DISENTRAPMENT Some form of escape from DEMOGRAPHIC ENTRAPMENT.

DISINFECTION Killing of infectious agents outside the body by direct exposure to chemical or physical agents.

Concurrent disinfection is the application of disinfective measures as soon as possible after the discharge of infectious material from the body of an infected person or after the soiling of articles with such infectious discharges, all personal contact with such discharges or articles being minimized prior to such disinfection.

Terminal disinfection is the application of disinfective measures after the patient has been removed by death or to a hospital, or has ceased to be a source of infection, or after other hospital ISOLATION practices have been discontinued. Terminal disinfection is rarely practiced; terminal cleaning generally suffices, along with airing and sunning of rooms, furniture, and bedding. Disinfection is necessary only for diseases spread by indirect contact; steam sterilization or incineration of bedding and other items is desirable after a disease such as plague or anthrax.[56,69,188]

DISINFESTATION Any physical or chemical process serving to destroy or remove undesired small animal forms, particularly arthropods or rodents, present upon the person, the clothing, or in the environment of an individual or on domestic animals. Disinfestation includes delousing for infestation with *Pediculus humanus humanus*, the body louse. Synonyms include the terms *disinsection* and *disinsectization* when insects only are involved.[8,20-22,56,188,217-219]

DISMOD A model designed to help disease experts arrive at internally consistent estimates of incidence, duration, and case fatality rates of BURDEN OF DISEASE. It uses a life-table approach in following an initially disease-free cohort over time while applying the risks (incidence, remission, case fatality rate) associated with a disease and the COMPETING RISK of all other diseases as represented by general mortality. Using a competing risk approach, it calculates the relative proportions of each cohort that will develop, recover from, or die from the disease, die from other causes of mortality, or continue to live disease-free. To the extent that it takes into account other competing risk factors of mortality, this approach may be more realistic than one that simply assumes that Prevalence = Incidence × Duration. Differences between the two approaches seem most marked in chronic diseases with low rates of remission and cause-specific mortality.[163]

DISORDER A disturbance or departure —e.g., of an organ or body system, of an institution—from normal balance or healthy function. See also DISEASE; DYSREGULATION; IMPAIRMENT; SYNDROME.

DISTAL DETERMINANT See DETERMINANT, DISTAL (DISTANT).

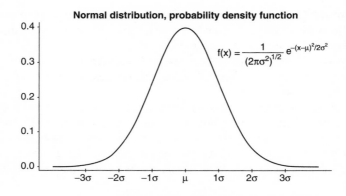

Normal distribution, probability density function

$$f(x) = \frac{1}{(2\pi\sigma^2)^{1/2}} \, e^{-(x-\mu)^2/2\sigma^2}$$

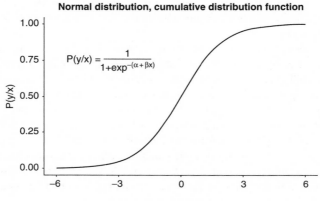

Normal distribution, cumulative distribution function

$$P(y/x) = \frac{1}{1+\exp^{-(\alpha+\beta x)}}$$

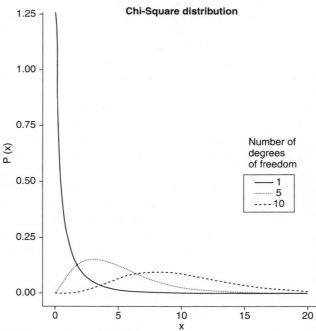

Chi-Square distribution

Number of degrees of freedom

——— 1
············ 5
- - - - 10

Common types of distribution functions (part 1 of 3).

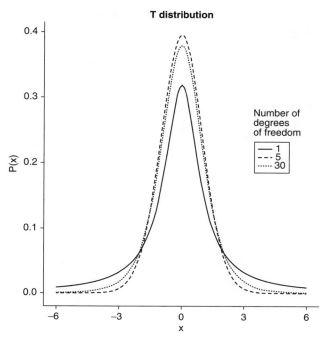

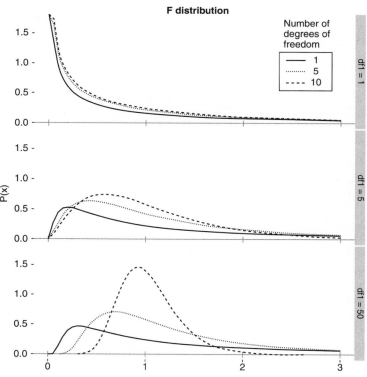

Common types of distribution functions (part 2 of 3).

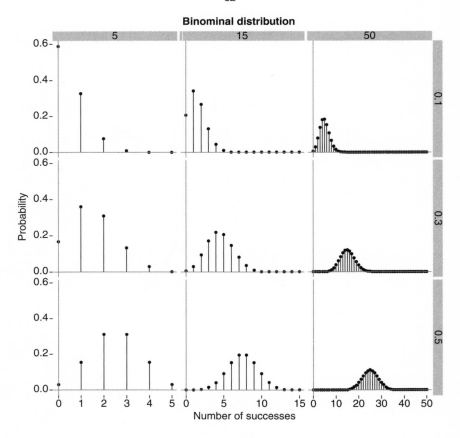

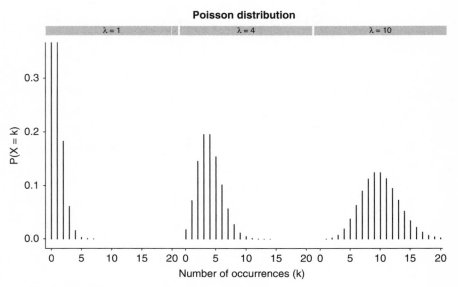

Common types of distribution functions (part 3 of 3).

DISTRIBUTION

1. (Syn: frequency distribution) The complete summary of the frequencies of the values or categories of a measurement made on a group of persons (or on an individual at different times). The distribution tells either how many or what proportion of the group was found to have each value (or each range of values) out of all the possible values that the measurement can have.[1,7,12,34,37]

2. In statistics, a DISTRIBUTION FUNCTION.

DISTRIBUTION-FREE METHOD (Syn: nonparametric method) A method that does not depend upon the form of the underlying distribution. Like all statistical methods, however, it depends on assumptions of randomness (in sampling or in allocation to exposure) and thus may be subject to BIAS.[1,7,34,37]

DISTRIBUTION FUNCTION (Syn: probability distribution) A mathematical function that gives the relative frequency or probability with which a random variable falls at or below each of a series of values. Examples include the NORMAL DISTRIBUTION, LOG-NORMAL DISTRIBUTION, CHI-SQUARE DISTRIBUTION, t-DISTRIBUTION, F DISTRIBUTION, LOGISTIC DISTRIBUTION, BINOMIAL DISTRIBUTION, POISSON DISTRIBUTION, and MULTINOMIAL DISTRIBUTION, all of which have applications in epidemiology and related sciences.[1,12,34,37]

DMF Decayed, missing, and filled teeth. Lowercase letters (i.e., dmf) are used for deciduous dentition, uppercase for permanent teeth. The DMF number is widely used in dental epidemiology.

DOMINANCE A concept from biological and urban ecology describing how one group or species has more influence or control than the others. In an urban community, dominance may be related to competition over land value, strategic geographical location, or a healthier environment.[31]

DOMINANT In genetics, alleles that fully manifest their phenotype when present in the heterozygous state. Contrast RECESSIVE.

DOSE The amount of a substance available for interaction with metabolic processes or biologically significant receptors after crossing the relevant boundary (epidermis, gut, respiratory tract). The absorbed dose is the amount crossing a specific absorption barrier.[5,12,14]

DOSE-RESPONSE RELATIONSHIP (Syn: dose-effect relationship) The relationship between a given dose or set of doses (i.e., amount, duration, concentration) of an agent or exposure and the magnitude of a graded effect in an individual (for whom repeated measurements are available) or a population. The relationship of observed responses or outcomes in a population to varying levels of a beneficial or harmful agent. Commonly displayed as a graph, sometimes as a HISTOGRAM. Important related aspects include: the rate of effects at zero dose or at low doses (baseline, or control); the existence of a truly unexposed subgroup, of a subgroup with truly low exposure, and the range of exposures; the presence or absence of a THRESHOLD DOSE; whether the relationship is MONOTONIC or NONMONOTONIC; and the form of the mathematical expression that better fits the relationship between the dose and the response (linear, logarithmic, etc.).[1,3,5-7,12-14,24,26,270,342] Monotonic relationships and TRENDS can be linear and nonlinear. Other relevant features include the time element (e.g., how soon after the dose is the response observed? is there a latent period?), and the range of individual variation (what proportion of those exposed experience no response, and a slight, moderate, or severe response?).

DOT CHART, DOT PLOT A display (plot) of the individual values of a set of numbers. The x axis represents categories of a noncontinuous variable, and the y axis represents the values displayed by the observations.[102-106] See also CHART.

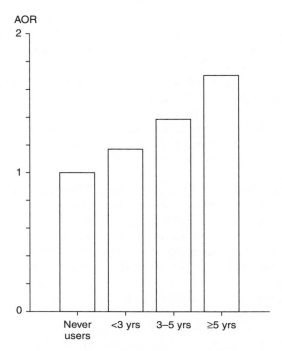

Dose-response relationship. The adjusted odds ratio (AOR) of invasive breast cancer among postmenopausal women using sequential estradiol-progestagen therapy by duration (Finland, 1995–2007). Source: Lyytinen HK et al.[343]

DOUBLE-BLIND TRIAL A procedure of blind assignment to study and control groups and blind assessment of outcome, designed to ensure that ASCERTAINMENT of outcome is not biased by knowledge of the group to which an individual was assigned. *Double* refers to both parties –the subjects in the study and control groups, and the observer(s) in contact

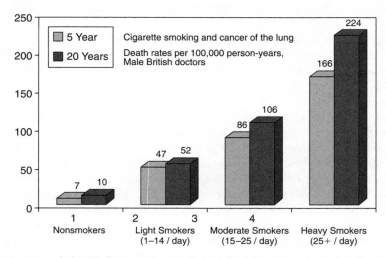

Dose-response relationship. Lung cancer and other causes of death in relation to smoking among male British doctors. Source: Doll and Peto.[344] With permission.

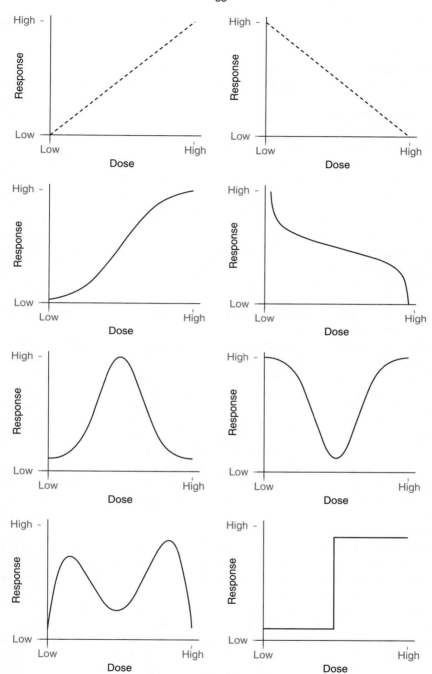

Dose-response curves in the health sciences. Source: Vandenberg LN et al.[342]

with the subjects; those describing a RANDOMIZED CONTROLLED TRIAL should provide a specific description of who among those involved in the trial were blinded.[1,6,58,73-77,270] See also BLINDED STUDY.

DOUBLING TIME The average time taken for a population to double in numbers.

DOUBLY ROBUST ESTIMATOR An estimator for an effect which, when two different statistical models are specified (e.g., one for the exposure and one for the outcome), is CONSISTENT for the effect of interest whenever at least one of the two statistical models is correctly specified.[1,101,345,346] See also MULTIPLY ROBUST ESTIMATOR.

DRIFT See GENETIC DRIFT; SOCIAL DRIFT.

DROPLET NUCLEI A type of particle implicated in the spread of airborne infection. Droplet nuclei are tiny particles (1–10 μm diameter) that represent the dried residue of droplets. They may be formed by (1) evaporation of droplets coughed or sneezed into the air or (2) aerosolization of infective materials. See also TRANSMISSION OF INFECTION.

DROPOUT A person enrolled in a study who becomes inaccessible or ineligible for follow-up for intentional reasons (e.g., because of unwillingness to undergo invasive diagnostic procedures).[6,26] The occurrence of dropouts can lead to severe BIAS. See also ATTRITION BIAS; CENSORING; LOST TO FOLLOW-UP; SELECTION BIAS.

DRUG RESISTANCE The ability of an organism to develop strains that are impervious to specific threats to their existence.[13,347]

DRUG RESISTANCE, MULTIPLE (MDR) Simultaneous resistances to several structurally and functionally distinct drugs.

DRUG-RESISTANT TUBERCULOSIS, MULTIPLE (MDR TUBERCULOSIS) A form of tuberculosis that is resistant to two or more of the primary drugs used for the treatment of tuberculosis (at least isoniazid and rifampin). It occurs when bacteria develop the ability to withstand antibiotic attack and relay that ability to newly produced BACTERIA. It can spread from one person to another. On an individual basis, improper use of the antituberculosis medications remains an important cause of drug-resistant tuberculosis. Treatment of MDR tuberculosis requires second-line drugs (SLDs) that are less effective, more toxic, and costlier than first-line isoniazid- and rifampin-based regimens.[56,69,188,217-219]

DRUG-RESISTANT TUBERCULOSIS, EXTENSIVELY (XDR) A form of tuberculosis caused by a strain of *Mycobacterium tuberculosis* resistant to isoniazid and rifampin, to any fluoroquinolone, and to at least one of the three following injectable drugs: capreomycin, kanamycin, and amikacin.[56,188,217-219,348]

DUMMY VARIABLE See INDICATOR VARIABLE.

DYNAMIC POPULATION A population that gains and loses members. All natural populations are dynamic—a fact recognized by the term *population dynamics,* which is used by demographers to denote changing composition.[1] See also OPEN POPULATION; POPULATION DYNAMICS; STABLE POPULATION; FIXED COHORT.

DYSREGULATION Relative or complete failure to regulate (check, control, enforce, adjust, lead) an organization, system, area, or process to preserve its nature, balance, aims, or functions (such as homeostasis, immunity, metabolism, health, validity, accountability, cohesion, freedom, equity, efficiency, wealth). Examples include many types of physiological, mental, emotional, economic, political, technological, and genetic dysregulation, leading to responses and effects that are poorly modulated, disruptive, costly, inefficient, unjust, corrupt, unsustainable, unhealthy, or pathological.[13,32,33,38,40,58,78,80,83,120,121,128,140,150,164,169,183-186,213,246,249,267,286,290,313-320,323,333,339,342,799] See also EPIGENETICS; EPIGENOME; GLOBALIZATION; MULTISTAGE MODELS.

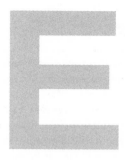

e Symbol for the base of natural or Napierian logarithms. It may be defined mathematically as the sum of the exponential series

$e^x = 1 + x + x^2/2! + x^3/3! + \ldots x^n/n!$ where $x = 1$ and n approaches infinity, i.e.,

$e = 1 + 1 + 1/2 + 1/6 + 1/24 + \ldots = 2.71828\ldots$

EARLY CLINICAL DETECTION Early detection of disease in a clinical setting among persons presenting to a clinician or using medical services (by contrast with early detection of disease through a population-based screening program). In principle the term includes both symptomatic and asymptomatic individuals, but in practice most individuals who undergo early clinical detection show signs and symptoms of the disease to be detected or have precursor lesions (i.e., alterations that have conclusively been demonstrated to increase risk of the target disease).[6,9,58] See also CASE FINDING.

EARLY DETECTION OF DISEASE Identification of a specific disease at an early stage in the NATURAL HISTORY OF THE DISEASE. Detection before the usual clinical diagnosis does not guarantee diagnosis at an early stage, nor does it assure a more effective treatment. Sometimes an ambiguous and misleading expression because of the term *detection*, because it may imply that the disease would otherwise be diagnosed "late," and because often no disease is diagnosed: only the possibility is raised—to be confirmed by proper diagnostic means—of a putatively precursor lesion (perhaps, naturally reversible), or of a genetic variant, or of a biochemical difference. Furthermore, the actual risk of disease conferred by the latter may not have been demonstrated by valid longitudinal studies.[5-9,58,203,349] Since detection is not a synonym of diagnosis, confirmation of the suspected diagnosis will require additional tests, properly diagnostic. By definition, early detection of disease does not prevent disease occurrence. It may do so only if early detection of a precursor lesion leads to complete and definitive removal of all such lesions; otherwise long-term medical surveillance of precursor lesions or other alterations (and, as usual, of overt disease) will be required, and no gain will exist over diagnosis of disease through customary clinical paths.

Early detection may be accomplished both by EARLY CLINICAL DETECTION and by population-based SCREENING programs. It includes both symptomatic and asymptomatic individuals. It may be a form of SECONDARY PREVENTION; in certain diseases it may contribute to TERTIARY PREVENTION. Early detection of disease will usually appear to improve survival, even when it is ineffective (e.g., because treatment is not administered earlier, treatment is not more effective when administered earlier, or no effective treatment is available). Early detection (of disease, of precursor lesions, of genetic factors putatively conferring disease susceptibility, and even of classic RISK FACTORS) is not an aim in itself: it is justified only if it improves outcomes meaningful to individuals or communities. See also CASE-FINDING; LEAD-TIME BIAS; SCREENING.

EARLY-WARNING SYSTEM In disease SURVEILLANCE, a specific procedure to detect as early as possible any departure from usual or normally observed frequency of phenomena. For example, the routine MONITORING of numbers of deaths from pneumonia and influenza in large American cities has been used as an early warning system for the identification of influenza epidemics. In developing countries, a change in children's average weights is an early warning signal of nutritional deficiency.[12,13,48,69,83,160,267] See also CASE REPORT.

EBM See EVIDENCE-BASED MEDICINE.

EBPH See EVIDENCE-BASED PUBLIC HEALTH.

ECLOSION Emergence of imago (adult) from pupal case, hatching of larva from egg; a term descriptive of life stages of insect vectors.

ECOEPIDEMIOLOGY A paradigm proposing that the appropriate epidemiological approach is to analyze determinants and outcomes at different levels of organization, emphasizing contextual analysis within and across levels.[350,351] In the early 1980s this term was applied to the study of ecological influences on human health, whether related to environmental pollutants or biological interactions as life cycles of parasites. Mervyn Susser (b. 1921) and Ezra Susser[350,351] used the term within a conceptual approach that unifies MOLECULAR, CLINICAL, and SOCIAL EPIDEMIOLOGY in a multilevel application of methods aimed at identifying causes, categorizing risks, and controlling public health problems.[31,33,279,308,350-352] See also GLOBAL HEALTH; MULTILEVEL ANALYSIS.

ECOLOGICAL CASE-REFERENT STUDY A type of study suitable for use in the evaluation of community-wide interventions and characterized by measurement of the exposure on a ecological scale and of the outcome on an individual scale.

ECOLOGICAL ANALYSIS Analysis based on aggregated or grouped data; errors in inference may result because associations may be artifactually created or masked by the aggregation process.[1,3,24,295] See also AGGREGATIVE FALLACY; ECOLOGICAL FALLACY.

ECOLOGICAL BIAS See AGGREGATIVE FALLACY; CROSS-LEVEL BIAS; ECOLOGICAL FALLACY.

ECOLOGICAL CORRELATION A correlation in which the units studied are populations or groups rather than individuals. Correlations found in this manner may not hold true for the individual members of the same populations. See also ECOLOGICAL FALLACY.

ECOLOGICAL DEPTH A criterion used for assessing the impact or penetration of an intervention into the local system; it includes the intervention scope (number of levels) and the duration of effect. An epidemiological program with high ecological depth yields an effect at multiple levels (individual, environmental) that endures over time.[31]

ECOLOGICAL FALLACY (Syn: aggregation bias, ecological bias)

1. An erroneous inference that may occur because an association observed between variables on an aggregate level does not necessarily represent or reflect the association that exists at an individual level; a causal relationship that exists on a group level or among groups may not exist among the group individuals.[1,3,5,6,24,26,31,38,295]

2. An error in inference due to failure to distinguish between different levels of organization. A correlation between variables based on group (ecological) characteristics is not necessarily reproduced between variables based on individual characteristics; an association at one level may disappear at another or even be

reversed. Example: At the ecological level, a correlation has been found in several studies between the quality of drinking water and mortality rates from heart disease; it would be an ecological fallacy to infer from this alone that exposure to water of a particular level of hardness necessarily influences the individual's chances of dying from heart disease. Policies, decisions, and actions at a given level (individual, municipal, regional, etc.) must be based on evidence—on causal relationships at that level. See also AGGREGATIVE FALLACY; ATOMISTIC FALLACY; CROSS-LEVEL BIAS; MODIFIABLE AREAL UNIT PROBLEM.

ECOLOGICAL FOOTPRINT The dimensions and composition of the ecosystem required to sustain the actions or goods of a population, such as a hospital, a factory, a holiday resort, an aircraft. An estimate of the impact of an individual, group, or organization on the environment based on consumption and pollution. The term is applied mainly to the required input of resources and output of waste products. Ecological footprint analysis compares human demand and consumption of natural resources with the system's ecological capacity to regenerate them.[13,33]

ECOLOGICAL STUDY In epidemiology, a study in which the units of analysis are populations or groups of people rather than individuals.[1,8] An example is the study of the relationship between the distribution of income and mortality rates in states or provinces. Conclusions of ecological studies may not apply to individuals; thus caution is needed to avoid the ECOLOGICAL FALLACY. Ecological studies can reach valid CAUSAL INFERENCES on causal relationships at the ecological (aggregate, group) level—i.e., on causal processes that occur at the group level or among groups.[295] Ecological studies have a role when implementing and evaluating policies that affect entire groups or regions. See also AGGREGATIVE FALLACY, ATOMISTIC FALLACY, CROSS-LEVEL BIAS.

ECOLOGICAL TRANSITION Within a framework of human development, ecological transitions are shifts in roles or settings that occur across the LIFE COURSE (e.g., arrival of a new sibling, entering school, finding a job, getting married, moving one's household, retiring). These transitions usually entail a change in a person's role or behavioral expectations.[31]

ECOLOGY The study of the relationships among living organisms and their environment. The comprehensive science of the relation of the organism to the environment. See also HUMAN ECOLOGY.

ECONOMIC APPRAISAL (Syn: economic evaluation) A general term for the economic evaluation of options. This can be done from a variety of perspectives.[38,92,285,353-356] See also ASYMMETRY OF INFORMATION; COST-BENEFIT ANALYSIS; COST-EFFECTIVENESS ANALYSIS; COST-UTILITY ANALYSIS.

ECOSOCIAL THEORY OF DISEASE DISTRIBUTION One of the multilevel epidemiological frameworks that seek to integrate social and biological reasoning and a historical and ecological perspective to gain new insights into determinants of population distributions of disease and social inequalities in health.[279,357,358] See also ECOEPIDEMIOLOGY.

ECOSYSTEM Plant and animal life systems considered in relation to the environmental factors and processes that influence them. The fundamental unit in ecology, comprising the living organisms and the nonliving elements that interact in a defined region. This region may be any size, from a drop of pond water to the entire biosphere. A comparatively stable and enduring arrangement of a population with mutual dependencies, including all living and nonliving (e.g., water, climate) elements within an area. The population operates collectively as a unit in ways that maintain a viable relationship with the environment. Edges of ecosystems are seldom clearly defined.[13,31,33,139,213,279,359,360]

EFFECT The result of a cause or of another intervening variable. See also CAUSALITY; EFFECT MEASURE.

EFFECTIVENESS The extent to which a specific intervention, procedure, regimen, or service, when deployed in the usual circumstances of living and practice, does what it is intended to do for a specified population.[6,9,17,26,58,67,110,231,232] A measure of the extent to which an intervention or policy fulfills its objectives in practice. Contrast with EFFICACY and EFFICIENCY. If possible, the determination of effectiveness should be based on pragmatic RANDOMIZED CONTROLLED TRIALS. See also INTENTION-TO-TREAT ANALYSIS; PRAGMATIC STUDY.

EFFECTIVE POPULATION SIZE The average number of individuals in a population that contribute genes to the next generation.

EFFECTIVE SAMPLE SIZE Sample size after dropouts, deaths, and other specified exclusions from an original sample.

EFFECT MEASURE A quantity that measures the effect of a factor on the frequency or risk of a health outcome or effect. Such measures include the ATTRIBUTABLE FRACTION, which measure the fraction of cases due to a factor; RISK DIFFERENCES and RATE DIFFERENCES, which measure the amount a factor adds to the RISK or RATE of a disease; and RISK RATIOS, ODDS RATIOS, and RATE RATIOS, which measure the amount by which a factor multiplies the risk, ODDS, or rate of disease. The identification of these quantities with effect measures presumes that there is no BIAS in the quantity.[1,3,270]

EFFECT MODIFICATION (Syn: effect-measure modification) Variation in the selected effect measure for the factor under study across levels of another factor.[1-3,7,8,66,270,798] See also HETEROGENEITY; INTERACTION.

EFFECT MODIFIER (Syn: modifying factor)
1. A pre-exposure factor across whose levels the value of the effect measure of interest varies.[1-3,270]
2. A factor that biologically, clinically, socially, or otherwise alters the effects of another factor under study. For example, age-related decline in liver function can lead to stronger effects of toxins in the elderly; immunization reduces or eliminates the adverse consequences of exposure to pathogenic organisms. See also CAUSALITY; CONFOUNDING; INTERACTION.

EFFICACY the extent to which a specific intervention, procedure, regimen, or service produces a beneficial result under ideal conditions; the benefit or UTILITY to the individual or the population of the service, treatment regimen, or intervention.[5-9,17,110] If possible, the determination of efficacy should be based on the results of RANDOMIZED CONTROLLED TRIALS. Contrast with EFFECTIVENESS and EFFICIENCY.

EFFICIENCY
1. The effects or end results achieved in relation to the effort expended in terms of money, resources, and time. The extent to which the resources used to provide a specific intervention, procedure, service, or policy of known efficacy or effectiveness are minimized. A measure of the economy (or cost in resources) with which a procedure of known EFFICACY and EFFECTIVENESS is carried out. The process of making the best use of scarce resources. If possible, the determination of efficiency should be based on the results of RANDOMIZED CONTROLLED TRIALS.[5,17,232]
2. In statistics, the relative PRECISION with which a particular study design or estimator will estimate a parameter of interest (i.e., relative to the maximum attainable precision); the extent to which a study design maximizes the precision of effect estimates obtained from a given number of subjects or a given amount of PERSON-TIME.[7]

3. In health economics[354] the main types of efficiency are:

TECHNICAL EFFICIENCY refers to the relationship between resources (capital and labor) and health outcomes.

PRODUCTIVE EFFICIENCY refers to maximizing health outcomes for a given cost or minimizing cost for a given outcome.

ALLOCATIVE EFFICIENCY is maximizing community health at given levels of technical and productive efficiency.

EGG COUNT See WORM COUNT.

ELASTICITY The measurement of how changing an economic variable affects others. The responsiveness of a dependent variable (output, demand) to changes in one of the variables influencing it (e.g., an input, price, or income). It may be positive or negative. Numerically it is given by

Elasticity = % change in dependent variable / % change in the determining variable

The most common elasticities are *income elasticity* (the responsiveness of consumption to changes in income) and *demand elasticity* or *own-price elasticity* (the responsiveness of the consumption of a good or service to a change in its price).[355] See also MORAL HAZARD.

ELIGIBILITY CRITERIA An explicit statement of the conditions under which persons are admitted to an epidemiological study, such as a case-control study or a randomized controlled trial.

ELIMINATION Reduction of case transmission to a predetermined very low level; e.g., elimination of tuberculosis as a public health problem was defined by the WHO (1991) as reduction of prevalence to a level below one case per million population. Compare ERADICATION (OF DISEASE).

EMBODIMENT

1. Processes through which extrinsic factors experienced at different life stages are inscribed into an individual's body functions or structures, and the result of such processes.[23] How humans biologically *incorporate* the world in which we live, including aspects of the societal and ecological CONTEXT. Corporal embedding of social factors. Recognizing that humans are simultaneously social beings and biological organisms, the concept aims to highlight that bodies tell stories (1) about the conditions of human existence; (2) which often match people's stated accounts; and (3) which people cannot or will not tell. A multilevel phenomenon integrating soma, psyche, and society in historical and ecological contexts; hence an antonym to disembodied genes, minds, and behaviors. Pathophysiological responses and clinical expressions of social inequalities result from and reflect how people literally embody and express their experiences of INEQUALITY.[19,43,158,248,279,333-336,357,361-365]

2. A tangible or visible form of an idea, quality, or feeling. The representation or expression of something in such a form.[234] The subjective experience of one's own body is different from the scientific picture of a body in physiological terms. The specific ways in which we experience ourselves as embodied are thus essential for analyses about knowledge and experience[235,335] See also DISEASE.

EMBRYO Biologically, in the human, the stage of the conceptus from uterine implantation (about 7 days after fertilization) to completion of organ development (about 54–60 days); conventionally, 8 weeks after conception, 10 weeks after the last menstrual period. The distinction between an embryo and a FETUS can be important in law and in perinatal epidemiology.

EMERGENCY

1. A state in which normal procedures are suspended and extra-ordinary measures are taken in order to avert a DISASTER.
2. In epidemiology, a situation that threatens personal and population health, habitat, safety, peace, or human rights, often associated with an environmental or political crisis. It is usually sudden in onset but may also develop gradually. Examples include floods, droughts, earthquakes, or armed conflicts.[13,69,116,366]

EMERGING INFECTIONS (Syn: emerging pathogens) Infectious diseases that have recently been identified and taxonomically classified. Many of them are capable of causing dangerous epidemics. They include human immunodeficiency virus (HIV) infection, Ebola virus disease, hantavirus pulmonary syndrome and other viral hemorrhagic fevers, *Campylobacter* infection, transmissible spongiform encephalopathies, Legionnaires' disease, and Lyme disease. Some appear to be new diseases of humans (e.g., HIV infection). Others, such as the viral hemorrhagic fevers, may have existed for many centuries and have been recognized only recently, because ecological or other environmental and demographic changes have increased the risk of human infection. *Reemerging infections* are certain "old" diseases, such as tuberculosis and syphilis, that have experienced a resurgence because of changed host-agent-environment conditions.[56,69,217-219,367,368]

EMPIRICAL Based directly on experience (e.g., observation or experiment) rather than on reasoning or theory alone.

EMPIRICAL-BAYES METHODS Statistical methods that have the mathematical form of BAYESIAN STATISTICS but that estimate the prior distributions from the data being analyzed instead of deriving them from external data or expert judgment.[1,7] Such methods are especially useful for addressing MULTIPLE COMPARISONS PROBLEMS, as they arise, for example, in genomewide "scans." See also SHRINKAGE ESTIMATION.

EMPLOYMENT CONDITION A situation or characteristic related to employment with an influence on well-being and health in the population, including unemployment, informal employment, precariousness, wages, or benefits (permits, vacations, pensions, workers' compensation schedules). These terms are linked to the concept of "fair employment," which complements the concept of "decent work" of the International Labour Organization.[13,267,358,369,370]

EMPORIATRICS The specialty of travel medicine.[371] From the Greek *emporion* (trade). See also TRAVEL MEDICINE.

ENABLING FACTORS See CAUSATION OF DISEASE, FACTORS IN.

ENCOUNTER A face-to-face transaction between a personal health worker and a patient or client. Not limited to health care settings.

ENDEMIC DISEASE The constant OCCURRENCE of a disease, disorder, or noxious INFECTIOUS AGENT in a geographic area or population group; it may also refer to the chronic high PREVALENCE of a disease in such area or group. See also HOLOENDEMIC DISEASE; HYPERENDEMIC DISEASE; HYPOENDEMIC DISEASE.

ENDOBIOTIC An endogenous substance that produces a toxic metabolite when it is metabolized. A substance or organism that grows within a living organism. Contrast XENOBIOTIC.

END RESULTS See OUTCOMES.

ENTOMOLOGICAL INOCULATION RATE (EIR) An indicator related to the number of infectious bites from a malaria mosquito an individual is exposed to in a given time period. It allows a direct estimation of transmission which is easy to understand and to compare, and is theoretically one of the best ways to define malaria endemicity.[56,372,373]

ENTROPY In thermodynamics, entropy is a measure of the disorder in a system. In statistics, entropy means the same; it is a measure of disorder, uncertainty, or chaos or, more loosely, randomness.[374]

ENVIRONMENT All that which is external to the individual human host. Physical, biological, social, cultural, and other dimensions of the environment commonly interact, and all can influence the health status of individuals and populations.[12,13,33,80,139,169,211,267,309,350,351,359,365,375] "The environment provides the food people eat, the water they drink, the air they breathe, the energy they command, the plagues and pests they combat and the mountains, seas, lakes, streams, plants and animals that they enjoy and depend upon."[376]

ENVIRONMENTAL EPIDEMIOLOGY A branch or subspecialty of EPIDEMIOLOGY that uses epidemiological principles, reasoning, and methods to study and control the health effects on populations of physical, chemical, and biological processes and agents external to the human body (e.g., climate change, air pollution, dietary pollutants, urbanization, energy production and combustion). Recognition of health hazards posed by large-scale environmental and ecological changes added extra dimensions to the field.[12,13,14,33,213,309,375,377]

ENVIRONMENTAL HEALTH CRITERIA DOCUMENT Official publication containing a review of existing knowledge about chemicals, radiation, etc., and their identifiable immediate and long-term effects on health. Environmental health criteria documents are produced by the WHO, the International Agency for Research on Cancer (IARC), and many national agencies, such as the National Institute for Occupational Safety and Health (NIOSH) in the United States.

ENVIRONMENTAL HEALTH IMPACT ASSESSMENT A statement of the beneficial or adverse health effects or risks due to an environmental exposure or likely to follow an environmental change. Such statements may contain or refer to results of epidemiological and/or toxicological studies of environmental health hazards.[13]

ENVIRONMENTAL HYPERSENSITIVITY An ill-defined concept that refers to a set of poorly understood conditions and syndromes that some authors deem potentially related to exposure to low concentrations of chemical, physical, or other environmental agents. Related conditions might include the sick building syndrome, the chronic fatigue syndrome, and multiple chemical sensitivity.

ENVIRONMENTAL TOBACCO SMOKE (ETS) A specific form of air pollution due to burning tobacco, especially SIDESTREAM SMOKE. ETS is carcinogenic to humans; e.g., it is classified in group 1 by the International Agency for Research on Cancer (IARC). Closely related terms are INVOLUNTARY SMOKING or *passive smoking* and *secondhand smoke*.[13,27,179]

EPIDEMIC [from the Greek *epi* (upon), *dēmos* (people)] The occurrence in a community or region of cases of an illness, specific health-related behavior, or other health-related events clearly in excess of normal expectancy. The community or region and the period in which the cases occur must be specified precisely. The number of cases indicating the presence of an epidemic varies according to the agent, size, and type of population exposed; previous experience or lack of exposure to the disease; and time and place of occurrence. Epidemicity is thus relative to usual frequency of the disease in the same area, among the specified population, at the same season of the year.

A single case of a COMMUNICABLE DISEASE long absent from a population or first invasion by a disease not previously recognized in that area requires immediate reporting and full field investigation; two cases of such a disease associated in time and place may be sufficient evidence to be considered an epidemic. Classic epidemics initially identified following the occurrence of small numbers of cases include the epidemic of vaginal cancer in daughters of women who took diethylstilbestrol during pregnancy,[378] and the PANDEMIC of AIDS, which was heralded by a report[379] of cases of *Pneumocystis carinii* pneumonia among gay men in Los Angeles in 1981.

The purpose of SURVEILLANCE systems is to identify epidemics as early as possible so that effective control measures can be put in place. This remains a most important task for epidemiology. The word may be used also to describe outbreaks of disease in animal or plant populations.[48] See also EPIZOOTIC; EPORNITHIC.

EPIDEMIC, COMMON SOURCE (Syn: common vehicle epidemic, holomiantic disease) Outbreak due to exposure of a group of persons to a noxious influence that is common to the individuals in the group. When the exposure is brief and essentially simultaneous, the resultant cases all develop within one incubation period of the disease (a "point" or "point source" epidemic).[56,160] The term *holomiantic disease* was used to describe outbreaks of this type, but as with several other terms created from Greek or Latin roots, transmission to epidemiologists who lacked a classical education did not take place.

EPIDEMIC, MATHEMATICAL MODEL OF See MATHEMATICAL MODEL.

EPIDEMIC, POINT SOURCE See EPIDEMIC, COMMON SOURCE.

EPIDEMIC CURVE A graphic plotting of the distribution of cases by time of onset.[8]

EPIDEMIOLOGICAL INTELLIGENCE (Syn: epidemic intelligence) The process of detecting, verifying, analyzing, assessing, and investigating signals that may represent a threat to public health.[160,366,380] Activities aimed at managing epidemiological crises, biochemical threats, radiological risks, natural disasters, or the public health impact of terrorist attacks and wars. A government body engaged in collecting secret or sensitive information related to epidemic outbreaks. The Global Public Health Intelligence Network (GPHIN) of the World Health Organization is an Internet-based multilingual early-warning tool that continuously searches news wires and websites to identify information about disease outbreaks and other events of potential international public health concern. To ensure a comprehensive picture of the epidemic threat to global health security, WHO also gathers epidemic intelligence from informal sources. With the advent of modern communication technologies, many initial outbreak reports now originate in the electronic media and electronic discussion groups.[381] See also DIGITAL EPIDEMIOLOGY.

EPIDEMICS, HISTORY OF A domain of history that deals with the effects of diseases on the course of history.[39-42,69,324,382-386] A rather comprehensive monograph is Thomas McKeown's *The Origins of Human Disease*.[387] Partial accounts include histories of the impact on societies of syphilis,[388] tuberculosis,[389] smallpox,[390] typhus,[391] AIDS,[392] diseases in ancient Greece,[393,394] and many other conditions.[395]

EPIDEMIC THRESHOLD The number or density of susceptibles required for an epidemic to occur. According to the MASS ACTION PRINCIPLE, the epidemic threshold is the reciprocal of the INFECTION TRANSMISSION PARAMETER.

EPIDEMIOLOGICAL COHERENCE See COHERENCE, EPIDEMIOLOGICAL.

EPIDEMIOLOGICAL RESEARCH Scientific research among human populations and defined groups of individuals into the frequency of occurrence, distribution and causes of phenomena of public health, clinical, social, or biological RELEVANCE, with valid selection of subjects and measurements, and formal CAUSAL INFERENCES on the DETERMINANTS of such phenomena.[1-3,5-9,24-26,39-42,58,85,128,202,270,279] See also CREATIVITY; INTEGRATIVE RESEARCH.

EPIDEMIOLOGICAL TRANSITION THEORY Traditionally,[396] the mortality component of the DEMOGRAPHIC TRANSITION was considered to have three phases: (1) The "age of pestilence and famine"; (2) the "age of receding pandemics"; (3) the "age of degenerative and man-made diseases." [396] It was previously thought that as countries develop NON-COMMUNICABLE DISEASES replaced COMMUNICABLE DISEASES as the main causes of the BURDEN OF DISEASE. It is now evident that the poorest countries face a multiple burden of communicable disease and non-communicable diseases, including their related social and individual DETERMINANTS.[397]

EPIDEMIOLOGIST A professional who to different degrees strives to study and control factors that influence the occurrence and distribution of disease and other health-related conditions and processes in defined groups, populations, and societies, has an expertise in POPULATION THINKING and epidemiological methods, and is knowledgeable about public health, CAUSAL INFERENCE in health, and the substantive matter relevant to the specific job. The control of disease and related RISK FACTORS in populations is often considered to be a core task for the epidemiologist involved in the provision of public health services. The *diversity* of training, skills, tasks, interests, contexts, and professional and ideological profiles is similar to many other professions: we thus find slightly more or less emphasis in practice or theory; on service, planning, policy, advocacy, research, teaching; on individual and collective exposures and other causes, or on outcomes and other effects; methods, environment, social factors, biology, clinical medicine; specialty or transdisciplinarity. Epidemiologists show a rich plurality of scientific cultures and practices.

EPIDEMIOLOGY The study of the occurrence and distribution of health-related events, states, and processes in specified populations, including the study of the DETERMINANTS influencing such processes, and the application of this knowledge to control relevant health problems.

Study includes surveillance, observation, screening, hypothesis testing, analytic research, experiments, and prediction. *Distribution* refers to analysis by time, place (or space), and population (i.e., classes or subgroups of persons affected in an organization, population, or society, or at regional and global scales). *Determinants* are the geophysical, biological, behavioral, social, cultural, economic, and political factors that influence health. *Health-related events, states, and processes* include outbreaks, diseases, disorders, causes of death, behaviors, environmental and socioeconomic processes, effects of preventive programs, and use of health and social services. *Specified populations* are those with common contexts and identifiable characteristics. *Application to control…* makes explicit the aim of epidemiology—to promote, protect, and restore health, and to advance scientific knowledge.

The primary "knowledge object" of epidemiology as a scientific discipline are causes of health-related events, states, and processes in groups and populations. In the past 90 years, the definition has broadened from concern with communicable disease epidemics to include all phenomena related to health in populations.[1-3,5,24,25,28,39-42,85,128,211, 214,270,279,398-408] Therefore, epidemiology is much more than a branch of medicine treating of epidemics. Epidemiology may also study disease in populations of animals and plants. See also CAUSALITY; GROUP COMPARISON; POPULATION THINKING STRATEGY.

EPIDEMIOLOGY, DEMARCATION OF Marking or fixing the boundaries or limits—and networks— of epidemiology as a scientific discipline and profession; assessing epidemiology's aims, roles, methodologies, objects of research, legitimate uses and applications (e.g., in public health policy and services, clinical practice, basic research, social media, regulation, environmental and social policies), achievements and failures; examining its distinctiveness, similarities, and relationships with other scientific disciplines and professions. Defense of scientific identity and solidarity, disciplinary autonomy, and EPISTEMIC authority of epidemiology are also important elements of boundary work.[398] These forms of scientific and social discourse are important components of the process by which various sciences establish their scientific and intellectual nature, moral order, social status, and mission. Epidemiology benefits from a rich plurality of scientific cultures and practices; it thus naturally enjoys diverse demarcation discourses.[1-3,5,24,25,28,39-42,83,85,128,171,211,215,268-270,279,306,310,352,398-408]

EPIDEMIOLOGY, ANALYTIC See ANALYTIC STUDY.

EPIDEMIOLOGY, APPLIED See APPLIED EPIDEMIOLOGY.

EPIDEMIOLOGY, BLACK-BOX See "BLACK-BOX EPIDEMIOLOGY."

EPIDEMIOLOGY, CANCER See CANCER EPIDEMIOLOGY.

EPIDEMIOLOGY, CARDIOVASCULAR See CARDIOVASCULAR EPIDEMIOLOGY.

EPIDEMIOLOGY, DESCRIPTIVE See DESCRIPTIVE EPIDEMIOLOGY.

EPIDEMIOLOGY, DEVELOPMENTAL See DEVELOPMENTAL AND LIFE COURSE EPIDEMIOLOGY.

EPIDEMIOLOGY, DIGITAL See DIGITAL EPIDEMIOLOGY.

EPIDEMIOLOGY, DISASTER See DISASTER EPIDEMIOLOGY.

EPIDEMIOLOGY, ENVIRONMENTAL See ENVIRONMENTAL EPIDEMIOLOGY.

EPIDEMIOLOGY, EXPERIMENTAL See EXPERIMENTAL EPIDEMIOLOGY.

EPIDEMIOLOGY, FIELD See FIELD EPIDEMIOLOGY.

EPIDEMIOLOGY, FORENSIC See FORENSIC EPIDEMIOLOGY.

EPIDEMIOLOGY, HEALTH CARE See HOSPITAL EPIDEMIOLOGY.

EPIDEMIOLOGY, HOSPITAL See HOSPITAL EPIDEMIOLOGY.

EPIDEMIOLOGY, LANDSCAPE See LANDSCAPE EPIDEMIOLOGY.

EPIDEMIOLOGY, LIFE COURSE See DEVELOPMENTAL AND LIFE COURSE EPIDEMIOLOGY.

EPIDEMIOLOGY, MECHANISTIC See MECHANISTIC EPIDEMIOLOGY.

EPIDEMIOLOGY, OBSERVATIONAL See OBSERVATIONAL EPIDEMIOLOGY.

EPIDEMIOLOGY, OCCUPATIONAL See OCCUPATIONAL EPIDEMIOLOGY.

EPIDEMIOLOGY, PRIMARY CARE See PRIMARY CARE EPIDEMIOLOGY.

EPIDEMIOLOGY, PSYCHOSOCIAL See SOCIAL EPIDEMIOLOGY.

EPIDEMIOLOGY, SATELLITE See SATELLITE EPIDEMIOLOGY.

EPIDEMIOLOGY, SOCIAL See SOCIAL EPIDEMIOLOGY.

EPIDEMIOLOGY, SOCIOLOGY OF See SOCIOLOGY OF EPIDEMIOLOGY.

EPIDEMIOLOGY, SPATIAL See SPATIAL EPIDEMIOLOGY

EPIDEMIOLOGY, THEORETICAL See THEORETICAL EPIDEMIOLOGY.

EPIGENETIC INHERITANCE A set of reversible heritable changes in gene function or other cell phenotypes that occur without a change in the genotype. Such changes may be spontaneous, in response to environmental factors, or in response to other genetic events.[78,80,86,316-321,409] Epigenetic processes include PARAMUTATION, GENE SILENCING, IMPRINTING, REPROGRAMMING, bookmarking, X chromosome inactivation, position effect, or transvection.

EPIGENETICS The study of heritable changes that are not the result of changes in the DNA sequence. Information heritable during cell division other than the DNA sequence itself. Changes in GENE EXPRESSION that are not regulated by the DNA nucleotide sequence (e.g., GENE SILENCING by promoter HYPERMETHYLATION or HISTONE MODIFICATION). In spite of not being coded in the DNA, some epigenetic changes are heritable across generations. Such changes have been observed in biological systems exposed to nickel, cadmium, or arsenic. DISEASES OF COMPLEX ETIOLOGY arise from environmentally induced genetic dysregulation and the accumulation of genetic and epigenetic alterations that confer upon an incipient neoplastic cell (a "clone") the properties of unlimited, self-sufficient growth and resistance to normal homeostatic regulatory mechanisms.[32,78,80,183-185,245,316-321,409-416,799]

EPIGENOME The overall epigenetic state of a cell. At the intersection between environment and genetic variation, the epigenome is an important target of environmental factors. According to the COMMON DISEASE GENETIC AND EPIGENETIC (CDGE) HYPOTHESIS, the epigenome may modulate the effect of genetic variation either by affecting the gene's expression through the action of chromatin proteins or DNA methylation or by modulating protein folding of the gene product. The epigenome may, in turn, be affected by sequence variation in the genes encoding chromatin or chaperone proteins. Environmental factors (e.g., toxins, growth factors, dietary methyl donors, and hormones) can affect the GENOME and the epigenome. Although the epigenome is particularly susceptible to dysregulation during gestation, neonatal development, puberty, and old age, it is most vulnerable to environmental exposures during embryogenesis. Many XENOBIOTICS may modify the epigenome.[321,417] See also DEVELOPMENTAL ORIGINS OF HEALTH AND DISEASE; METAGENOME.

EPI INFO Free software developed by the CDC for epidemiologists and other health professionals. Supports development of a questionnaire or form, the data entry process, and data analysis, including epidemiological measures, tables, graphs, and maps.[418]

EPISODE Period in which a health problem or illness exists, from its onset to its resolution. See also ENCOUNTER.

EPISTASIS Gene interaction; particularly, interaction between different alleles at different genes (e.g., the suppression by a gene of the effect of another gene). It can occur at the same step or at different stages of the same biochemical pathway.[57]

EPISTEMIC Relating to knowledge or to the degree of its validation.

EPISTEMIC COMMUNITIES

1. Transnational networks of scientists and of other knowledge-based professionals. Scientific associations have features of epistemic communities; subgroups within them may act as epistemic communities.[40]

2. NETWORKS of experts who define for policy makers what the problems they face are and what they should do about them.

3. A group of people who do not have any specific history together but share ideas and customs. Those who accept one version of a story that is particularly meaningful for their communities.

EPISTEMIC CULTURES Sets of practices, arrangements, and mechanisms bound together by necessity, affinity, interest, and historical coincidence that, in a given scientific field or area of professional expertise, make up how we know what we know.[419] Cultures of pursuing and warranting knowledge; they are pursued by specialists separated off from other specialists by long training periods, stringent division of labor, distinctive technological tools and methodologies, financing sources, scientific associations, journals,... and dictionaries. Interiorized processes of knowledge creation. They build the epistemic subject and referents, the meaning of empirical, methods of consensus formation, or forms of engagement with the social world.[135,398] They draw on different background knowledges, which become merged in knowledge work. They are forms of life and agree on acceptable forms of life (e.g., what it is to be a "postdoc" in epidemiology). See also KNOWLEDGE CONSTRUCTION; SOCIOLOGY OF SCIENTIFIC KNOWLEDGE.

EPISTEMOLOGY
1. The theory of knowledge. Epistemological questions include the origin of knowledge, the place of experience and reason in generating knowledge, the relationship between knowledge and certainty and between knowledge and the impossibility of error, and the changing forms of knowledge as societies change. These issues are linked with others, such as the nature of truth and the nature of experience and meaning.[235]
2. The study of the relation between the knower (or would-be knower) and what can be known. Answers to these questions are constrained by answers to ontological questions.[420]

In epidemiology and other sciences, debates have benefited from clarifying the methodological, epistemological, and ontological nature of the issues under analysis.[25,39-42,270,398,421,422] For instance, the proposition that methods used in an epidemiological study must be coherent with the "knowledge object"[421] of the study does not primarily address a methodological issue but an epistemological one; also of an essentially epistemological nature are criticisms of studies that suffer from a hypertrophy or a dissonance of the methodological apparatus vs. the study hypotheses, of studies based on a poor conception of the hypotheses, or of statistical analyses unguided by knowledge available on the study subject.[1,2,26,53,100,268,270] See also ONTOLOGY.

EPIZOOLOGY See VETERINARY EPIDEMIOLOGY.

EPIZOOTIC An outbreak (epidemic) of disease in an animal population; often with the implication that it may also affect human populations.[20-22,188]

EPIZOOTIOLOGY See VETERINARY EPIDEMIOLOGY.

EPORNITHIC An outbreak (epidemic) of disease in a bird population.

EQUATOR A network that aims to help improve the reliability and value of medical research literature by promoting transparent and accurate reporting of research studies. Its library contains a searchable database of reporting guidelines and links to other resources relevant to research reporting. Guidelines include CONSORT, STROBE, PRISMA, STARD, COREQ, ENTREQ, SQUIRE, CHEERS, CARE, or SAMPL.[266,423]

EQUIPOISE A state of genuine uncertainty about the benefits or harms that may result from different exposures or interventions. A state of equipoise is an indication for a RANDOMIZED CONTROLLED TRIAL, because there are no ethical concerns about one regimen being better for a particular patient.[6,26]

EQUITY Fairness, impartiality. An important concept in epidemiology, public health, and bioethics, especially in relation to human rights and HEALTH DETERMINANTS.[17,19,28,117,118,248,249,260,263,279,302,304,424-427] See also HEALTH EQUITY.

EQUIVALENCE TESTS Significance tests in which the TEST HYPOTHESIS is that sampled populations or outcomes under different treatments differ to a prescribed degree. A significant result of an equivalence test comparing the effects of two treatments would support the alternative to the test hypothesis, i.e., that the effects are equivalent. The size of the differences tested is generally the upper limit of dissimilarity that is considered trivial or not clinically significant.[6,26]

EQUIVALENCE TRIAL A trial designed to test that two or more treatments are "equivalent" to each other; e.g., when a new therapy is expected to bring certain advantages over the current standard (less side effects, easier administration, lower cost), but not anticipated to be more effective on the most relevant or primary outcomes.[73,76,77,428]

ERADICATION (OF DISEASE) Termination of all TRANSMISSION OF INFECTION by extermination of the INFECTIOUS AGENT through surveillance and containment. Eradication, as in the instance of smallpox, is based on the joint activities of control and surveillance. Regional eradication has been successful with poliomyelitis and in some countries appears close to succeeding for measles. The term ELIMINATION is sometimes used to describe eradication of diseases such as measles from a large geographic region or political jurisdiction. In 1992, the WHO put it this way: "Eradication is defined as achievement of a status whereby no further cases of a disease occur anywhere, and continued control measures are unnecessary." Smallpox was eradicated in 1977, based on joint control and SURVEILLANCE activities.[56,69,160,188,196,217-219]

ERROR A false or mistaken result of a measurement. Any other false or mistaken result obtained in a study or experiment.[1-3,7,25,270] Two broad kinds of error can occur in studies in the health, life, and social sciences:

1. Random error: the portion of variation in a measurement that has no apparent connection to any other measurement or variable, generally regarded as due to CHANCE.
2. Systematic error: error that is consistently wrong in a particular direction; it often has a recognizable source (e.g., a faulty measuring instrument). See BIAS.

ERROR, TYPE I (Syn: alpha error) The error of wrongly rejecting a test hypothesis; e.g., in null testing, declaring that a difference exists when it does not.[1,7,37] See also MULTIPLE COMPARISON PROBLEM; p VALUE; SIGNIFICANCE, STATISTICAL; STATISTICAL TEST.

ERROR, TYPE II (Syn: beta error) The error of failing to reject a false TEST HYPOTHESIS; e.g., in null testing, declaring that a difference does not exist when in fact it does.[1,7,37] See also POWER; STATISTICAL TEST.

ERROR, TYPE III Wrongly assessing the causes of interindividual variation within a population when the research question requires an analysis of causes of differences between populations or time periods. When the objects of the study are risk differences between groups or periods, the study must examine multiple groups or periods; otherwise a type III error can result. Risk differences between individuals within a particular population may not have the same causes as differences in the average risk between two different populations.[429] See also ATOMISTIC FALLACY; EPISTEMOLOGY; ONTOLOGY; STRATEGY, "POPULATION."

ERROR BAR A graphical display of the statistical uncertainty of an estimate, displayed as lines having the length of one or more standard deviations, standard errors, or confidence intervals for the estimate that extend out from the plotted estimated value.

ESTIMABILITY See IDENTIFIABLITY.

ESTIMATE A measurement or a statement about the value of some quantity is said to be an estimate if it is known, believed, or suspected to incorporate some degree of error.

ESTIMATOR In statistics, a function (formula) for computing estimates of a parameter from observed data (e.g., the MANTEL-HAENSZEL ODDS RATIO).

ETHICS The branch of philosophy that deals with distinctions between right and wrong—with the moral consequences of human actions. Ethical principles govern the conduct of epidemiology, as they do all human activities.[5,6,26,117,118,248-250,427] The ethical issues that arise in epidemiological practice and research include informed consent, confidentiality, respect for human rights, and scientific integrity. Epidemiologists and others have developed guidelines for the ethical conduct of epidemiological studies.[259-265] See also INFORMED CONSENT.

ETHICS (ETHICAL) REVIEW COMMITTEE See INSTITUTIONAL REVIEW BOARD.

ETHNIC GROUP, ETHNICITY

1. A social group characterized by a distinctive social and cultural tradition maintained within the group from generation to generation, a common history and origin, and a sense of identification with the group. Members have distinctive features in their way of life, shared experiences, and often some common genetic heritage. These features may be reflected in their health and disease experience.

2. The social group a person belongs to and either identifies with or is identified with by others as a result of a mix of cultural and other factors, including language, religion, ancestry, diet, and physical features traditionally associated with RACE. Sometimes the concept is used synonymously with race, but such custom is more pragmatic than scientific.[5,292,365,430]

ETHNOEPIDEMIOLOGY Epidemiological study of causal factors for health and disease among different ethnic groups, with development of intervention strategies that take culture into account.[431]

ETIOLOGICAL FRACTION AMONG THE EXPOSED The fraction of exposed cases for which exposure played a role in the development of their disease. It should not be confused with the ATTRIBUTABLE FRACTION AMONG THE EXPOSED.[1] See PROBABILITY OF CAUSATION.

ETIOLOGICAL FRACTION FOR THE POPULATION The fraction of all cases for which exposure played a role in the development of their disease. It should not be confused with the ATTRIBUTABLE FRACTION FOR THE POPULATION.[1] See PROBABILITY OF CAUSATION.

ETIOLOGICAL STUDY A study that aims to unveil, quantitatively analyze, and scientifically interpret causal relationships. Although most ANALYTICAL STUDIES may have such an aim, the term may be useful to emphasize that the purpose is not just to analyze relationships but to interpret relationships in causal terms. An intervention study is an example.[1-3,25,39-42,270] See also CAUSAL INFERENCE.

ETIOLOGY Literally, the science of causes; CAUSALITY. In common usage, cause, the causal process. See also PATHOGENESIS.

EVALUATION A process that attempts to determine as systematically and objectively as possible the relevance, effectiveness, and impact of activities in the light of their objectives. Several varieties of evaluation can be distinguished (e.g., evaluation of structure, process, and outcome).[12,17,28,165,202,232,285,329,353,432] See also CLINICAL TRIAL; EFFECTIVENESS; EFFICACY; EFFICIENCY; HEALTH SERVICES RESEARCH; PROGRAM EVALUATION AND REVIEW TECHNIQUES; QUALITY OF CARE.

EVANS'S POSTULATES Expanding biomedical knowledge led to revision of the HENLE-KOCH POSTULATES.[42] Alfred Evans (1917-1996)[433] developed those that follow:

1. Prevalence of the disease should be significantly higher in those exposed to the hypothesized cause than in controls not so exposed.

2. Exposure to the hypothesized cause should be more frequent among those with the disease than in controls without the disease—when all other RISK FACTORS are held constant.

3. Incidence of the disease should be significantly higher in those exposed to the hypothesized cause than in those not so exposed, as shown by prospective studies.

4. The disease should follow exposure to the hypothesized causative agent with a normal or log-normal DISTRIBUTION of incubation periods.

5. A spectrum of host responses should follow exposure to the hypothesized agent along a logical biological gradient from mild to severe.

6. A measurable host response following exposure to the hypothesized cause should have a high probability of appearing in those lacking this before exposure (e.g., antibody, cancer cells) or should increase in magnitude if present before exposure. This response pattern should occur infrequently in persons not so exposed.

7. Experimental reproduction of the disease should occur more frequently in animals or humans appropriately exposed to the hypothesized cause than in those not so exposed; this exposure may be deliberate in volunteers, experimentally induced in the laboratory, or may represent a regulation of natural exposure.

8. Elimination or modification of the hypothesized cause should decrease the incidence of the disease (e.g., attenuation of a virus, removal of tar from cigarettes).

9. Prevention or modification of the host's response on exposure to the hypothesized cause should decrease or eliminate the disease (e.g., immunization, drugs to lower cholesterol, specific lymphocyte transfer factor in cancer).

10. All of the relationships and findings should make biological and epidemiological sense.

See also CAUSALITY; HILL'S CONSIDERATIONS FOR CAUSATION; MILL'S CANONS.

EVIDENCE

1. Scientific knowledge. Results of research used to support decision-making.

2. Any form of knowledge—including but not confined to research—of sufficient quality to inform decisions.[17]

EVIDENCE-BASED MEDICINE (EBM) The consistent use of knowledge derived from biological, clinical, and EPIDEMIOLOGICAL RESEARCH in the management of patients, with particular attention to the balance of benefits, risks, and costs of diagnostic tests, screening programs, and treatment regimens, taking account of each patient's circumstances, including baseline risk, comorbid conditions, culture, and personal preferences.[6,9,58,202,203,302] There are no major intellectual reasons either against Evidence-Based (EB) nursing, EB health care planning,[58] EB proteomics,[91,434,435] or, for that matter, EB justice and EB economics.

EVIDENCE-BASED PUBLIC HEALTH (EBPH)

1. Application of the most valid, precise, and relevant scientific knowledge in setting PUBLIC HEALTH policies and practices. The evidence may be derived from epidemiological, statistical, medical, economic, demographic, sociological, and several other scientific disciplines. Sources of evidence should preferably be published, peer-reviewed, and critically appraised articles and reports. Implementation of public health policies, programs, and interventions requires good evidence on FEASIBILITY, EFFICACY, EFFECTIVENESS, EFFICIENCY, COST, COSTS OF INACTION, acceptability to the target population, and careful analysis of ethical, cultural, and political implications.[117,118,248-250,259-265,436-439] Some of such evidence may also be obtained from FOCUS GROUPS.

2. The development, implementation, and evaluation of effective programs and policies in public health through application of the principles of scientific reasoning, including systematic uses of data and information systems and appropriate use of behavioral and social science theory and program planning models. In EBPH, public health activities are explicitly linked with the underlying scientific evidence that suggests relevance and purpose and which demonstrates effectiveness.[12,13,17,28,83,210,214,290,302,436,440]

EVIDENCE-INFORMED HEALTH POLICYMAKING An approach to policy decisions that aims to ensure that decision-making is well informed by scientific evidence. It is characterized by the systematic and transparent access to, and appraisal of, evidence as an input into the policymaking process.[14,17,24,38,83,267,302,366,426,441] See also POLICY BRIEF.

EXACT METHOD A statistical method based on the actual (i.e., "exact") probability distribution of the study data rather than on an approximation, such as a normal or a CHI-SQUARE DISTRIBUTION (e.g., FISHER'S EXACT TEST).[1,7]

EXACT TEST A statistical test based on the actual null probability DISTRIBUTION of the study data (rather than, say, a normal approximation). Examples include the Fisher-Irwin test for fourfold tables (or FISHER'S EXACT TEST) and Student's *t*-test for normal distributions with unknown variances.

EXCEPTION FLAGGING (REPORTING) SYSTEM An automated system of data analysis that calculates thresholds for unusual events. Used in SURVEILLANCE.

EXCESS RATE (EXPOSED) See RATE DIFFERENCE.

EXCESS RATE (POPULATION) A measure of the number of disease cases associated with exposure to a putative cause of the disease in the population. It is the difference between the rates of disease in the entire population and among the unexposed. See also ATTRIBUTABLE FRACTION.

EXCESS RISK A term sometimes used to refer to the population excess rate and sometimes to the RISK DIFFERENCE or ABSOLUTE RISK REDUCTION.[1]

EXCHANGEABILITY, EXCHANGEABLE (Syn: permutable, symmetric) Two groups are exchangeable with respect to certain variables if group membership labels can be interchanged (exchanged) without altering any probability statement involving the variables. For example, suppose two groups A and B are exchangeable with respect to their POTENTIAL OUTCOMES (outcomes under alternative exposures). Then the probability that group A has a better outcome than group B when A is exposed and B is not is equal to the probability that group B has a better outcome than group A when B is exposed and A is not. Here, exchanging A and B does not change the probability of the statement, or the probability of any other statement involving A, B, their exposures, and their outcomes. Exchangeability implies that no CONFOUNDING is present. Groups can also be conditionally exchangeable if there is no RESIDUAL CONFOUNDING; in this case, their exchangeability is conditional on adjusting for the set of measured confounders.[2,7,101]

EXPANDED PROGRAMME ON IMMUNIZATION (EPI) A program of immunizing against diphtheria, tetanus, measles, pertussis, poliomyelitis, and tuberculosis conducted especially in developing countries.[56,188,240]

EXPANSION OF MORBIDITY As life expectancy increases, the prevalence of long-term disease, especially among older persons, increases. Mental disorders such as dementia may be an example.[442] Thus this is the opposite of COMPRESSION OF MORBIDITY. Both phenomena may coexist in the same population, some disorders becoming less prevalent, others more so.

EXPECTATION OF LIFE (Syn: life expectancy or expectation) The average number of years an individual of a given age is expected to live if current mortality rates continue to apply. A statistical abstraction based on existing age-specific death rates.

Life expectancy at birth ($\overset{o}{e}_{0}$): Average number of years a newborn baby can be expected to live if current mortality TRENDS continue. Corresponds to the total number of years a given BIRTH COHORT can be expected to live divided by the number of children in the cohort. Life expectancy at birth is partly dependent on mortality in the first year of life; therefore it is lower in poor than in rich countries because of the higher infant and child mortality rates in the former.

Life expectancy at a given age, age x ($\overset{o}{e}_{x}$): The average number of additional years a person of age *x* will live, based on the age-specific death rates for a given year, if current mortality trends continue to apply.

Life expectancy is a hypothetical measure and indicator of current health and mortality conditions. It is not a rate.

EXPECTED YEARS OF LIFE LOST

1. The expected years of life lost (EYLL) from a harmful exposure or treatment is the difference between the life expectancy of persons subjected to the exposure or treatment and the life expectancy they would have had if they had not experienced that exposure or treatment.

2. A measure of the impact of a disease on society as a result of early death. The expected years of life lost due to a particular cause is the sum, over all persons dying from that cause, of the additional years these persons would have lived had they experienced normal life expectancy. Life expectancies are usually taken from the population concerned, but another population can be used (e.g., the one with the highest life expectancy), which yields the *standard expected years of life lost*. See also BURDEN OF DISEASE; POTENTIAL YEARS OF LIFE LOST.

EXPERIMENT The core of an experimental study. Manipulation of one or more exposure variables (e.g., treatments, health promotion programs, public health policies) and control of potential confounders by the investigator in order to estimate an effect size or test a specific hypothesis involving the causal effect of the exposure variables on prespecified outcomes.

EXPERIMENT, NATURAL See NATURAL EXPERIMENT.

EXPERIMENTAL STUDY A study in which the investigator intentionally alters one or more factors and controls the other study conditions in order to analyze the effects of so doing. A study in which conditions are under the direct control of the investigator.[7,101]

EXPERIMENTAL EPIDEMIOLOGICAL STUDY An epidemiological study with a clear experimental component; usually, a large phase III or a phase IV RANDOMIZED CONTROLLED TRIAL or a COMMUNITY TRIAL.[795] See also CLINICAL TRIAL (phase IV); OBSERVATIONAL STUDY; RANDOM ALLOCATION.

EXPERIMENTAL EPIDEMIOLOGY The application of epidemiological reasoning, knowledge, and methods to experiments, particularly to large phase III and phase IV RANDOMIZED CONTROLLED TRIALS, and to COMMUNITY TRIALS. Clinical or community-based studies merit the term *experiment* or *quasi-experiment* only if it is possible to modify conditions (e.g., exposures) during the study.[1-3,795] See also NATURAL EXPERIMENT.

EXPERIMENTAL TREATMENT ASSIGNMENT ASSUMPTION See POSITIVITY.

EXPLANATORY STUDY, EXPLANATORY TRIAL A study (including observational studies and randomized clinical trials) whose main objective is to explain—rather than essentially describe—a process or mechanism by isolating the effects of specific variables, pathways and mechanisms of action.[6,9,24,272,443-445,641,800] Contrast with the decision-oriented PRAGMATIC STUDY.

EXPLANATORY VARIABLE

1. A variable that causally explains the association or outcome under study.
2. In statistics, a synonym for INDEPENDENT VARIABLE.[7]

EXPLORATORY STUDY A study whose main objective is to examine or ascertain some preliminary facts or to familiarize researchers with a problem or technology, often without clear or precise hypotheses; or, sometimes, to screen several hypotheses at once in a preliminary fashion.[1] It may be even more preliminary than a PILOT INVESTIGATION. See also AGNOSTIC ANALYSIS; DATA DREDGING; DATA MINING; FISHING EXPEDITION; SERENDIPITY.

EXPOSED In epidemiology, the exposed group (or simply, *the exposed*) is often used to connote a group whose members have been exposed to a supposed cause of a disease or health state of interest or possess a characteristic that is a determinant of the health outcome of interest.

EXPOSED CASES IMPACT NUMBER See IMPACT NUMBERS.

EXPOSOME A potential measure of the effects of life course exposures on health. It comprises the totality of exposures to which an individual is subjected from conception to death, including those resulting from environmental agents, socioeconomic conditions, lifestyle, diet, and endogenous processes. Characterization of the exposome could permit addressing possible associations with health outcomes and their SIGNIFICANCE, if any, alone or in combination with genomic factors.[80,91,153,186,187,446-448,799]

EXPOSURE

1. The variable whose causal effect is to be estimated. Examples of exposures assessed by epidemiological studies are environmental and lifestyle factors, socioeconomic and working conditions, medical treatments, and genetic traits. Exposures may be harmful or beneficial—or even both (e.g., if an immunizable disease is circulating, exposure to immunizing agents helps most recipients but may harm those with adverse reactions to the vaccine).[1,12,14,67,240,270]
2. Proximity and/or contact with a source of a disease agent in such a manner that effective transmission of the agent or harmful effects of the agent may occur.
3. The amount of a factor to which a group or individual was exposed; sometimes contrasted with dose, the amount that enters or interacts with the organism.
4. The process by which an agent comes into contact with a person or animal in such a way that the person or animal may develop the relevant outcome, such as a disease.

EXPOSURE ASSESSMENT Process of estimating concentration or intensity, duration, and frequency of exposure to an agent that can affect health.[1,12,14,24,25,377,449,450]

EXPOSURE CONTROL See RISK MANAGEMENT.

EXPOSURE IMPACT NUMBER See IMPACT NUMBERS.

EXPOSURE LIMIT General term defining the regulated level of exposure that should not be exceeded.[449]

EXPOSURE-ODDS RATIO See ODDS RATIO.

EXPOSURE RATIO The ratio of rates at which persons in the case and control groups of a CASE-CONTROL STUDY are exposed to the RISK FACTOR (or to the protective factor) of interest.

EXPRESSION, GENE See GENE EXPRESSION.

EXPRESSIVITY In genetics, the extent to which a gene is expressed, i.e., demonstrated in the phenotype.

EXTENDED TRIAL A study using additional data collected from the same patients after completion of a formal Phase III randomized controlled trial. Analysis of such data allows researchers to collect additional information on toleration and efficacy. See also CLINICAL TRIAL.

EXTENSIVELY DRUG-RESISTANT TUBERCULOSIS (XDR) See DRUG-RESISTANT TUBERCULOSIS, EXTENSIVELY.

EXTERNAL EFFECTS (Syn: externalities) The negative or positive UTILITIES accruing to an individual from another person's consumption or choices. Also known as *spillover effects*, externalities are costs and benefits incurred in the consumption or production of goods and services that are not borne by the individual consumer or producer. While some are pecuniary, affecting only the value of other resources, other effects affect physically other people; communicable diseases are a classic example of this type of (negative) externality. Other examples include the health risks to others of alcohol use, which are not included in the purchase price of the alcohol; antimicrobial resistance; the adverse health effects from industrial pollution not included in the price of the industrial products manufactured, nor in charges imposed on the producer; and the impact on the economy of depleting natural resources not included in the calculation of national income or national product. There may be external costs and external benefits. HERD IMMUNITY from vaccination is a positive example: if the majority of a community is vaccinated against an infectious disease, the resulting herd immunity benefits those who have not been vaccinated.[67,69,355]

EXTERNALITIES, EXTERNALITY See EXTERNAL EFFECTS.

EXTERNAL VALIDITY See VALIDITY.

EXTRAPOLATE, EXTRAPOLATION To predict the value of a variate outside the range of observations; the resulting prediction. See also INTERPOLATE.

EXTREMAL QUOTIENT The ratio of the rate in the geographic region with the highest rate of interventions, such as surgical procedures, to the rate in the region with the lowest rate.[451]

EXTRINSIC INCUBATION PERIOD Time required for development of a disease agent in a vector from the time of uptake of the agent to the time when the vector is infective.[56,188,217-219] See also INCUBATION PERIOD; VECTOR-BORNE INFECTION.

F$_1$ ("F one") Term used in genetics to describe first-generation progeny of a mating.

FACE VALIDITY See VALIDITY, MEASUREMENT.

FACTOR

1. An event, characteristic, or other definable entity that leads to a change in a health condition or other defined outcome. See also CAUSALITY; CAUSATION OF DISEASE, FACTORS IN.

2. A synonym for (categorical) independent variable, or, more precisely, an independent variable used to identify, with numerical codes, membership of qualitatively different groups. A causal role may be implied, as in "overcrowding is a factor in disease transmission," where overcrowding represents the highest level of the factor "crowding." [7]

FACTOR ANALYSIS A set of statistical methods for analyzing the correlations among several variables in order to estimate the number of fundamental dimensions that underlie the observed data and to describe and measure those dimensions. Used frequently in the development of scoring systems for rating scales and questionnaires.[7,30]

FACTORIAL DESIGN A method of setting up an experiment or study to ensure that all levels of each intervention or classificatory factor occur with all levels of the others.[7,37]

FALSE DISCOVERY RATE (FDR) The expected proportion of incorrectly rejected null hypotheses. A method to account for multiple comparisons.[452] For any large number of tests, the FDR represents the expected proportion of rejected null hypotheses that might be FALSE POSITIVES (i.e., false discoveries). The conditional probability that the NULL HYPOTHESIS of no association is true, when the data are statistically significant and cause the null hypothesis to be rejected: $\Pr\{H_0$ is true | Rejection of $H_0\}$. There are numerous statistical algorithms for estimating or controlling the FDR.[453] See also Q-VALUE.

FALSE NEGATIVE

1. A negative test result in a person who possesses the attribute (e.g., the disease) for which the test is conducted. The labeling of a diseased person as healthy when SCREENING in the detection of disease.[6,9,58] See also SENSITIVITY.

2. An incorrect acceptance of the NULL HYPOTHESIS of no effect or no association in an intervention or association study.[1]

FALSE POSITIVE

1. A positive test result in a person who does not possess the attribute (e.g., the disease) for which the test is conducted. The labeling of a healthy person as diseased in SCREENING.[6,9,58] See also SPECIFICITY.

2. An incorrect rejection of the NULL HYPOTHESIS of no effect or no association in an intervention or association study.[1,13,83,87,178] See also EXPLORATORY STUDY.

FAMILIAL AGGREGATION A tendency of some diseases to cluster in families, which may be the result of genetic and epigenetic mechanisms, shared environmental exposures (e.g., diet), or both. ASCERTAINMENT BIAS should be considered. See also EMBODIMENT.

FAMILIAL DISEASE Disease that exhibits a tendency toward familial occurrence or aggregation. Familial occurrence of disease may be due to genetic transmission, intrafamilial TRANSMISSION OF INFECTION or culture, interaction within the family, or the family's shared experience, including its exposure to common environmental factors.[1,5,7,57,80,153,187,349,413,454-456]

FAMILY A group of two or more persons united by blood, adoptive or marital ties, or the common-law equivalent; the family may include members who do not share the household but are united to other members by blood, adoptive or marital ties, or equivalent ties. Epidemiological studies may be concerned with family members or with those who share the same household or dwelling unit.

FAMILY, EXTENDED A group of persons comprising members of several generations united by blood, adoptive and marital ties, or equivalent ties.

FAMILY, NUCLEAR A group of persons comprising members of a single or at most two generations, usually husband-wife-children, united by blood, adoptive or marital ties, or equivalent ties.

FAMILY CONTACT DISEASE Disease that occurs among members of the family of a worker who is exposed to a toxic substance such as asbestos dust and carries this home on his or her person or clothing, causing exposure to other family members.

FAMILY MEDICAL HISTORY The medical history of individual family members and the genetic relationships within a family. When the latter are represented in diagram form using standardized symbols and terminology, it is usually referred to as a PEDIGREE or family tree. The family medical history can be used for identifying persons at increased risk for some diseases, which may be prevented or where EARLY DETECTION may result in delayed onsets or improved outcomes. FAMILIAL AGGREGATION of disease can be due to shared lifestyle, environmental, genetic, epigenetic, social, cultural, and psychological factors.[80,183-185,245,316-321,409-417,455,457,799]

FAMILY OF CLASSIFICATIONS The Conference for the Tenth Revision of the INTERNATIONAL STATISTICAL CLASSIFICATION OF DISEASES AND RELATED HEALTH PROBLEMS recommended adopting the concept of the family of disease and health-related classifications.[458] This "family" comprises ICD-10 (the ICD three-character core classification), its short tabulation lists, and the ICD four-character classification; lay reporting and other community-based information schemes in health; specialty-based adaptations for oncology, psychiatry, etc.; other health-related classifications, such as the INTERNATIONAL CLASSIFICATION OF FUNCTIONING, DISABILITY AND HEALTH (ICF); and the International Nomenclature of Diseases (IND).

FAMILY PEDIGREE See FAMILY HISTORY.

FAMILY STUDY An epidemiological study of a family or a group of families; used to describe SURVEILLANCE of family groups (e.g., for tuberculosis). In genetics, investigation of families showing an unusual characteristic in order to determine whether the characteristic clusters in certain families, and if so, why.[5]

FAMILY TREE See FAMILY HISTORY.

FARR'S LAWS OF EPIDEMICS William Farr (1807–1883), who was the first Compiler of Abstracts in the General Register Office of England and Wales, enunciated several "laws" of epidemics.[460] He observed that epidemics appear to be generated in

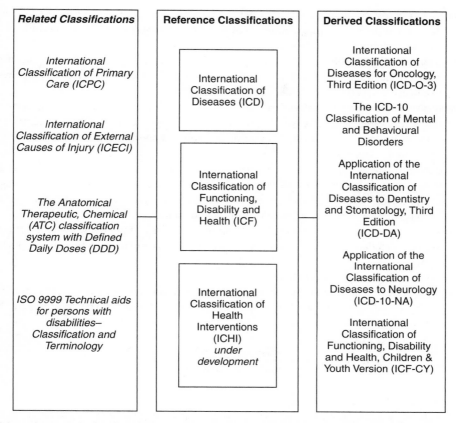

Schematic representation of the family of international classifications of the World Health Organization.
Source: World Health Organization.[459] With permission.

unhealthy places, go through a regular course, and decline. In his Second Annual Report (1840), he demonstrated mathematically that the decline in mortality of a waning epidemic occurs at a uniformly accelerating rate. He constructed mathematical models to explain the natural history of epidemic diseases, often correctly and elegantly.

FATALITY RATE The death rate observed in a designated series of persons affected by a simultaneous event (e.g., victims of a disaster). A term to be avoided, because it can be confused with CASE FATALITY RATE.

F DISTRIBUTION (Syn: variance ratio distribution) The DISTRIBUTION of the ratio of two independent quantities each of which is distributed like a variance in normally distributed samples.[7,37] So named in honor of R. A. Fisher, who first described it.

FEASIBILITY (of a study, program, intervention) The viability, practicability, or workability of the study, program, or intervention. How possible or practicable it is to carry it out. The feasibility of clinical and epidemiological research studies is strongly influenced by clinical, ethical, cultural, logistic, and economic factors. In assessing the weaknesses of a study in terms of internal and external VALIDITY and statistical PRECISION, the feasibility of the theoretically better alternatives must be considered.[1,6,26,58]

FEASIBILITY STUDY Preliminary study to determine the practicability of a proposed health program or procedure or of a larger study and to appraise the factors that may influence its practicability. See also PILOT INVESTIGATION, STUDY.

FECUNDABILITY The probability of pregnancy in each menstrual cycle in healthy non-contracepting sexually active couples. Estimates of fecundability can be derived from TIME-TO-PREGNANCY data.

FECUNDITY The ability to produce live offspring. Fecundity is difficult to measure, since it refers to the theoretical ability of a woman to conceive and carry a fetus to term. If a woman produces a live birth, it is known that she and her consort were fecund during some time in the past.

FEMALE-MALE GAP A set of national, regional, or other estimates—for example, of health status or literacy—in which all the figures for females are expressed as a percentage of the corresponding figures for males, which are indexed to 100. In some countries, a useful indicator of selective female abortion and infanticide.

FERTILITY The actual production of live offspring. STILLBIRTHS, fetal deaths, and abortions are not included in the measurement of fertility in a population.[1] See also GRAVIDITY; PARITY.

FERTILITY RATE See GENERAL FERTILITY RATE.

FERTILITY RATIO A measure of the fertility of the population that restricts the denominator to the female population of appropriate age for childbearing. The fertility ratio is defined as

$$\text{Fertility ratio} = \frac{\text{Number of girls under 15 years of age}}{\text{Number of women in } 15-49 \text{ age group}} \times 1000$$

See also GENERAL FERTILITY RATE.

FETAL DEATH (Syn: stillbirth) Death prior to the complete expulsion or extraction from its mother of a product of conception, irrespective of the duration of pregnancy. The death is indicated by the fact that, after such separation, the fetus does not breathe or show any other evidence of life, such as beating of the heart, pulsation of the umbilical cord, or definite movement of voluntary muscles. Defined variously as death after the 20th or 28th week of gestation. (The definition of the length of gestation varies between different jurisdictions, making this event difficult to compare internationally.) The WHO Conference for the Tenth Revision of the INTERNATIONAL CLASSIFICATION OF DISEASES (ICD-10) recommended that the definition of fetal death should remain unchanged. See also LIVE BIRTH.

FETAL DEATH CERTIFICATE (Syn: certificate of stillbirth) A vital record registering a fetal death, or STILLBIRTH. Some health jurisdictions require the use of a fetal death certificate for all products of conception, whereas others require its use only in cases in which gestation has reached a particular duration, usually the 20th or the 28th week.

FETAL DEATH RATE (Syn: stillbirth rate) The number of fetal deaths in a year expressed as a proportion of the total number of births (live births plus fetal deaths) in the same year.

$$\text{Fetal death rate} = \frac{\text{Number of fetal deaths in a year}}{\text{Number of fetal deaths plus live}} \times 1000$$
$$\text{births in the same year}$$

Note that the denominator is larger than for the FETAL DEATH RATIO and that the fetal death rate is therefore lower than the fetal death ratio, which is used in some jurisdictions. International comparisons of STILLBIRTH or fetal death statistics will be flawed if the distinction is not appreciated.

FETAL DEATH RATIO A measure of fetal wastage, related to the number of live births. Defined as

$$\text{Fetal death ratio} = \frac{\text{Number of fetal deaths in a year}}{\text{Number of live births in the same year}}$$

(Can be expressed as a rate per 1000.)

FETAL ORIGINS HYPOTHESIS See DEVELOPMENTAL ORIGINS OF HEALTH AND DISEASE.

FETUS Biologically, the stage of the conceptus after organ development is complete; in humans, 8 weeks after conception, 10 weeks after the last menstrual period. Vital statistical and medicolegal usage is less precise. Sometimes it means any stage of the conceptus between fertilization and expulsion; more often it means a gestational age less than 26 weeks from conception, 28 weeks from the last menstrual period. Recently it has come to mean less than 18 or 20 weeks, respectively, reflecting the current capability of perinatology to enhance survival prospects for a very immature developing conceptus.

FIELD EPIDEMIOLOGY The practice of epidemiology in the field—in the community—commonly in a public health service (i.e., a unit of government or a closely allied institution). Field epidemiology is how epidemics and outbreaks are investigated, and it is a tool for implementing measures to protect and improve the health of the public. Field epidemiologists must deal with unexpected, sometimes urgent problems that demand immediate solution. Its methods are designed to answer specific epidemiological questions in order to plan, implement, and/or evaluate public health interventions. These studies must consider the needs of those who will use the results. The task of a field epidemiologist is not complete until results of a study have been clearly communicated in a timely manner to those who need to know and an intervention has been made to improve the health of the people.[28,191] See also APPLIED EPIDEMIOLOGY.

FIELD SURVEY The planned collection of data in "the field," usually among noninstitutionalized persons in the GENERAL POPULATION.[72,160,167] A method of establishing a relationship between two or more variables in a population in numerical terms by eliciting and collating information from existing sources (not only records but people who can say how they feel or what happened). See also CROSS-SECTIONAL STUDY.

FIELD TRIAL Epidemiological or clinical study (including some RANDOMIZED CONTROLLED TRIALS) conducted outside clinical and laboratory settings, in the GENERAL POPULATION, or in primary care.[1,67,110] See also COMMUNITY TRIAL; PRAGMATIC STUDY.

FISHER'S EXACT TEST The test for association in a two-by-two table that is based upon the exact HYPERGEOMETRIC DISTRIBUTION of the frequencies within the table when both margins are treated as fixed (unvarying).[7,37] See also EXACT TEST.

FISHING EXPEDITION An EXPLORATORY STUDY without coherent hypotheses to find clues and leads for further study. The term is sometimes rightly used to disapprove poorly conceived studies; however, such analytic "expeditions" may be done for worthwhile causes (e.g., to seek clues to the cause of a major outbreak, or in GWAS).[53,87-89] See also AGNOSTIC ANALYSIS; DATA DREDGING; DATA MINING.

FITNESS This word has specific meanings in several fields related to epidemiology.

1. In population genetics, a measure of the relative survival and reproductive success of a given phenotype or population subgroup.
2. In HEALTH PROMOTION and health risk appraisal, physical fitness is a set of attributes that people have or achieve that relate to their ability to perform physical activity. Intellectual and emotional fitness can also be described and to some extent measured.

FIXED COHORT A cohort in which no additional membership is allowed—that is, it is fixed by being present at some defining event ("zero time"); an example is the cohort comprising survivors of the atomic bomb exploded at Hiroshima.[1,8,24] See also DYNAMIC POPULATION.

FLOW CHART See FLOW DIAGRAM.

FLOW DIAGRAM (Syn: logic model, flow chart) A diagram comprising blocks connected by arrows representing steps in a process. An ALGORITHM used in decision analysis. Flow diagrams have many uses (e.g., to show eligibility, recruitment, and losses in design and execution of a study or to show how a program is intended to work).[26,102-106]

FOCUS GROUP A Small convenience sample of people brought together to discuss a topic or issue with the aim of ascertaining the range and intensity of their views rather than arriving at a consensus. This sociological method is used by epidemiologists to, for example, appraise perceptions of health problems, assess acceptability of a field study, or refine the questions to be used in a field study. The distinction between a focus group and a DELPHI survey is that the latter does aim to reach a consensus, is more formal, is usually made up of experts, generally functions by mail or telephone, and the identities of members preferably are unknown to one another. In a focus group, persons meet face to face, although it is possible for their identities to remain unknown to one another.[26]

FOCUS OF INFECTION A defined and circumscribed locality containing the epidemiological factors needed for transmission: a human community, a source of infection, a vector population, and appropriate environmental conditions.[56]

FOLLOW-UP Observation over a period of time of an individual, group, or an initially defined population whose relevant characteristics have been assessed in order to observe changes in health status or health-related variables.[1,3,270] See also ATTRITION BIAS; COHORT; LOST TO FOLLOW-UP.

FOLLOW-UP STUDY

1. A study in which individuals or populations—selected on the basis of whether they have been exposed to risk, received a specified preventive or therapeutic procedure, or possess a certain characteristic—are followed to assess the outcome of exposure, the procedure, or effect of the characteristic (e.g., occurrence of disease).[1]
2. Synonym for COHORT STUDY.

FOMITES (singular, fomes) Articles that convey infection to others because they have been contaminated by pathogenic organisms. Examples include a handkerchief, drinking glass, door handle, clothing, and toys.

FORCE OF MORBIDITY (Syn: hazard rate, instantaneous incidence rate, PERSON-TIME INCIDENCE RATE) A theoretical measure of the number of new cases that occur per unit of population-time (e.g., person-years at risk).[1] This is a measure of the occurrence of disease at a point in time, t, defined mathematically as the limit, as Δt approaches zero, of

$$\frac{\text{Probability that a person well at time } t \text{ will develop the disease in the interval } t + \Delta t}{\Delta t}$$

The average value of this quantity over the interval t to $(t + \Delta t)$ can be estimated as

$$\frac{\text{Incident cases observed from } t \text{ to } (t + \Delta t)}{\text{Number of person} - \text{time units of experience observed}}$$
$$\text{from } t \text{ to } (t + \Delta t)$$

FORCE OF MORTALITY (Syn: actuarial [death] rate) The hazard rate of the occurrence of death at a point in time t—the limit as Δt approaches zero—of the probability that an individual alive at time t will die by time $t + \Delta t$, divided by Δt. Distinct from cumulative death rate.

FORECASTING A method of estimating what may happen in the future that relies on extrapolation of existing trends (demographic, epidemiological, etc.). It may be less useful than SCENARIO BUILDING, which has greater flexibility. For example, extrapolation of mortality TRENDS for coronary heart disease in the early 1960s in the United States suggested that the mortality rates would continue to rise, whereas in fact the rates began to fall soon after that time.

FORENSIC EPIDEMIOLOGY The use of epidemiological reasoning, knowledge, and methods in the investigation of public health problems that may have been caused by or associated with intentional and/or criminal acts.[461]

FOREST PLOT A plot that summarizes different estimates of the same quantity, such as results of different studies included in a META-ANALYSIS.[6,9,229,230] The name was introduced at a time when the graph had vertical lines representing the studies.

FORTUITOUS RELATIONSHIP See ASSOCIATION, FORTUITOUS.

FORWARD SURVIVAL ESTIMATE A procedure for estimating the age distribution at some later date by projecting forward an observed age distribution. The procedure uses survival ratios, often obtained from model life tables.[11]

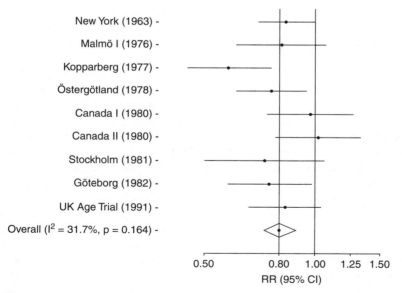

Forest plot. Meta-analysis of breast cancer mortality after 13 years of follow-up in breast cancer screening trials. The graph shows the relative risk of dying from breast cancer in nine randomized controlled trials evaluating the reduction in mortality from breast cancer in women offered screening compared with those who were not. Source: Independent UK Panel on Breast Cancer Screening.[462] With permission.

FOURFOLD TABLE See CONTINGENCY TABLE.

"FOURTH WORLD" The environmental and socioeconomic situation of decayed urban neighborhoods in affluent nations, resembling the conditions encountered in the poorest developing countries. It includes homeless people, who are among an underclass (often disenfranchised) found in urban communities in rich countries. This term should not be used without explanation in scientific writing.

FRACTALS Mathematical patterns in which smaller parts have the same shape as larger parts, indefinitely down to ever finer levels of magnification. Blood vessels and the bronchial tree behave according to fractal theory down to microscopic levels.[463] Fractals have been applied in studies of the way human and other populations grow and spread, and of the spread of some infections and neoplasms.

"FRAGILE" DATA Data derived from a well-designed study that do not quite reach a level of STATISTICAL SIGNIFICANCE but provide a basis to suggest an unexpected or potentially relevant conclusion. Alternatively, data that suggest important conclusions from a poorly designed study. Hence, a potentially misleading term.

FREQUENCY See OCCURRENCE.

FREQUENCY DISTRIBUTION See DISTRIBUTION; DISTRIBUTION FUNCTION.

FREQUENCY MATCHING See MATCHING.

FREQUENCY POLYGON A graphic illustration of a distribution, made by joining a set of points, for each of which the abscissa is the midpoint of the class and the ordinate, or height, is the frequency.

FREQUENTIST STATISTICS The most common type of statistical method during the 20th century and continuing today. Called *frequentist* to reflect the fact that the probability statements in the models it uses, and in the inferences it produces, refer to the relative frequencies of observations or data under different possibilities for or hypotheses about the underlying parameters under study (such as exposure effects). The most prominent examples are *P* VALUES and CONFIDENCE INTERVALS. A procedure is sometimes said to be properly *calibrated* or *frequency valid* if its stated frequency properties (e.g., 95% confidence) match its actual frequency performance (e.g., 95% coverage frequency).[1,7,34,37] See also CALIBRATION.

Frequentist statistics are usually contrasted to BAYESIAN STATISTICS, which use and produce probability statements about possible values for or hypotheses about study parameters. During most of the 20th century, frequentist and Bayesian statistics were considered competing schools of inference. There has been increasing recognition, however, that many Bayesian methods often display excellent frequency properties when used as frequentist statistics and, conversely, that most frequentist procedures have illuminating Bayesian interpretations. As a result, frequentist and Bayesian methods have increasingly come to be viewed as complementary rather than competing approaches to statistical analysis, especially in observational research.

F TEST Most commonly, a test used to test that several groups come from populations with the same variance. The "F" is taken to stand for R. A. Fisher (1890–1962), who is generally credited with inventing the ANALYSIS OF VARIANCE.[7]

FUNDING BIAS Bias in characterizing an association (usually between an exposure and a set of outcomes) owing to the absence or withdrawal of financial and other types of

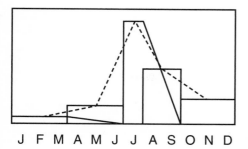

J F M A M J J A S O N D   **Frequency polygon**. Numbers of notified cases in
specified months. Source: Abramson JH.[464]

support. Lack of support obstructs or discourages the conduct of research. It may lead
to PUBLICATION BIAS.[267] See also CONFLICT OF INTEREST.

FUNNEL PLOT A type of graph used in META-ANALYSIS to detect PUBLICATION BIAS. The estimate
of risk is plotted against sample size or a measure of the within-study variance. If there is
no publication bias, the plot is funnel-shaped; but if studies showing positive results are
more likely to be published than NULL STUDIES, there is a "hole in the lower left corner"
of the funnel. The "contour-enhanced funnel plot" is thought to aid in differentiating
asymmetry due to publication bias from that due to other factors.[9,26,87,226,229,230,294,465-467]

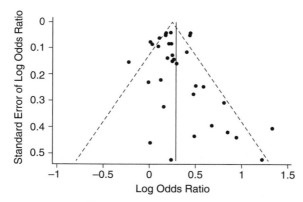

Funnel plot. Funnel plot with pseudo 95% confidence limits for publication bias in studies of the association
between overweight (14 studies) or obesity (19 studies) and low back pain. Source: Shirl R, et al.[468]

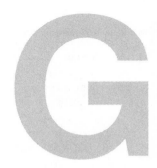

GAMBLER'S FALLACY (Syn: Monte-Carlo fallacy) The notion that the probability of an event occurring increases with the length of time since the event previously occurred when no such relation exists (e.g., as with properly randomized games of chance).[38]

GAME THEORY A branch of mathematical logic concerned with the range of possible reactions to a particular strategy; each reaction can be assigned a probability, and each reaction can lead to further action by the "adversary" in the game. Used in systems analysis. It has occasional applications in disease SURVEILLANCE and control. It is one of the underlying theories used in CLINICAL DECISION ANALYSIS and in determining utilities (e.g., in calculating QALYs).

GAMETE A mature sex cell: the ovum of the female or the spermatozoon of the male. Gametes are haploid, each containing half the normal number of chromosomes of a somatic cell and fusing with its counterpart at fertilization to produce a zygote, which has the normal number of diploid CHROMOSOMES and develops into an embryo.

GAMETOCYTE
1. A cell that is in the process of developing into a GAMETE by undergoing gametogenesis.
2. The sexual stage of malaria parasites. Male gametocytes (microgametocytes) and female gametocytes (macrogametocytes) are inside red blood cells in the bloodstream. If they are ingested by a female *Anopheles* mosquito, they undergo sexual reproduction, which starts the extrinsic (sporogonic) cycle of the parasite in the mosquito.[56]

GATEKEEPER A person or system that selectively regulates ACCESS to a HEALTH CARE service. A health care provider at the first contact level who has responsibilities for the provision of PRIMARY CARE as well as for the coordination of specialized care and referral.[17]

GAUSSIAN DISTRIBUTION See NORMAL DISTRIBUTION.

G-COMPUTATION See G-FORMULA.

GENDER
1. In grammar, the term to designate a noun (person, animal, or object) as masculine, feminine, or neuter.
2. The totality of culturally constructed awareness, attitudes, beliefs, emotions, and behaviors about males and females, and sometimes their sexual orientation. A social construct regarding culture-bound conventions, roles, and behaviors for—as well as relationships between and among—women and men, boys and girls.[248,336,357,407,469]

GENE A sequence of DNA that codes for a particular protein product or that regulates other genes. A DNA segment that is transcribed into messenger RNA and translated into a protein. Traditionally, genes have been deemed to comprise the exons that are actually translated plus the intervening introns.[57] Today, the nature, properties, and effects of genes are in the midst of a profound reassessment by science.[145,349,454,470-472]

GENE-ENVIRONMENT INTERACTIONS Any type of INTERACTION (at any level: physical, chemical, biological, physiological, statistical, clinical, epidemiological) between one or more genetic variants and one or more environmental factors. Gene-environment interactions (G*E) can be described, analyzed, and interpreted by several types of models, which take into account the various ways in which genetic effects can be modified by environmental exposures (and vice versa), the levels of such exposures, and the model on which the genetic effects are based.[473] Studies on G*E need not be restricted to inherited alterations in low penetrance, SUSCEPTIBILITY genes: G*E also encompass the fact that certain environmental factors and mixtures *interact* biologically with the genetic material and cause MUTATIONS or influence GENE EXPRESSION.[78,80-82,174,175] While the physico-chemical interaction between an environmental factor and DNA or RNA that contributes to cause or to maintain an acquired genetic alteration (or a change in gene expression) is a real biological interaction,[415] statistically it is not treated as an interaction but as a MAIN EFFECT. See also NONGENOTOXIC CARCINOGENS.

Some diseases have a different probability of occurrence, severity, or prognosis in individuals with a genetic variant (or with other, more complex genetic characteristics) when the individual is exposed to some environmental RISK FACTORS. Identification of the relevant genetic information and exposures can help implement interventions that reduce disease burden in high-risk populations (e.g., by eliminating or otherwise preventing exposure to the environmental factor).[57,174,473]

GENE EXPRESSION The amount and timing of appearance of the functional product of a gene. The process by which the DNA sequence of a gene is converted into functional proteins. Non-protein-coding genes (e.g., rRNA genes, tRNA genes) are not translated into protein. Gene expression is a multistep process that begins with the transcription of DNA (of which genes are made) into messenger RNA. It is then followed by posttranscriptional modification and translation into a gene product, followed by folding, posttranslational modification, and targeting. The amount of protein that a cell expresses depends on the tissue, the developmental stage of the organism, and the physiologic state of the cell. The expression of many genes is known to be regulated after transcription; thus, an increase in the concentration of mRNA may not increase expression. See also EPIGENETICS.

GENE POOL The total of all genes possessed by reproductive members of a population.

GENERAL FERTILITY RATE A more refined measure of fertility than the crude birthrate. The denominator is restricted to the number of women of childbearing age (i.e., 15–44 or 15–49. Defined as

$$\text{General fertility rate} = \frac{\text{Number of live births in an area during a year}}{\text{Midyear female population age } 15 - 44 \text{ in same area in same year}}$$

The upper age limit for this rate is 44 –sometimes 49– years in most jurisdictions.

GENERALIZABILITY The degree to which results of a study may apply, be relevant, or be generalized to populations or groups that did not participate in the study. In etiological research, such inferences are not merely statistical in nature but must be based on theory, judgment, and evidence external to the study (e.g., on available knowledge on biological, clinical, or social mechanisms linking an exposure to an outcome); inferences may partly be subjective but not arbitrary. REPRESENTATIVENESS of the study sample may enhance generalizability in studies with strong descriptive components; yet, knowledge of subject matter, context, and study conditions enables generalization in studies of etiologic nature that are not based on a strictly representative sample. Scientific and statistical inferences build on different types of logic.[1,3,6,24-26,270,474] See also VALIDITY.

GENERALIZATION The elaboration of the reasons and circumstances in which a scientific finding is valid and relevant beyond a specific study. It often requires the INTEGRATION of knowledge from several branches of science.[1,25,270,474] See also CAUSAL INFERENCE.

GENERALIZED LINEAR MODEL See LINEAR MODEL, GENERALIZED.

GENERAL POPULATION All members of a human population, defined essentially on the basis of geographical location, as in a country, region, city, etc. All inhabitants of some given area. Everyone in the POPULATION being studied, irrespective of race, ethnicity, or professional status.[211,430] Individuals admitted to hospitals, other health care facilities, and prisons are usually considered not to be part of the general population. The term is often used to underline the different results that studies tend to obtain in the general population and in specific populations, subgroups, or settings (e.g., in a working population, a hospitalized population).

GENERATION EFFECT (Syn: cohort effect) Variation in health status that arises from the different causal factors to which each BIRTH COHORT in the population is exposed as the environment and society change. Each consecutive birth cohort is exposed to a unique environment that coincides with its life span.

GENERATION TIME The interval between receipt of infection by the host and the latter's maximal infectivity. This applies to both clinical cases and inapparent infections. With person-to-person TRANSMISSION OF INFECTION, the interval between cases is determined by the generation time. See also SERIAL INTERVAL; INCUBATION PERIOD.

GENE SILENCING One of the EPIGENETIC processes that regulate gene expression. Commonly used to describe that instead of being expressed ("turned on"), a gene is "switched off" by an epigenetic mechanism.

GENETIC ASSOCIATION STUDY See ASSOCIATION STUDY; GWAS.

GENETIC DIVERSITY The variety of different types of genes in a species or population. A form of BIODIVERSITY.

GENETIC DRIFT Random variation in gene frequency from generation to generation, most often observed in small populations. The process of evolution through random statistical fluctuation of genetic composition of populations.

GENETIC ENGINEERING Manipulation of the GENOME of a living organism.

GENETIC EPIDEMIOLOGY The specialty that investigates the genetic bases of disease-related phenotypes and any kind of health-related TRAIT in groups of people (e.g., relatives), and genetic and EPIGENETIC INHERITANCE of disease in populations. The study of the role of genetic factors and their interaction with environmental factors in the occurrence of disease in human populations.[8,57,78,86,146,349,454,475-477,799] In recent years it has experienced a substantial convergence and integration with MOLECULAR EPIDEMIOLOGY.

GENETIC LINKAGE The phenomenon whereby phenotypes and alleles at one or more marker alleles tend to be inherited together. Particular genes occupy specific sites in chromosomes, one member of each pair of chromosomes coming from each parent. When two genes are fairly close to each other in the same chromosome pair, they tend to be inherited together. Such genes are said to be linked, and the phenomenon is called genetic linkage.[54,57,86] See also GENETIC PENETRANCE; LINKAGE ANALYSIS; LINKAGE DISEQUILIBRIUM; MOLECULAR EPIDEMIOLOGY.

GENETIC PENETRANCE The frequency with which a characteristic or TRAIT that a genetic variant controls (the phenotype) is seen in people who carry the variant. The extent to which a genetically determined condition is expressed in an individual. The proportion of individuals with a given GENOTYPE that show the PHENOTYPE under specific environmental conditions. When all individuals carrying a dominant mutation show the mutant phenotype, the gene is said to show complete penetrance. The relation between the frequency of a variant and its penetrance is often inverse: the more penetrant (e.g., deleterious) a variant, the less frequent it is in the population. Only highly penetrant mutations may act with no INTERACTION with external factors. GENE-ENVIRONMENT INTERACTIONS are intrinsic to the mode of action of low-penetrant genes. Current knowledge suggests that low-penetrant genetic traits cause a smaller fraction of the BURDEN OF DISEASE than certain environmental agents (e.g., smoking, air pollution, chemical carcinogens).[13,54,80,169,174,175,478-480,799] See also EPIGENETICS; HEREDITY; MONOGENIC DISEASES; POLYGENIC DISEASES.

GENETIC POLYMORPHISM See POLYMORPHISM, GENETIC.

GENETIC PREDISPOSITION See GENETIC SUSCEPTIBILITY.

GENETICS The branch of biology dealing with genetic heredity and variation of individual members of a species. Its branches include population genetics, which partly overlaps with genetic and molecular epidemiology.

GENETIC SCREENING The use of genetic, clinical, and epidemiological knowledge, reasoning, and techniques to detect genetic variants that have been demonstrated to place an individual at increased risk of a specific DISEASE. Ethical problems may arise in genetic screening; e.g., when the evidence on clinically relevant benefits is weak, regarding the provision of information to persons of their putative increased risk when there is no effective treatment, potential loss of eligibility for employment and insurance benefits.[9,58,302,349,454,478] See also ETHICS; NUMBER NEEDED TO SCREEN.

GENETIC SUSCEPTIBILITY (Syn: genetic predisposition) Increased (or decreased) probability of developing a particular condition or disease due to the presence of one or more genetic variants and/or a family history that indicates an increased (decreased) risk of the disease.

GENETIZATION The process by which issues considered to be medical but not necessarily genetic become defined as problems with a strong genetic component or as having a genetic cause. The attribution of physiological, pathological, behavioral, or social conditions to genetic causes, often at the expense of clinical, environmental, cultural, economic, or social explanations. The expansion of genetics into the life and health sciences and professions (e.g., the genetization of prenatal medicine, oncology, primary care), and into everyday existence. In genetization processes "genetic" is often considered to be synonymous with *inherited*, and vice versa, thus neglecting somatic (acquired) genetic alterations and cultural inheritance.[80,187,292,323,361-364,470,481,482] See also HEREDITY; INTEGRATION; MEDICALIZATION; REDUCTIONISM.

GENOME The array of genes carried by an individual. The total genetic material of an organism. The whole set of the DNA of a species. See also EPIGENOME; EXPOSOME; METAGENOME.

GENOME-WIDE ASSOCIATION STUDY (GWAS) (Syn: whole genome association study, WGA study) An ASSOCIATION STUDY in which numerous genetic variants across the genome are analyzed to measure differences associated with a TRAIT (e.g., height), DISEASE, or PHENOTYPE. The most common GWAS design compares the DNA of people with the disease under investigation (cases) and a suitable group of people without the disease (controls). Alternative GWAS designs can be used to analyze quantitative traits such as height, blood pressure, or biomarker levels. GWAS "AGNOSTIC" ANALYSIS primarily examines differences in SINGLE NUCLEOTIDE POLYMORPHISMS (SNPs) between individuals with a specific disease and non-diseased controls. In contrast to the CANDIDATE GENE APPROACH, which specifically tests one or a few genetic regions, a GWAS investigates most of or the whole genome. The approach is therefore said to be non-candidate-driven or "AGNOSTIC." GWAS identifies SNPs and other variants in DNA that are associated with a condition but cannot distinguish between causal variants and those that are simply correlated (i.e., in LINKAGE DESIQUILIBRIUM) with the true causal variants. Pathway-based analysis of GWAS can detect associations that might be missed by focusing on single loci or even genes.[483] So far, GWAS-discovered variants are weak RISK FACTORS (most with relative risks of 1.05 to 1.50 per allele). Variants are not modifiable and, thus, do not have direct potential to reduce disease incidence. A remarkable number of associations reported by GWAS have been replicated, but only some have yet consistently demonstrated RELEVANCE and SIGNIFICANCE.[51-55,87-89,91,273,484,485]

GENOTOXIC A substance, setting, or process that is toxic or harmful to the genetic material. An agent or process that interacts with cellular DNA, either directly or after metabolic biotransformation, resulting in alteration of DNA structure. DNA-adduct formation is one type of genotoxicity.[78,80-82,415] See also CARCINOGEN.

GENOTOXIC CARCINOGENS Chemical carcinogens capable of causing damage to DNA. They can be mutagenic, clastogenic, or aneugenic. Inside the cell, carcinogens or their metabolic products can either directly or indirectly affect the regulation and expression of genes involved in cell-cycle control, DNA repair, cell differentiation, or apoptosis. Some carcinogens act by genotoxic mechanisms, such as forming DNA adducts or inducing CHROMOSOME breakage, fusion, deletion, missegregation, and nondisjunction; for example, carcinogenic ions or compounds of nickel, arsenic, and cadmium can induce structural and numerical chromosomal aberrations. DNA binding and induction of mutations in cancer-related genes, such as TP53 and K-*ras*, are important genotoxic mechanisms of tumor initiation. Also important in causing diseases of complex etiology, such as cancer, is the accompanying ability of many compounds to promote the outgrowth of transformed cell clones through NONGENOTOXIC mechanisms.[13,78,80-82,178,416]

GENOTYPE The genetic constitution inherited by an organism or a person, as distinct from the physical characteristics and appearance that emerge with development (i.e., the PHENOTYPE). The genetic constitution of an organism; modulated by the environment, it is then expressed as a phenotype.

GEOGRAPHICAL INFORMATION SYSTEM (GIS) An information system that incorporates digitally constructed maps and uses sophisticated modeling techniques to analyze and display information patterns. Satellite imaging and remote sensing have greatly expanded the scope of GISs (e.g., TRENDS in specific diseases are suggested after analyzing the composition of vegetation and the amounts of precipitation in tropical regions, which relate to changes in the distribution and abundance of predators and insect vectors). Another application is digitally prepared spot maps of disease clusters using postal codes and notified cases.[1,8,14,24,486] An important application is in GEOMATICS. See also DISEASE MAPPING; MEDICAL GEOGRAPHY; SATELLITE EPIDEMIOLOGY.

GEOMATICS The collection, processing, storage, and analysis of geographical information. An important application is sequentially generated computer maps to show regional and temporal trends and variations in various sectors of society, including the health sector. Uses include the assessment of time trends in the geographical distribution of diseases such as malaria.

GEOMETRIC MEAN See MEAN, GEOMETRIC.

GESTATIONAL AGE Strictly speaking, the gestational age of a fetus is the elapsed time since conception. However, as the moment when conception occurred is rarely known precisely, the duration of gestation is measured from the first day of the last normal menstrual period. Gestational age is expressed in completed days or completed weeks (e.g., events occurring 280–286 days after the onset of the last normal menstrual period are considered to have occurred at 40 weeks of gestation).

Measurements of fetal growth, as they represent continuous variables, are expressed in relation to a specific week of gestational age (e.g., the mean birth weight for 40 weeks is that obtained at 280–286 days of gestation on a weight-for-gestational-age curve). Some specified variations of gestational age are: *Preterm*, less than 37 completed weeks (less than 259 days); *Term*, from 37 to less than 42 completed weeks (259–293 days); *Postterm*, 42 completed weeks or more (294 days or more).

GESTATION LENGTH An ambiguous term for the duration of pregnancy because it can be calculated in different ways:

1. Biologically, as used by embryologists and teratologists, the time from fertilization (conception) to expulsion of the fetus; in humans the mean is 266 days (38 weeks).
2. In obstetrics and often in epidemiology, gestation is dated from the last menstrual period, on average 2 weeks earlier than the time of fertilization, i.e., mean 280 days (40 weeks).

G-ESTIMATION A method to estimate the parameters of structural nested models (SNMs). It requires the assumption of no RESIDUAL CONFOUNDING, or the slightly weaker assumption of known magnitude of the residual confounding.[1,2] The general version of g-estimation was proposed by Robins.[487-489] The standard INSTRUMENTAL VARIABLE estimator is a particular case of g-estimator. Other methods to estimate the causal effect of a time-varying treatment in the presence of time-varying confounders are the parametric G-FORMULA and INVERSE PROBABILITY WEIGHTING (IPW) of MARGINAL STRUCTURAL MODELS (MSMs).[1,2,11,101,110]

G-FORMULA A formula representing the causal effect of any generalized, time-varying treatment under the assumption of no RESIDUAL CONFOUNDING. It expresses the causal effect in terms of a standardized outcome difference across exposure groups conditional on the covariates and is applicable whenever the covariates block all BACKDOOR PATHS. It was discovered by Robins in 1986 and subsequently rediscovered by other researchers.[488] Also known as the g-computation algorithm formula. It is the foundation for the theory for CAUSAL INFERENCE in settings with time-varying treatments and confounders. In the simple non-time-varying setting, the g-formula reduces to STANDARDIZATION. The g-formula is a nonparametric method; in practice a fully parametric version (the parametric g-formula) is used.[2]

GINI COEFFICIENT A measure of dispersion in a set of values. Devised by Corrado Gini (1884–1965), demographer and economist.[490] A common measure of income INEQUALITY derived from the LORENZ CURVE. The coefficient has also been used to measure the DISTRIBUTION of health and health care resource consumption. The Lorenz curve shows the percentage of total income earned by the cumulative percentage of the population.

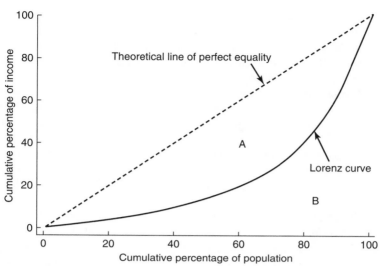

Gini coefficient.

In a "perfectly equal society," the poorest 15% of the population would earn 15% of the total income, the poorest 65% of the population would earn 65% of the total income, and the Lorenz curve would equal the 45-degree "theoretical line of perfect equality." As inequality increases in a community, the Lorenz curve deviates from the "line of equality." The Gini coefficient is the size of the area between the "line of equality" and the Lorenz curve (area A in the figure) divided by the total area under the line of equality (A+B). Thus, the more the Lorenz curve departs from the theoretical line, the higher the Gini coefficient is. The coefficient can take a value between 0 and 1: a 0 would be obtained in a society where all income was equally shared, and a 1 (or 100%) in a totally unequal society. Assumptions and properties of the Lorenz curve and the Gini coefficient must be assessed before comparing values across different groups.[1,7,491] See also CONCENTRATION INDEX; SLOPE INDEX OF INEQUALITY; RELATIVE INDEX OF INEQUALITY.

GLOBAL BURDEN OF DISEASE See BURDEN OF DISEASE.

GLOBAL HEALTH The international, transdisciplinary, and intersectoral research, knowledge, and policies for improving population health and health determinants on a planetary scale. It sets health equity, sustainable development, and efficiency as worldwide priorities; focuses on transregional health issues; and seeks to influence SYSTEMIC causal pathways and policies.[48,113,163-169,213,360,492-494,799]

GLOBALIZATION The process toward a world with highly dense, fast, and integrated local/planetary networks (economic, industrial, financial, cultural, sanitary, political), deeply influenced and challenged by new forms of trade, governance (including lack of democratic rights and institutions), communications, transportation, information, entertainment, biomedical and computer technologies, markets, dysregulation, migrations, depletion of natural resources, and climate change, as well as by the coexistence of old and emerging health risks and problems.[17,213,215,309,426,494-498,799]

GLOVER PHENOMENON An old term referring to the wide variation in rates at which many common medical procedures are conducted in seemingly comparable communities with similar morbidity rates—a phenomenon analyzed by J. A. Glover and many others.

GOAL A desired state to be achieved within a specified time. See also TARGET.

"GOLD STANDARD" A method, procedure, or measurement that is widely accepted as being the best available. Often used to compare with new methods of unknown effectiveness (e.g., a potential new diagnostic test is assessed against the best available diagnostic test).[3,6,9,26,58]

GOMPERTZ-MAKEHAM FORMULA A formula describing the relationship of mortality rate to age. There is an age-independent component and a component that increases exponentially with age. Benjamin Gompertz, a nineteenth-century demographer, first identified the proportionate relationship of mortality to age. This was refined by W. M. Makeham in 1867 to provide a better model of the age-specific pattern of the instantaneous death rate. If q_x is the probability of dying at age x and A, B, and C are constants, $q_x = A + BC^x$. For ages beyond childhood, the Gompertz-Makeham formula closely fits observed patterns.

GONADOTROPHIC CYCLE One complete round of ovarian development in the mosquito (or other insect vector) from the time when the blood meal is taken to the time when the fully developed eggs are laid.

GOBI/FFF Growth monitoring, oral rehydration, breast-feeding, immunization/family planning, food production, female education (WHO/UNICEF/World Bank).

GOOD CLINICAL PRACTICE (GCP) An international set of ethical and scientific quality standards for designing, conducting, recording, and reporting trials that involve participation of human subjects.[26] It originates from the International Conference for Harmonization (ICH)[499] and derives from the Helsinki Declaration of the World Medical Association on Ethical Principles for Medical Research Involving Human Subjects.[500] The GCP standards are implemented, among others, by the European Medicines Agency,[501] and the U.S. Food and Drug Administration.[502,503]

GOOD MANUFACTURING PRACTICE (GMP) That part of quality assurance which ensures that products are consistently produced and controlled to the quality standards appropriate to their intended use and as required by the marketing authorization. GMPs are aimed primarily at diminishing the risks inherent in the production of goods as drugs and vaccines. Such risks include cross-contamination, and mix-ups (confusion) caused by, for example, false labels being put on containers.

GOODNESS OF FIT Degree of agreement between an empirically observed distribution and a mathematical or theoretical DISTRIBUTION.[1,2,78,796]

GOODNESS-OF-FIT TEST A statistical test of the hypothesis that data have been randomly sampled or generated from a population that follows a particular theoretical distribution or model. Among the most common such tests is the CHI-SQUARE TEST.[34,37]

GPHIN Global Public Health Intelligence Network of the World Health Organization. See also EPIDEMIOLOGICAL INTELLIGENCE.

GRAB SAMPLE See SAMPLE.

GRADE GUIDELINES The Grading of Recommendations Assessment, Development, and Evaluation system of rating quality of evidence and grading strength of recommendations in systematic reviews, health technology assessments, and clinical practice guidelines.[504]

GRADIENT OF INFECTION The variety of host responses to infection ranging from inapparent infection to fatal illness.[56]

GRAPH (Syn: chart, plot) A general term for the visual representation of the relationship between variables. Three-dimensional graphs of relationships between three variables can be represented and comprehended visually in two dimensions. The relationship between x and y may be linear, exponential, logarithmic, etc. Other types of graphs include histograms and BAR CHARTS.[7,102-108,505] See also ABSCISSA, ORDINATE; AXIS.

GRAVIDITY The number of pregnancies (completed or incomplete) experienced by a woman. See also PARITY.

"GRAY LITERATURE" (Syn: fugitive literature) Technical reports, studies, and essays that are not specifically aimed for conventional publication, have restricted distribution, and are hence seldom included in the bibliographic retrieval systems commonly available to scholars, officers, and the public. They may be commissioned, sponsored, or owned by companies, academic units, financial institutions, or government agencies, including local or regional health departments. This literature used to include many unpublished masters or doctoral dissertations, but these and many other papers are nowadays enjoying wider access in digital formats. Scientific articles published in journals using languages other than English do not per se have the features mentioned above (e.g., they have wide circulations among scholars and health professionals). Gray literature, including epidemiological studies, may not be PEER REVIEWED. Nonetheless, such literature may contain highly valid and relevant scientific findings, including information useful in META-ANALYSIS and in PUBLIC HEALTH IMPACT ASSESSMENT.[17,229,230,302]

GROSS REPRODUCTION RATE (Syn: raw coefficient of reproduction) The average number of female children a woman would have if she survived to the end of her childbearing years and if, throughout that period, she were subject to a given set of age-specific fertility rates and a given sex ratio at birth. It provides a measure of REPLACEMENT-LEVEL FERTILITY (or of the *replacement of the generations*) in the absence of mortality. In a hypothetical generation, it is equal to the number of girls born to a woman until the end of the reproduction period at a given (current year) age-specific fertility. See also NET REPRODUCTION RATE.

GROUP COMPARISONS Comparisons that consist in contrasting what is observed in a group of people in the presence of exposure to what would have occurred had the group of interest not been exposed to the postulated cause. Differences in frequency of disease occurrence between groups can logically be interpreted as being caused by the

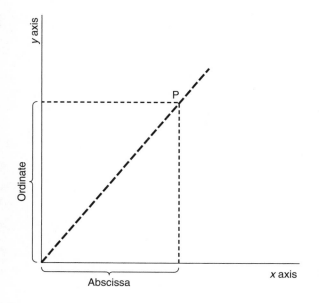

Graph showing abscissa, ordinate, and locus of a point, P, in relation to x and y AXIS.

exposure.[42] Integratedly with POPULATION THINKING, this is the main mode of knowledge acquisition in epidemiology.[1-3,5,6,9,24-26,38-41,63,85,101,201,203,206,211,224,250,269,270,400]

GROWTH RATE OF POPULATION A measure of population growth (in the absence of migration) comprising addition of newborns to the population and subtraction of deaths. The result, known as *natural rate of increase*, is calculated as

$$\frac{\text{Live births during the year} - \text{deaths during the year}}{\text{Midyear population}} \times 1000$$

Alternatively, it is the difference between crude birthrate and crude death rate.

GUIDELINES A formal statement about a defined task or function. Examples include clinical practice guidelines, guidelines for application of preventive screening procedures, and guidelines for ethical conduct of epidemiological practice and research.[6,9,58,117,248,260-265,506] Contrast with CODE OF CONDUCT, in which the rules are intended to be strictly adhered to and may include penalties for violation. In the terminology developed by the European Community, *directives* are stronger than *recommendations*, which are stronger than *guidelines*. In North America, *guidelines* is normal usage also for recommendations.[17]

GUTTMAN SCALE A MEASUREMENT SCALE that ranks response categories to a question, with each unit representing an increasingly strong expression of an attribute, such as pain or disability, or an attitude.[7]

GWAS See GENOME-WIDE ASSOCIATION STUDY.

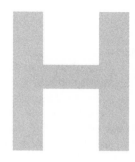

HALF-LIFE Time in which the concentration of a substance is reduced by 50%.

HALO EFFECT

1. The influence upon an observation of the observer's perception of the characteristics of the individual observed (other than the characteristic under study). The influence of the observer's recollection or knowledge of findings on a previous occasion.[38]

2. The effect (usually beneficial) that the manner, attention, and caring of a provider have on a patient during a medical encounter regardless of what medical procedures or services the encounter involves. See also PLACEBO EFFECT.

HANDICAP Reduction in a person's capacity to fulfill a social role as a consequence of an IMPAIRMENT or disability, inadequate training for the role, or other circumstances. Applied to children, the term usually refers to the presence of an impairment or other circumstance that is likely to interfere with normal growth and development or with the capacity to learn. See also DISABILITY; IMPAIRMENT; INTERNATIONAL CLASSIFICATION OF IMPAIRMENTS, DISABILITIES, AND HANDICAPS.

HANDICAP-FREE LIFE EXPECTANCY The average number of years an individual is expected to live free of handicap if current patterns of mortality and handicap continue to apply.[328] See also DISABILITY-FREE LIFE EXPECTANCY; HEALTH EXPECTANCY.

HAPHAZARD SAMPLE Sample selected based on criteria as convenience or accessibility, without regard of REPRESENTATIVENESS, GENERALIZABILITY, or even VALIDITY.

HAPMAP The International HapMap (distribution of common genetic variants in the genome).[53]

HARDY-WEINBERG EQUILIBRIUM State in which the allele and genotype frequencies do not change from one generation to the next in a population.[54,57,475] Although conditions for Hardy-Weinberg equilibrium are seldom strictly met, genotype frequencies are often consistent with the Hardy-Weinberg law. Several software packages exist to test whether a set of genotypic frequencies are in Hardy-Weinberg equilibrium.

HARDY-WEINBERG LAW The principle that both gene and genotype frequencies will remain in equilibrium in an infinitely large population in the absence of mutation, migration, selection, and nonrandom mating. If p is the frequency of one allele and q is the frequency of another and $p + q = 1$, then p^2 is the frequency of homozygotes for the allele, q^2 is the frequency of homozygotes for the other allele, and $2pq$ is the frequency of heterozygotes.

HARMONIC MEAN See MEAN, HARMONIC.

HAWTHORNE EFFECT The effect (usually positive or beneficial) of being under study upon the persons being studied; their knowledge of the study often influences their behavior. The name derives from work studies in the Western Electric Plant, Hawthorne, Illinois.[8,507-509]

HAZARD

1. The inherent capability of a natural or human-made agent or process to adversely affect human life, health, property, or activity, with the potential to cause a DISEASE, EPIDEMIC, ACCIDENT, or DISASTER.[14,38]

2. Synonym for HAZARD RATE.

HAZARD RATE (Syn: force of morbidity, instantaneous incidence rate) A theoretical measure of the probability of occurrence of an event per unit time at risk; e.g., death or new disease, at a point in time, t, defined mathematically as the limit, as Δt approaches zero, of the probability that an individual well at time t will experience the event by $t + \Delta t$, divided by Δt. It equals the PROBABILITY DENSITY of the event divided by the SURVIVAL FUNCTION for the event.[1,3,7,8,11,24]

HAZARD IDENTIFICATION See RISK ASSESSMENT.

HEALTH

1. The World Health Organization describes it in the preamble to its constitution as: "A state of complete physical, mental, and social well-being and not merely the absence of disease or infirmity."

2. The extent to which an individual or a group is able to realize aspirations and satisfy needs, and to change or cope with the environment. Health is a resource for everyday life, not the objective of living; it is a positive concept, emphasizing social and personal resources as well as physical capabilities.

3. A state characterized by anatomical, physiological, and psychological integrity; ability to perform personally valued family, work, and community roles; ability to deal with physical, biological, psychological, and social stress; a feeling of well-being; and freedom from the risk of disease and untimely death.[510]

4. A state of equilibrium between humans and the physical, biological, and social environment compatible with full functional activity.[360] A sustainable state in which humans and other living creatures with which they interact can coexist indefinitely in equilibrium. *Health* is derived from the Old English *hal*, meaning whole, sound in wind and limb. See also SUSTAINABILITY.

HEALTH-ADJUSTED LIFE EXPECTANCY Life expectancy expressed in quality-adjusted life years. See HEALTH EXPECTANCY.

HEALTH BEHAVIOR The actions we take regarding health motivated by knowledge, attitudes, practices, norms, available options, and CONTEXT. Health behavior may promote and preserve good health or be a DETERMINANT of disease.[158,511] See also DISEASE; ILLNESS BEHAVIOR; SICKNESS "CAREER."

HEALTH CARE Services provided to individuals or communities by agents of the health services or professions to promote, maintain, monitor, or restore health. Health care is not limited to medical care, which implies action by or under the supervision of a physician.[6,9,15,16,19,58,59] See also ACCESS; HEALTH EQUITY.

HEALTH CARE EPIDEMIOLOGY See HOSPITAL EPIDEMIOLOGY.

HEALTH DETERMINANTS See DETERMINANT.

HEALTH DEVELOPMENT A collective effort to improve health and well-being in all individuals and communities of a society, taking into account prevailing political, cultural, social, and economic features.

HEALTH EDUCATION Learning resources and teaching programs concerned with health—its protection and promotion. It often begins in the family and continues through primary and secondary education, with emphasis on exercise, diet, care of teeth, avoidance of sexually transmitted disease, sexuality, social relationships, smoking, alcohol, and other drugs, accidents, violence, etc. Health education may be provided by school teachers and nurses as well as by specially trained educators or physicians. It is also conducted in the community and with subsets of the population, including pregnant women, workers, people about to retire, or the elderly. See also ACQUAINTANCE NETWORK; CONTEXT; PREVENTION.

HEALTH EQUITY Fairness and impartiality in any health-related DETERMINANT or outcome. Equity in epidemiologic risk management aims to ensure that communities near sites hazardous to health are not more exposed to such risks than are more affluent communities. Achieving equity of ACCESS to public health and health care services regardless of social, ethnic, and cultural status remains a priority in many countries.[17,19,248-250,279,303-308,357-359,407,424-427,469,491] See also HEALTH INEQUITY.

HEALTH EXPECTANCY A general term for several health indicators in which LIFE EXPECTANCY is weighted for health status. The term refers to the average amount of time a person is expected to live in a given health state if current patterns of mortality and health states continue to apply; the patterns are derived from epidemiological and vital statistics data. Health expectancy is therefore a statistical estimate based on existing age-specific death rates and age-specific prevalences for health states, or on age-specific transition rates between health states.[512] Specific health expectancies are based on health states, such as those defined by the INTERNATIONAL CLASSIFICATION OF FUNCTIONING, DISABILITY AND HEALTH (ICF). Examples include DISABILITY-FREE LIFE EXPECTANCY and HANDICAP-FREE LIFE EXPECTANCY. *Health expectancy*—also called *life expectancy in good health* or *healthy life expectancy* and *disability-free life expectancy*—considers only the time spent in good health. *Health-adjusted life expectancy* and *disability-adjusted life expectancy* assign values to ranges of health states.

HEALTH FOR ALL The cultural, social, and political objective of health policy, endorsed in the WHO Declaration of Alma-Ata (1978). It was interpreted as a goal to be achieved by the year 2000, as a slogan, and as an aspiration that might be realized by implementing primary health care for all citizens of a country.

HEALTH GAP General term for a group of health indicators in which lost life expectancy is weighted by health status. They may be distinguished on the basis of a specified or implied health target or norm for a population, definition and weighting of health states, and inclusion or exclusion of values other than health. Unlike health expectancies, they can be computed for specific causes of mortality and morbidity. POTENTIAL YEARS OF LIFE LOST and EXPECTED YEARS OF LIFE LOST use a target selected arbitrarily or drawn from a life table and give all remaining years of life equal weight; DISABILITY-ADJUSTED LIFE YEARS (DALYs) assign weights to years of life remaining.

HEALTH IMPACT ASSESSMENT (HIA) An analysis, evaluation, and assessment of the consequences and implications for public health of specific social or environmental interventions or processes (e.g., construction of a power plant, a housing development or a road, legal status of immigrants). A combination of procedures, methods, and tools by which a policy, program, or project may be judged as to its potential effects on the health of a population. Considered an opportunity to integrate health into all policies, HIA aims to influence the decision-making process, addressing all determinants of health, tackling inequities, and promoting participation and empowerment in health.[13,28,210,267,302,424-426,513] See also IMPACT ASSESSMENT.

HEALTH IN ALL POLICIES (HIAP) A theme or slogan for INTERSECTORAL ACTION, horizontal health policies, and HEALTHY PUBLIC POLICIES. A strategy to help strengthen links between

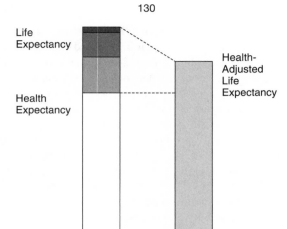

Relationships between life expectancy, health expectancy, and health-adjusted life expectancy. The shaded areas in the left bar indicate varying degrees of illness or disability. The right bar is a weighted average of all the components of the left bar and is necessarily greater than health expectancy but less than life expectancy. Source: Spasoff RA.[96] With permission.

health and other policies. HiAP addresses the effects on health across all policies (such as agriculture, education, the environment, fiscal policies, housing, and transport).[121,514] It seeks to improve health and at the same time contribute to the well-being and the wealth of the nations through structures, mechanisms, and actions planned and managed mainly by sectors other than health. An approach that promotes coordination mechanisms to ensure that the health dimension is integrated into activities of all government agencies and services. While the health sector has gradually increased its cooperation with other government sectors, industry, and nongovernmental organizations in the past four decades, other sectors have increasingly taken health and the well-being of citizens into account in their policies. The key factor enabling such a development has been that health and well-being are shared values across societal sectors. HiAP is a political result of the growing recognition of the importance of health for the overall objectives of a society: health is a key foundation stone of strategies of growth, competitiveness, and sustainable development. The HiAP approach uses an integrated approach to HEALTH IMPACT ASSESSMENT (HIA).[13,17,302,426,515] See also COSTS OF INACTION.

HEALTH INDEX A numerical indication of the health of a given population derived from a specified composite formula. The components of the formula may be INFANT MORTALITY RATES, INCIDENCE RATE for particular disease, or other HEALTH INDICATOR.

HEALTH INDICATOR A variable, susceptible to direct measurement, that reflects the state of health of a population. Examples include infant mortality rates, incidence rates based on notified cases of disease, disability days, etc. These measurements may be used as components in the calculation of a HEALTH INDEX.

HEALTH INEQUALITIES Differences in health status or in the distribution of health determinants between different population groups. Some are attributable to biological variations or free choice, and others to the external environment and social conditions outside the control of individuals. In the latter case, they may be unnecessary and avoidable as well as unjust and unfair, and cause or reflect HEALTH INEQUITY.[19,43,248,252,302,304-308,424-427,469] Health inequalities have been documented since at least the analyses of the vital statistics of

England and Wales by William Farr. See also GINI COEFFICIENT; LORENZ CURVE; SLOPE INDEX OF INEQUALITY; RELATIVE INDEX OF INEQUALITY.

HEALTH INEQUITY Systematic health inequalities that are a result of modifiable social and economic policies and practices that create barriers to opportunity. An antonym of HEALTH EQUITY.

HEALTH OUTCOMES ASSESSMENT See PATIENT-REPORTED OUTCOMES.

HEALTH PROMOTION The process of enabling people to increase control over their health and improve it. It involves the population as a whole in the context of their everyday lives rather than focusing on people at risk for specific diseases and is directed toward action on the DETERMINANTS or causes of health.[516] See also PREVENTION; PREVENTIVE MEDICINE.

HEALTH RELATED-PATIENT REPORTED OUTCOMES (HR-PRO) INSTRUMENT See MEASUREMENT, TERMINOLOGY OF; MINIMALLY IMPORTANT DIFFERENCE; PATIENT-REPORTED OUTCOMES; RELIABILITY; RESPONSIVENESS.

HEALTH RISK APPRAISAL (HRA) (Syn: health hazard appraisal) A generic term applied to methods for describing an individual's chances of becoming ill or dying from selected causes. The many versions available share several features: Starting from the average RISK of death for the individual's age and sex, a consideration of various lifestyle and physical factors indicates whether the individual is at greater or less than average risk of death from the commonest causes of death for his or her age and sex. All methods also indicate what reduction in risk could be achieved by altering any of the causal factors (e.g., cigarette smoking) that the individual could modify. The premise underlying such methods is that information on the extent to which an individual's characteristics, habits, health practices, and CONTEXT are influencing her risk of disease will assist health professionals in counseling.[12,14,27,158,212,361] See also RISK FACTOR.

HEALTH SECTOR The sector of society that is concerned with and deals with all issues and services related to health, sickness, and the provision of health care to the population.[358] See also DETERMINANT.

HEALTH SERVICES Services performed by health professionals or by others under their direction for the purpose of promoting, maintaining, or restoring health. In addition to personal health care, health services include measures for health protection, health promotion, and disease prevention.[17,307,358,432]

HEALTH SERVICES RESEARCH The integration of knowledge from clinical, epidemiological, sociological, economic, management, and other sciences in the study of the organization, functioning, and performance of health services. Health services research is usually concerned with relationships between NEEDS, DEMAND, supply, use, and OUTCOMES of health services.[5,17,26,202,270,303,499,517] The aim of health services research is evaluation. Several components of evaluative health services research are distinguished, namely:

1. Evaluation of *structure*, concerned with resources, facilities, and manpower.
2. Evaluation of *process*, concerned with matters such as where, by whom, and how health care is provided.
3. Evaluation of *output*, concerned with the amount and nature of health services provided.
4. Evaluation of *outcome*, concerned with the results—i.e., whether persons using health services experience measurable benefits, such as improved survival or reduced disability.

HEALTH STATISTICS Aggregated data describing and enumerating attributes, events, behaviors, services, resources, outcomes, or costs related to health, disease, and health services.

The data may be derived from survey instruments, medical records, and administrative documents.[24] VITAL STATISTICS are a subset of health statistics.

HEALTH STATUS The degree to which a person is able to function physically, emotionally, and socially with or without aid from the health care system. Compare QUALITY OF LIFE.

HEALTH STATUS INDEX A set of measurements designed to detect short-term fluctuations in the health of members of a population; these measurements include physical function, emotional well-being, activities of daily living, feelings, etc. Most indexes require the use of carefully composed questions designed with reference to matters of fact rather than shades of opinion. The results are usually expressed by a numerical score that gives a profile of the well-being of the individual.

HEALTH SURVEY A survey designed to provide information on the health status of a population. It may be descriptive, exploratory, or explanatory.[17,24,38,160,167,518,519] See also BIOMONITORING; CROSS-SECTIONAL STUDY; MORBIDITY SURVEY.

HEALTH SYSTEM The human and material resources that a nation or community deploys to preserve, protect, and restore health and to minimize suffering caused by disease and injury, and the corresponding administrative and organizational arrangements. The main components of the system are primary community-oriented personal health care, hospital-based specialized care, and public health services.[17,28,116,520]

HEALTH SYSTEMS RESEARCH (Syn: health research) The multidisciplinary study of health systems, including HEALTH SERVICES RESEARCH, supported by data on DETERMINANTS of health and accurate health statistics.[17,232,432,521]

HEALTH TECHNOLOGY ASSESSMENT (HTA) The formal evaluation of technologies used in health care, including medicine, and in public health. It explicitly involves not only EFFICACY but also COST-EFFECTIVENESS, COST-UTILITY, and all other aspects of technology that may be important for society. HTA supports evidence-based decision-making in health care policy and practice.[323,432,504]

HEALTHY LIFESTYLE A pattern of behavior that maximizes health protective behaviors while minimizing health risk behaviors. Such patterns of BEHAVIOR are influenced by individual, social, and environmental factors. See also BEHAVIORAL MEDICINE; LIFESTYLE MODIFICATION.

HEALTHY PUBLIC POLICIES Policies that improve the conditions under which people live, including housing, education, nutrition, access to information, child care, transportation, and necessary community and personal social and health services.[522] POLICY adequacy may be measured by its impact on POPULATION HEALTH.[13,17,24,210,279,302,366,426,438,514,515] See also COSTS OF INACTION; HEALTH IN ALL POLICIES; PREVENTION.

HEALTHY WORKER EFFECT A phenomenon observed initially in studies of occupational diseases: workers often exhibit lower overall death rates than the GENERAL POPULATION, because persons who are severely ill and chronically disabled are ordinarily excluded from employment or leave employment early.[24,523] Death rates in the general population may be inappropriate for comparison if this effect is not taken into account. Similar effects are known for military personnel, migrants, and other groups. See also OCCUPATIONAL EPIDEMIOLOGY.

HEALTHY YEARS EQUIVALENTS (HYES) A measure of health-related quality of life that incorporates two sets of preferences; one set reflects individuals' preferences for life years or duration of life, and the other reflects preferences for states of health.[524]

HEALY (healthy life years) A composite indicator that incorporates mortality and morbidity in a single number.[525] See also BURDEN OF DISEASE; DISABILITY-ADJUSTED

LIFE YEARS (DALYs); DISABILITY-FREE LIFE EXPECTANCY; LIFE EXPECTANCY FREE FROM DISABILITY (LEFD); MINIMALLY IMPORTANT DIFFERENCE; PATIENT-REPORTED OUTCOMES; QUALITY-ADJUSTED LIFE YEARS (QALY).

HELMINTH A parasitic worm that lives inside its host. Many live only in the intestinal tract of a parasitized host, while others may invade organs.[526]

HENLE–KOCH POSTULATES A set of CAUSAL CRITERIA for making judgments about microorganisms as causes of infectious diseases. They were first formulated by F. G. Jacob Henle and adapted by Robert Koch in 1877 and 1882. Koch stated that these postulates should be met before a causal relationship can be accepted between a particular bacterial parasite or disease agent and the disease in question:

1. The agent must be shown to be present in every case of the disease by isolation in pure culture.
2. The agent must not be found in cases of other disease.
3. Once isolated, the agent must be capable of reproducing the disease in experimental animals.
4. The agent must be recovered from the experimental disease produced.

Postulates 1 and 2 require complete specificity in a unique and unconfounded bacterial cause; 3 demands biological coherence; and 4 requires performance as predicted in experimental tests. Insistence on the invariable presence of the organism (postulate 1) conforms with Galileo's original notion of necessary and SUFFICIENT CAUSE. For the more recently recognized viruses and prions, which lack independent life and often specificity also, the generalizations of the postulates do not hold. Nor do they hold for DISEASES OF COMPLEX ETIOLOGY, which cause most of the BURDEN OF DISEASE in many areas of the world.[1-3,5,8,39,42,69,84,101,206-210,406,407,433,798] See also CAUSAL INFERENCE.

HERD IMMUNITY The immunity of a group or community. The resistance of a group to invasion and spread of an INFECTIOUS AGENT, based on the resistance to infection of a high proportion of individual members of the group. The resistance is a result of the number susceptible and the probability that those who are susceptible will come into contact with an infected person. Resistance of a population to invasion and spread of an infectious agent, based on the agent-specific immunity of a high proportion of the population. The proportion of the population required to be immune varies according to the agent, its transmission characteristics, the distribution of immunes and susceptibles, and other (e.g., environmental) factors.[1,24,56,67,110,188,240,527]

HERD IMMUNITY THRESHOLD The proportion of immunes in a population, above which the incidence of the infection decreases.[385] This can be mathematically expressed as

$$H = 1 - 1/R_0 = (R_0 - 1)/R_0 = (rT - 1)/rT$$

where H is the herd immunity threshold, R_0 is the BASIC REPRODUCTIVE RATE, *r is the* TRANSMISSION PARAMETER, and T is the total population.

HEREDITY The passing on of biological (including genetic) characteristics from one generation to the next. The transmission of characters and dispositions in the process of organic reproduction. Non-biological TRAITS and attributes may also be passed on from parents to offspring through education and culture (e.g., religious or health beliefs). Introduced in the biomedical sciences from the legal sphere, where it was used synonymously with INHERITANCE and *succession*.[528,529]

HERITABILITY The degree to which a TRAIT is deemed to be inherited, either through genetic means or through the shared environment. It is commonly estimated from family studies, including twin studies, based on the comparison of the variation in disease among different members of the families. However, population variation does not equal causation, nor does heritability equal genetic determination. Heritability studies do not provide valid estimates of the proportion of cases of disease that are attributable to genetic factors, neither can they estimate the proportion of cases that are due to environmental factors.[57,530] See also ATTRIBUTABLE FRACTION.

HERITABILITY, "MISSING" The large proportion of the heritability that is estimated to exist for most diseases which is not explained by the genetic variants identified so far (e.g., by GWAS). There is a wide gap between the population variation in disease explained by the results of GWAS (usually less than 10%) and estimates of heritability (often more than 50%). Most known variants confer only small increments in risk and explain a small proportion of familial clustering, leading to question how the remaining, "missing" heritability can be explained.[51,53,484] Population variation should not be confused with the proportion of disease explained by a genetic TRAIT or an environmental exposure. The genetic and environmental components are inseparable; and, as more is learned about a particular disease, it becomes inevitable that the attributable proportions for different risk factors sum to more than 100%, whereas the proportions of population variation cannot add up to more than 100%.[530]

HETEROGENEITY

1. In a broad sense, diversity, variety; e.g., of the characteristics of a population, of causes of an outcome (*etiological heterogeneity*), of clinical results.[258]
2. (Syn: effect-measure modification) Differences in stratum-specific effect measures. When such measures are not equal it is said that the effect measure is *heterogeneous* or *modified* or *varies* across strata.[1-3] See also EFFECT MODIFICATION; INTERACTION.
3. In a META-ANALYSIS, the variability in the intervention effects being evaluated in the different studies. It may be a consequence of clinical diversity (sometimes called *clinical heterogeneity*) or of methodological diversity (*methodological heterogeneity*), or both, among the studies. It manifests in the observed intervention effects being more different from each other than one would expect due to random error (chance) alone.[229,230] See also I^2; LATENT HETEROGENEITY.

HETEROSCEDASTICITY Nonconstancy of the variance of a measure over the levels of the factors under study.

HETEROZYGOUS GENOTYPE Occurs when the two alleles at a particular gene locus are different. It may include one normal allele and one mutation, or two different mutations.

HEURISTIC METHOD A method of reasoning that relies on a combination of empirical observations and unproven theories to produce a solution that may be approximately correct, useful, and defensible, but cannot be proven sound under the given conditions of application.[138] In common parlance, "rule of thumb."

HIBERNATION Survival of organisms (including arthropod vectors) during cold periods by reducing the metabolic rate.

HIERARCHICAL ANALYSIS See MULTILEVEL ANALYSIS.

HIERARCHICAL MODEL See MULTILEVEL MODEL.

HIERARCHY OF EVIDENCE A classification that attempts to order the potential quality of scientific evidence on the basis of asserted quality or value.[9,58,202] As an example, evidence was appraised by the Canadian Task Force on the Periodic Health Examination[531] and the U.S. Preventive Services Task Force[532] as a prerequisite to their recommendations about SCREENING and preventive interventions. The classes of evidence that these groups used are:

I: Evidence from at least one properly designed randomized controlled trial.

II-1: Evidence from well-designed controlled trials without RANDOM ALLOCATION.

II-2: Evidence from well-designed cohort or case-control analytic studies, preferably from more than one center or research group.

II-3: Evidence obtained from multiple time series, with or without the intervention; dramatic results in uncontrolled experiments (e.g., first use of penicillin in the 1940s).

III: Opinions of respected authorities, based on clinical experience, descriptive studies, reports of expert committees, consensus conferences, etc.

Assessments of scientific quality must take into account ethics and feasibility; e.g., randomized controlled trials or cohort studies may be unethical or unfeasible. Even when such studies are available, the actual quality of evidence they supply may not in fact be better than other studies for the issue of interest.

"HIGH-RISK" PREVENTIVE STRATEGY See STRATEGY, "HIGH-RISK."

HILL'S CONSIDERATIONS FOR CAUSATION A series of theoretical and empirical properties that causal relations may or may not satisfy, proposed by Austin Bradford Hill (1897–1991)[533] and further elaborated by Mervyn Susser[207] and others.[1,2,6,25,39,42,69,206,208,270] Sometimes referred to as "Hill's criteria" (for causal inference, of causality), even though Hill did not use "criteria" (which might suggest each is necessary); instead, Hill described them as "considerations" or "viewpoints," stating that none was necessary (although the consensus is that temporality is indeed necessary). They are:

Strength: This is defined by the size of the risk as measured by appropriate statistical estimates. The stronger, the more likely to be causal, although weak relationships may also be causal.[145] See also ABSOLUTE RISK REDUCTION; RELATIVE RISK; RISK DIFFERENCE.

Consistency: The association is consistent when results are replicated in studies in different settings using different methods. Replicability and survivability.

Specificity: Present when a putative cause produces a specific effect, as hypothesized or predicted by background theory (e.g., exogenous estrogen usage is expected to show a relation to hormone-sensitive conditions but not to seat-belt use). The particularity with which one variable predicts the occurrence of another.

Temporality: Exposure always precedes the outcome. This is the only necessary criterion of causality. Assessing the TIME ORDER is not always straightforward (e.g., because of DISEASE PROGRESSION BIAS and other causes of REVERSE CAUSATION).

Dose-response relationship: Often, but not always, an increasing level of exposure (in amount and/or time) increases risk. More generally, the relation of exposure to risk follows the expected theoretical pattern (e.g., morbidity and mortality follow a U-shaped relation to some vitamins). Causal dose-response relationships need not be linear, neither need they be MONOTONIC.

Biological plausibility: The association is coherent with firmly established knowledge on pathobiological processes. Exceptional caution is needed in this consideration: when the understanding of biological mechanisms is incomplete, implausible and speculative biological explanations will seem plausible and even coherent. See also PLAUSIBILITY.

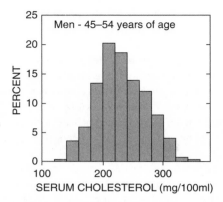

Histogram. Distribution of serum cholesterol levels in men aged 45–54 years.

Coherence: The association is compatible with existing theory and knowledge. It may be theoretical and factual, biological, clinical, epidemiological, social, or statistical. See also COHERENCE, EPIDEMIOLOGICAL.

Experiment: An experiment shows that the caused condition can be altered (e.g., prevented) by changing exposure to the putative cause.

Analogy: Similar relations have previously been established. For example, if a virus has been found to cause a particular sarcoma in dogs, it might be reasoned that a similar virus causes the analogous sarcoma in humans. This consideration is not clearly distinguishable from *plausibility* unless the latter is limited to biology and *analogy* to upper (clinical, epidemiological) levels.

See also ASSOCIATION; CAUSAL CRITERIA; CAUSALITY; CAUSATION OF DISEASE, FACTORS IN; COHERENCE; DISEASES OF COMPLEX ETIOLOGY; EVANS'S POSTULATES; HENLE-KOCH POSTULATES; MILL'S CANONS; NECESSARY CAUSE; PROBABILITY OF CAUSATION.

HISTOGRAM A graphic representation of the frequency DISTRIBUTION of a variable. Rectangles are drawn in such a way that their bases lie on a linear scale representing different intervals, and their areas are proportional to the frequencies of the values within each of the intervals.[37,102-107,505] See also BAR CHART; GRAPH.

HISTORICAL COHORT STUDY See COHORT STUDY, HISTORICAL.

HISTORICAL CONTROL Control subject(s) for whom data were collected at a time preceding that at which the data are gathered on the group being studied. Because of differences in exposure, etc., use of historical controls can lead to bias in analysis.[5]

HIV SEROCONCORDANT/-DISCORDANT Sexual partners having/not having the same HIV serological status.[56,188,217-219]

HOGBEN NUMBER A unique personal identifying number constructed by using a sequence of digits for birth date, sex, birthplace, and other identifiers. Suggested by the mathematician Lancelot Hogben (1895-1975). Used in PRIMARY CARE EPIDEMIOLOGY, usable in RECORD LINKAGE. See also IDENTIFICATION NUMBER; SOUNDEX CODE.

HOLOENDEMIC DISEASE A disease for which a high prevalent level of infection begins early in life and affects most of the child population, leading to a state of equilibrium such that the adults in a population show evidence of the disease much less commonly than do the children. In many communities malaria is a holoendemic disease.[56] See also HYPOENDEMIC DISEASE.

HOLOMIANTIC INFECTION See COMMON SOURCE EPIDEMIC.

HOMOSCEDASTICITY Constancy of the variance of a measure over the levels of the factors under study.

HOMOZYGOUS GENOTYPE Occurs when both alleles at a particular gene locus are the same. A person may be homozygous for the normal allele or for a mutation.

HORMESIS A term to define the observation of favorable biological responses at low dose exposures (i.e., in the case of chemicals, at concentrations below the toxicological threshold) to external stressors. As exposure to high concentrations of the same stressors causes detrimental biological responses, the result is a NONMONOTONIC dose response relationship characterized by a reversal of the biological response with increasing concentrations of the external stressors.[534,535] Hormesis is hypothesized for effects of radiation and a variety of endocrine-disrupting chemicals; beneficial effects of exercise, diets rich in certain plant foods, and calorie restriction, which also become harmful in extremes, might also be explained by hormetic effects.[342]

HOSPITAL-ACQUIRED INFECTION See NOSOCOMIAL INFECTION.

HOSPITAL DISCHARGE ABSTRACT SYSTEM Abstraction of MINIMUM DATA set from hospital charts for the purpose of producing summary statistics about hospitalized patients. Examples include the HOSPITAL INPATIENT ENQUIRY (HIPE) and Professional Activity Study (PAS). The statistical tabulations commonly include length of stay by final diagnosis, surgical operations, specified hospital service, and also give outcomes such as "death" and "discharged alive from hospital." This system cannot generally be used for epidemiological purposes as it is not possible to infer REPRESENTATIVENESS or to generalize; this is because the data usually lack a defined denominator and the same person may be counted more than once in the event of two or more HOSPITAL SEPARATIONS in the period of study. However, such data can be a fruitful source of cases for case-control studies. The systematic use of summary statistics on the process and outcome of hospital care began in the nineteenth century, pioneered in England by Florence Nightingale (1820–1910) and in Vienna by Ignaz Semmelweis (1818–1865). Nightingale was also a confrere of William Farr, Edwin Chadwick, and other great nineteenth-century reformers. Her *Notes on Hospitals* (1859) discussed and illustrated the importance of statistical analysis of hospital activity. Semmelweis studied the outcome of obstetric care, demonstrating that puerperal sepsis was associated with attendance on women in labor by doctors who had come from the necropsy room to the labor room without washing their hands.

HOSPITAL EPIDEMIOLOGY The application of epidemiological reasoning, knowledge, and methods in hospitals (and, by extension, in other health care settings), in order to address a wide range of preventive issues, and in particular to enhance the quality of patient care, the safety of health professionals, and the prevention of infections and other adverse outcomes.[56,69,188,217-219] See also NOSOCOMIAL INFECTION.

HOSPITAL INPATIENT ENQUIRY (HIPE) Statistical tables of a 10% sample of hospital patients in England and Wales, showing class of hospital, diagnosis, length of stay, outcomes, etc.

HOSPITAL SEPARATION A term used in commentaries on hospital statistics to describe the departure of a patient from hospital without distinguishing whether the patient departed alive or dead. The distinction is unimportant insofar as the statistics of hospital activity, such as bed occupancy, are concerned.

HOST

1. A person or other living animal, including birds and arthropods, that affords subsistence or lodgment to an INFECTIOUS AGENT under natural conditions. Some

protozoa and helminths pass successive stages in alternate hosts of different species. Hosts in which the PARASITE attains maturity or passes its sexual stage are primary or definitive hosts; those in which the parasite is in a larval or asexual state are secondary or intermediate hosts. A transport host is a CARRIER in which the organism remains alive but does not undergo development.[188]

2. In an epidemiological context, the host may also be the population or group; biological, social, and behavioral characteristics of this group relevant to health are called "host factors."

HOST, DEFINITIVE   In parasitology, the host in which sexual maturation occurs. In malaria, the mosquito (invertebrate host).[56]

HOST, INTERMEDIATE   In parasitology, the host in which asexual forms of the PARASITE develop. In malaria, this is a human or other vertebrate mammal or bird (vertebrate host).

HOT SPOT   A slang or jargon term for a problematic area (e.g., one where the disease or event is highly prevalent or severe), a nidus of infection, a section of an industrial or nuclear plant where a hazardous process is conducted or from which hazardous material can escape into the environment.[13,116,267]

HOUSEHOLD   One or more persons who occupy a dwelling (i.e., a place that provides shelter, cooking, washing, and sleeping facilities); this may or may not be a family. The term is also used to describe the dwelling unit in which the persons live.[469]

HOUSEHOLD SAMPLE SURVEY   A survey of persons in a sample of households. This, in many variations, is a favored method of gathering data for health-related and many other purposes. The households may be sampled in any of several ways—e.g., by cluster or use of random numbers in relation to numbered dwelling units. The survey may be conducted by interview, telephone survey, or self-completed responses to presented questions. The method is used in developing nations as well as in the industrial world.[110,160,167,518,519]

HuGENet   See HUMAN GENOME EPIDEMIOLOGY NETWORK.

HUMAN BLOOD INDEX   Proportion of insect vectors found to contain human blood.

HUMAN DEVELOPMENT   The process by which individuals, social groups, and populations achieve their potential level of health and well-being. Human development includes physical, biological, mental, emotional, educational, economic, social, and cultural components; some of these are expressed in the HUMAN DEVELOPMENT INDEX (HDI).[33,38,123,249]

HUMAN DEVELOPMENT INDEX (HDI)   A composite index combining indicators representing three dimensions—longevity (life expectancy at birth); knowledge (adult literacy rate and mean years of schooling); and income (real GDP per capita in purchasing-power-parity dollars) (Source: World Bank). The validity of the HDI has been questioned because it attempts to express multiple complex variables on a unidimensional scale.

HUMAN ECOLOGY   The study of human groups as influenced by environmental factors, including social and behavioral factors. A macrolevel, holistic approach to the study of human organization. See also ECOLOGY.

HUMAN GENOME EPIDEMIOLOGY NETWORK (HuGENet)   A collaboration committed to assess the impact of human genome variation on POPULATION HEALTH and how genetic information can be used to improve health and prevent disease, including assessment of the role and quality of genetic tests for screening.[1,91,536] See also GENETIC EPIDEMIOLOGY; MOLECULAR EPIDEMIOLOGY.

HUMAN IMMUNODEFICIENCY VIRUS (HIV)   The pathogenic organism responsible for the acquired immunodeficiency syndrome (AIDS). Formerly known as the lymphadenopathy virus (LAV), the name given by Montagnier et al., the original French discoverers, in 1983; it was also known as the human T-cell lymphotropic virus, type III (HTLV-III), the name given by Gallo et al. to the virus they reported in 1984. The retrovirus responsible for HIV disease, it is transmissible in blood, serum, semen, breast-feeding, body tissues, and other body fluids. The are two types: HIV-1 (responsible for the AIDS pandemic) and HIV-2; they compromise immune responses to organisms that are destroyed by a healthy immune system. The virus is immunologically unstable, but it produces antibodies that can be detected by Western blot and ELISA tests of blood, serum, semen, saliva, etc.[56,188,217-219]

HUMAN IMMUNODEFICIENCY VIRUS (HIV) INFECTION The SURVEILLANCE case definition for HIV infection uses either laboratory, clinical, or other criteria. The laboratory criteria include positive screening test for HIV antibody and other laboratory evidence of HIV infection. Additional criteria of the presence and absence of HIV infection are defined for infants.

HUMAN MICROBIOME The entirety of microorganisms living and interacting in and on the human body. The term broadly covers the human ecosystem of viruses, BACTERIA, archaea, and eukaryotes.

HYGIENE The principles and laws governing the preservation of health and their practical application. Practices conducive to good health. The sum of the procedures and techniques that promote human development and harmonious adaptation to the individual's milieu.[56,69]

HYPERENDEMIC DISEASE A disease that is constantly present at a high incidence and/or prevalence and affects most or all age groups equally.

HYPERGEOMETRIC DISTRIBUTION The exact probability DISTRIBUTION of the frequencies in a two-by-two contingency table, conditional on both the marginal frequencies being fixed at their observed levels.[1,7] Used for FISHER'S EXACT TEST.

HYPNOZOITE Dormant form of malaria PARASITES found in liver cells. After sporozoites (inoculated by the mosquito) invade liver cells, some sporozoites develop into dormant forms (the hypnozoites), which do not cause symptoms. Hypnozoites can become activated months or years after the initial infection, producing a RELAPSE.[56]

HYPOENDEMIC DISEASE A disease that is constantly present at a low incidence or prevalence and affects a small proportion of individuals in the area. A term commonly used in malaria literature to refer to regions with low transmission. See also HOLOENDEMIC DISEASE.

HYPOTHESIS, SCIENTIFIC

1. A supposition, arrived at from observation or reflection, that leads to refutable predictions.
2. Any conjecture cast in a form that will allow it to be tested and, possibly, refuted.[1,3,6,26,270] See also NULL HYPOTHESIS; TEST HYPOTHESIS.

HYPOTHESIS TESTING, STATISTICAL It usually refers to the procedure of comparing a P value to a pre-assigned ALPHA LEVEL (α; usually, α is taken to be 0.05) to determine whether to provisionally reject the TEST HYPOTHESIS (if $P < \alpha$); or, equivalently, of comparing a TEST STATISTIC to a value that the statistic has a probability α of exceeding. Statistical hypothesis testing is under criticism, in part because study analysis always requires broader considerations than whether $P < \alpha$, and also because evaluation of scientific hypotheses must consider and synthesize results from truly diverse lines of evidence.[1,3,7,34,37] See ALPHA LEVEL; CAUSAL INFERENCE; P VALUE; SIGNIFICANCE, STATISTICAL.

HYPOTHETICO-DEDUCTIVE METHOD Karl Popper's term (following Hume) for DEDUCTIVE LOGIC as applied to scientific research. For Popper, science is that which is testable.[537]

Therefore, a hypothesis must be stated a priori in order to test its *survivability* by efforts to reject it. Popper's underlying assumption is that no hypothesis can be truly verified and proved; at best, it can be *corroborated*. Many scientists reject Popper's assumption of *nonverifiability*. In order to verify ideas and hypotheses, scientists are often obliged to argue by induction.[1,2,39-42,538] That does not preclude using the hypothetico-deductive method as a testing procedure.[84] See also INDUCTION; INDUCTIVE REASONING; LOGIC.

I^2 A measure of HETEROGENEITY in a META-ANALYSIS.[229,230,258,300]

IATROGENESIS Literally, "doctor-generated"; often, broadly used to refer to adverse effects of preventive, diagnostic, therapeutic, surgical, and other medical, biotechnical, cosmetic, sanitary, and public health products, services, procedures, interventions, or policies. The process through which a professional activity generates an adverse health effect. There is a natural plurality of views on what constitutes iatrogenesis and its scope. Medicine and public health are obviously not the only professions that cause adverse health effects.[28,236,248,539] See also PREVENTION, QUATERNARY.

IATROGENIC EFFECT An adverse effect on health resulting from the activity of a health professional or organization. Adverse health effects are also caused by non-sanitary organizations (e.g., unjustified fear caused by DISEASE MONGERING by a marketing campaign).

ICD Acronym for the International Statistical Classification of Diseases and Related Health Problems. See INTERNATIONAL CLASSIFICATION OF DISEASES (ICD).

ICEBERG PHENOMENON That portion of disease which remains unrecorded or undetected despite physicians' diagnostic endeavors and community disease SURVEILLANCE procedures is referred to as the "submerged portion of the iceberg." Detected or diagnosed disease is the "tip of the iceberg." The submerged portion comprises disease not medically attended, medically attended but not accurately diagnosed, and diagnosed but not reported.[540] Other terms have been proposed to describe this concept in parts of the world where icebergs are unknown (e.g., "ears of the hippopotamus," "crocodile's nose").

ICF See INTERNATIONAL CLASSIFICATION OF FUNCTIONING, DISABILITY AND HEALTH.

ICHPPC See INTERNATIONAL CLASSIFICATION OF HEALTH PROBLEMS IN PRIMARY CARE.

IDENTIFIABLE, IDENTIFIABILITY (Syn: estimability)
1. A parameter is (consistently) identifiable from data and a probability model for the data if there is an estimator which is statistically CONSISTENT for the parameter when that model is correct.[1,101]
2. A parameter is (Fisher) identifiable if there is an estimator that gives back the parameter when applied to the data expected under the model.
3. A parameter is identifiable if the probability distribution for the data changes whenever the parameter changes, so that the distribution is always a one-to-one function of the parameter.[541]

IDENTIFICATION NUMBER, IDENTIFYING NUMBER Unique number given to every individual at birth or at some other milestone. The Nordic and Baltic nations have a system based on a sequence of digits for birth date, sex, birthplace, and additional digits for each individual. Other systems (e.g., National Insurance number in the United Kingdom, Social Security number in the United States, and Social Insurance number in Canada) are sometimes used but are neither universal nor unique, being sometimes applied to whole families or at least to more than one individual. See also HOGBEN NUMBER; SOUNDEX CODE.

IDIOSYNCRASY a distinctive characteristic or peculiarity of an individual. In PHARMA-COEPIDEMIOLOGY, it means an abnormal reaction, sometimes genetically influenced, following the administration of a medication.

IDU Injectiong drug user. See also IVDU.

IEA International Epidemiological Association, founded 1954. The aims of the IEA are to facilitate communication among those engaged in research and teaching in epidemiology throughout the world and to engage in the development and use of epidemiological methods in all fields of health including social, community, and preventive medicine and health services administration. These aims are achieved by holding scientific meetings and seminars, the publication of journals and reports, and by many other activities that take place every year on all continents. The official journal of the IEA is the *International Journal of Epidemiology*.[542]

IEA-EEF International Epidemiological Association European Epidemiology Federation. The European Epidemiology Federation (EEF) is an official group within the IEA. All members of the IEA in Europe are automatically members of the EEF. Most national associations of epidemiologists in the European region are also part of the EEF.[542]

IGNORABILITY

1. In CAUSAL ANALYSIS, the assumption that the POTENTIAL OUTCOMES under alternative possible exposure or treatment assignments are independent of the actual exposure or treatment assignments; if this independence holds within levels of covariates used for adjustment, the ignorability is said to be *conditional*. *Weak* or *marginal* ignorability is the assumption that each potential outcome (e.g., the outcome when exposed and the outcome when unexposed) is independent of actual exposure or treatment, while *strong* or *joint* ignorability is the assumption that the list of all the potential outcomes considered at once (i.e., the entire VECTOR of potential outcomes) is independent of actual exposure or treatment. Weak ignorability is equivalent to the assumption of no CONFOUNDING.[2,101]

2. In SAMPLING, the assumption that selection is independent of the study variables. Ignorable selection implies there will be no SELECTION BIAS in any measure of association computed from the data.

ILLNESS See DISEASE.

ILLNESS BEHAVIOR Conduct of persons in response to abnormal body signals. Such behavior influences the manner in which people monitor their bodies, define and interpret their symptoms, take remedial actions, and use the health care system. See also HEALTH BEHAVIOR.

IMMORTAL TIME BIAS A form of bias in which persons are credited with time at risk during which the effect cannot possibly occur (e.g., due to the PATHOPHYSIOLOGY of the disease or the clinical pharmacology of the drug); thus, such persons have an artificially low event rate. Inclusion of the "immortal" time is dependent on not having the outcome during that time. If persons cannot be defined as exposed until they reach a certain length of follow-up, and the same criterion is not applied to persons defined as unexposed, then "immortal time" will be included only for the exposed, resulting in a downward (negative) bias in the association between exposure and outcome.[1,543]

IMMUNITY, ACQUIRED Resistance acquired by a host as a result of previous exposure to a natural PATHOGEN or foreign substance for the host, e.g., immunity to measles resulting from a prior infection with measles virus.[56,67,188,196,217-219]

IMMUNITY, ACTIVE Resistance developed in response to stimulus by an antigen (infecting agent or vaccine) and usually characterized by the presence of antibody produced by the host.[67]

IMMUNITY, NATURAL Species-determined inherent resistance to a disease agent, e.g., resistance of humans to the virus of canine distemper.[67,69]

IMMUNITY, PASSIVE Immunity conferred by an antibody produced in another host and acquired naturally by an infant from its mother or artificially by administration of an antibody-containing preparation (antiserum or immune globulin).[67]

IMMUNITY, SPECIFIC A state of altered responsiveness to a specific substance acquired through immunization or natural infection. For certain diseases (e.g., measles, chickenpox), this protection generally lasts for the life of the individual.[56,67,69,188]

IMMUNIZATION (Syn: vaccination) The artificial induction of active immunity by introducing into a vulnerable host the specific antigen of a pathogenic organism. Protection of susceptible individuals from COMMUNICABLE DISEASE by administration of a living modified agent (as in yellow fever), a suspension of killed organisms (as in whooping cough), or an inactivated toxin (as in tetanus). Temporary passive immunization can be produced by administration of antibody in the form of immune globulin in some conditions.[56,67,69,110,188,240]

IMMUNIZATION, LATENT The process of developing immunity by a single or repeated inapparent asymptomatic infection. Not necessarily related to latent infection.[67,240] See also IMMUNITY, ACQUIRED.

IMMUNOGENICITY The ability of an INFECTIOUS AGENT to induce specific immunity.[67,69,240]

IMPACT EVALUATION

1. The measurement and assessment of changes in an outcome that are attributable to a defined intervention, program, or policy. Based on causal models, it requires to control for factors other than the intervention that might account for the observed changes.[13,17,426,544] See also ATTRIBUTABLE FRACTION; HEALTH IMPACT ASSESSMENT.

2. The application of experimental and quasi-experimental methods to approximate the COUNTERFACTUAL ideal in order to evaluate the impact of an intervention and attribute specific changes to a particular program or policy.[545]

IMPACT FACTOR See BIBLIOGRAPHIC IMPACT FACTOR (BIF).

IMPACT FRACTION A generalization of the ATTRIBUTABLE FRACTION FOR THE POPULATION that accommodates both hazardous and protective exposures, multiple levels of exposure, incomplete elimination of exposure, diffusion, or response to exposure. To define this measure, let IF be the impact fraction, let p' and p'' be the prevalences of an exposure level before and after an intervention program, and let RR be the Risk Ratio or Rate Ratio (properly adjusted for bias) relative to a common reference level, depending on whether impact on risks or rates is being estimated. Then the impact fraction is given by

$$IF = \frac{\Sigma(p' - p'')RR}{\Sigma p' RR} \text{ (with decreasing risk)}$$

$$\text{or } IF = \frac{\Sigma(p'' - p')RR}{\Sigma p' RR} \text{ (with increasing risk)}$$

where the sums are over all exposure categories; in the reference category, RR = 1. For a continuous exposure, the sums are replaced by integrals.[1]

IMPACT NUMBERS Four quantities related to the ATTRIBUTABLE FRACTION, used to communicate risk in terms relevant to four groups (total population, diseased, exposed, and exposed with disease). Expands the concept of NUMBER NEEDED TO TREAT. (1) Population Impact Number (PIN) is the number of subjects in the total population among whom one case is attributable to the RISK FACTOR. (2) Case Impact Number (CIN) is the number of people with the disease or outcome among whom one case is attributable to the risk factor. (3) Exposure Impact Number (EIN) is the number of people with the exposure among whom one case is attributable to the risk factor. (4) Exposed Cases Impact Number (ECIN) is the number of exposed people with the disease or outcome among whom one case is attributable to the risk factor.[546]

IMPAIRMENT A physical or mental defect at the level of a body system or organ.[26] See also DISABILITY; HANDICAP; INTERNATIONAL CLASSIFICATION OF FUNCTIONING, DISABILITY AND HEALTH (ICF).

IMPLEMENTATION SCIENCE The study and utilization of scientific methods to promote the INTEGRATION of research findings and evidence-based practices into policy and practice, thereby improving the EFFECTIVENESS of the health system.[547,548]

IMPRINTING

1. A form of learned behavior (e.g., the expression of affection) in a critical period of development early in a young animal's life, including a human; it may result from the interaction between mother and infant, or from exposure to one of a restricted set of stimuli.[549]

2. AN EPIGENETIC phenomenon in which the expression of a gene varies depending on whether it is inherited from the mother or the father.

IMPUTATION The process of replacing some missing values in a large-scale epidemiological or social research study, when all other relevant parameters and values are known for an individual, by inserting an AVERAGE or other plausible value. The process may be subject to biases and errors, and must be disclosed in reporting the results.[116]

INAPPARENT INFECTION (Syn: subclinical infection) The presence of infection in a host without occurrence of recognizable clinical signs or symptoms. Of epidemiologic significance because hosts so infected, although apparently well, may serve as silent or inapparent disseminators of the infectious agent.[20,22,56,69,188,217-219] See also DISEASE, PRECLINICAL; DISEASE, SUBCLINICAL; VECTOR-BORNE INFECTION.

INCEPTION COHORT A group of individuals identified and assembled for subsequent study at an early and uniform point in the course of the specified health condition; e.g., near the onset (inception) of symptoms, soon after diagnosis, at detection of a clinically significant pathological event. Thus, subjects who succumbed to or completely recovered from the disorder are included with those whose disease persisted.[6,203,239] Failure to select an inception cohort often severely biases studies on the NATURAL HISTORY OF DISEASE. See also STUDY BASE.

INCEPTION RATE The rate at which new spells of illness occur in a population. A term applied principally to short-term spells of illness, such as acute respiratory infections, and preferred by some epidemiologists because an annual incidence rate for such conditions may exceed the numbers in the population at risk.

INCIDENCE (Syn: incidence number) The number of instances of illness commencing, or of persons falling ill, during a given period in a specified population. More generally, the number of new health-related events in a defined population within a specified period of time. It may be measured as a frequency count, a rate, or a proportion.[1,3,24,270]

INCIDENCE DENSITY The average PERSON-TIME incidence rate. Sometimes used to describe the hazard.[1,3,8] See FORCE OF MORBIDITY; HAZARD RATE; INCIDENCE RATE.

INCIDENCE-DENSITY RATIO **(IDR)** The ratio of two incidence densities. See also RATE RATIO.

INCIDENCE PROPORTION (Syn: cumulative incidence, attack rate, RISK) Incidence expressed as a proportion of a cohort or group at risk. A measure of risk. The time period must be specified for it to be meaningful, although that period may be defined in a way that varies across individuals. For example, the proportion of childbirth labors that end with cesarean delivery is defined for the time period of labor, which may vary considerably. When the time period is constant across individuals and the incidence proportion is small, it is approximated by the INCIDENCE RATE multiplied by the length of the period. The proportion of a CLOSED POPULATION at risk for a disease that develops the disease during a specified interval.[1,3]

INCIDENCE RATE The RATE at which new events occur in a population. The numerator is the number of new events that occur in a defined period or other physical span.[1] Most often, the denominator is the PERSON-TIME at risk of the event during this period; it may instead be in other units, such as passenger-miles. The incidence rate most often used in public health practice is calculated from the formula

$$\frac{\text{Number of new events in specified period}}{\text{Average number of persons exposed to risk during this period}} \times 10^n$$

Strictly speaking, this ratio is neither a rate nor a proportion but is instead the rate multiplied by the length of the specified period. If the period is a year, the ratio is nonetheless often called the *annual incidence rate*. The average size of the population is often the estimated population size at the midperiod. The ratio divided by the length of the period is an estimate of the person-time incidence rate (i.e., the rate per 10^n person-years). If the ratio is small, as with many chronic diseases, it is also a good estimate of the CUMULATIVE INCIDENCE over the period (e.g., a year). If the number of new cases during a specified period is divided by the sum of the person-time units at risk for all persons during the period, the result is the PERSON-TIME INCIDENCE RATE.

INCIDENCE RATE RATIO The incidence rate in the exposed group divided by the incidence rate in the unexposed group. See also RATE RATIO.

INCIDENCE STUDY See COHORT STUDY.

INCIDENT NUMBER See INCIDENCE.

INCREMENTAL PROGNOSTIC IMPACT See DISCRIMINATORY ACCURACY.

INCUBATION PERIOD
1. The time interval between invasion by an INFECTIOUS AGENT and appearance of the first sign or symptom of the disease in question.[1,8,20,22,24,56,188,217-219] See also LATENT PERIOD.
2. In a VECTOR, the period between entry of the infectious agent into the vector and the time at which the vector becomes infective; i.e., transmission of the infectious agent from the vector to a fresh final host is possible (EXTRINSIC INCUBATION PERIOD).

INDEPENDENCE, STATISTICAL Two events are said to be (statistically) independent if the occurrence of one is in no way predictable from the occurrence of the other. Two variables are said to be independent if the distribution of values of one is the same for all values of the other. *Independence* is the antonym of ASSOCIATION.[1]

INDEPENDENT VARIABLE
1. In REGRESSION ANALYSIS, one of (commonly) several variables that appear as arguments on the right-hand side of a regression equation; a REGRESSOR or covariate.[1,3,7,36,244,270] In this usage there is no implication of CAUSALITY; in fact, the so-called indendent

variable might come after or even be affected by the DEPENDENT VARIABLE. See also REGRESSAND.

2. A variable that is hypothesized to influence an event or state (the dependent variable); i.e., the independent variable is not influenced by the event but may cause (or contribute to the occurrence of) the event, or contribute to change the (physiological, environmental, socioeconomic) status.

INDEX

1. In epidemiology and related sciences, this word usually means a rating scale, e.g., a set of numbers derived from a series of observations of specified variables. Examples include the many varieties of health status index, scoring systems for severity or stage of cancer, heart murmurs, mental retardation, etc.

2. One way to present a measurement with adjustment to the results of other measurements; e.g., the Quetelet Index II, now called body-mass index (BMI), is an index of this type (weight is corrected for height).

INDEX CASE The first case in a family or other defined group to come to the attention of the investigator. See also PRIMARY CASE; PROBAND.

INDEX GROUP (Syn: index series)

1. In an experiment, the group receiving the experimental regimen.
2. In a case-control study, the cases.
3. In a cohort study, the exposed group.[1-3,197,795]

INDICATOR VARIABLE In statistics, a variable taking only one of two possible values, one (usually 1) indicating the presence of a condition, and the other (usually zero) indicating absence of the condition. Used extensively in REGRESSION ANALYSIS.[1,244]

INDIRECT ADJUSTMENT See STANDARDIZATION.

INDIRECT BERKSON'S BIAS See BERKSON'S BIAS.

INDIRECT COSTS See COST, INDIRECT.

INDIRECT OBSTETRIC DEATH See MATERNAL MORTALITY.

INDIVIDUAL THINKING In medicine, it is the ability to make the best prediction and decision in terms of diagnosis, therapy, and prognosis for the health and well-being of the individual patient, and to adapt the management to the unique characteristics of a partly unpredictable person. Medicine is the art and science of individual thinking on health. True medicine is always personalized.[6,9,42,58,91,201,203] See also ATOMISTIC FALLACY; CLINICAL STUDY; ECOLOGICAL FALLACY; POPULATION THINKING; PREVENTION PARADOX; STRATEGY, "HIGH-RISK."

INDIVIDUAL VARIATION Two types are distinguished:

1. *Intraindividual variation:* The variation of biological variables within the same individual, depending upon circumstances such as the phase of certain body rhythms and the presence or absence of emotional stress. These variables do not have a precise value, but rather a range. Examples include diurnal variation in body temperature, fluctuation of blood pressure, blood sugar, etc.

2. *Interindividual variation:* As used by Darwin, the term means variation *between* individuals. This is the preferred usage; the first usage is better described as personal variation.

INDUCTION

1. Any method of rational or logical analysis that proceeds from the particular to the general. Although no infallible method of logical reasoning exists, general scientific theories require induction. Conceptually bright ideas and breakthroughs and

ordinary statistical inference belong to the realm of induction. Contrast DEDUCTION. See also HYPOTHETICO-DEDUCTIVE METHOD; INDUCTIVE REASONING; INFERENCE.

2. Causation of the initiating events of a disease process (e.g., induction of initiating mutations at the beginning of CARCINOGENESIS).

INDUCTION PERIOD The interval between initiation of exposure to the causal agent and initiation of the health process; e.g., from onset of exposure to the disease-causing agent to initiation of the disease.[1,24] See also CARCINOGEN; INCUBATION PERIOD; LATENCY PERIOD.

INDUCTIVE LOGIC See INDUCTIVE REASONING.

INDUCTIVE REASONING Argument that seeks to reach generalizations by reasoning from an assembly of particular observations. Francis Bacon was its first proponent as applied to science. It remains an important mode of (and a collection of methods for) scientific reasoning. Its status as a "logic" has long been debated, and many authors prefer to use the term INDUCTION instead of "inductive logic." Scholars have argued that statistical theories are attempts to put induction on a logically sound footing.[1,39-42,85,128] See also DEDUCTIVE LOGIC; HYPOTHETICO-DEDUCTIVE METHOD; INFERENCE.

INDUSTRIAL HYGIENE The science devoted to recognition, evaluation, and control of environmental factors or stresses arising from or in the workplace that may cause sickness or impaired health and well-being. The profession that anticipates and controls unhealthy conditions of work to prevent illness among employees. See also OCCUPATIONAL HEALTH.

INFANT MORTALITY RATE (IMR) A measure of the yearly frequency of deaths in children less than one year old. The denominator is the number of live births in the same year. Defined as

$$\text{Infant Mortality rate} = \frac{\text{number of deaths in a year of children less than 1 year of age}}{\text{number of live births in the same year}} \times 1000$$

It is often a useful indicator of the level of health in a population. The denominator is an approximation of the population at risk. This indicator is a ratio rather than a rate or a proportion.

INFECTIBILITY The host characteristic or state in which the host is capable of being infected.[56] See also INFECTIOUSNESS; INFECTIVITY.

INFECTION (Syn: colonization) The entry and development or multiplication of an INFECTIOUS AGENT in an organism, including the body of humans and animals. Infection is not synonymous with infectious disease; the result may be inapparent or manifest. The presence of living infectious agents on exterior surfaces of the body is called INFESTATION (e.g., pediculosis, scabies). Whereas infection implies multiplication of the infectious agent, contamination corresponds just to a contact with the agent. The presence of living infectious agents upon articles of apparel or soiled articles is not an infection, but CONTAMINATION of such articles.[20,22,48,56,69,160,188,217-219] See also INAPPARENT INFECTION; SURVEILLANCE; TRANSMISSION OF INFECTION.

INFECTION, CLINICAL Infection that causes clinical signs.[56,188,196,217-219]

INFECTION, GRADIENT OF The range of manifestations of illness in the host reflecting the response to an infectious agent, which extends from death at one extreme to inapparent infection at the other. The frequency of these manifestations varies with the specific infectious disease. For example, human infection with the virus of rabies is almost invariably fatal, whereas a high proportion of persons infected in childhood with the virus of hepatitis A experience a subclinical or mild clinical infection.[56,69,188,196,217-219]

INFECTION, LATENT PERIOD OF The time between initiation of infection and first shedding or excretion of the agent.

INFECTION RATE The incidence rate of manifest plus inapparent infections (the latter determined by seroepidemiology).[56,188,196]

INFECTION, SUBCLINICAL See INAPPARENT INFECTION.

INFECTION TRANSMISSION PARAMETER (r) The proportion of total possible contacts between infectious cases and susceptibles that lead to new infections.[56]

INFECTIOUS AGENT A microscopic element that is capable of causing a disease in a susceptible host. A non-eukaryotic microscopic element (prokaryotic, akaryotic) foreign to an organism, capable of multiplying in such organism. Examples include VIRUS, BACTERIA, fungus, PARASITES, and PRIONS. Infectious agents cause INFECTIONS and INFECTIOUS DISEASES.[20-22,56,188,217-219]

INFECTIOUS DISEASE A disease due to an infectious agent. While some infectious diseases are CONTAGIOUS, others are noncontagious. All INFECTIONS and INFESTATIONS are COMMUNICABLE DISEASES.

INFECTIOUS DISEASE CYCLE See CHAIN OF INFECTION.

INFECTIOUSNESS A characteristic of a disease that concerns the relative ease with which it is transmitted to other hosts. A droplet spread disease, for instance, is more infectious than one spread by direct contact. The characteristics of the portals of exit and entry are thus also determinants of infectiousness, as are the agent characteristics of ability to survive away from the host and of infectivity.[56]

INFECTIVITY

1. The characteristic of the disease agent that embodies capability to enter, survive, and multiply in the host.[56] A measure of infectivity is the SECONDARY ATTACK RATE.
2. The proportion of exposures, in defined circumstances, that result in infection.

INFERENCE The process of evolving from observations and axioms to generalizations. In statistics, the development of generalization from sample data, usually with calculated degrees of uncertainty. CAUSAL INFERENCE from observational data is a key task of epidemiology and other sciences as sociology, education, behavioral sciences, demography, economics, or health services research; these disciplines share methodological frameworks for causal inference.[1-3,50,84,101,206]

INFESTATION CONTAMINATION of a living organism by a PARASITE, and then the state of such hosting organism. The development on (rather than in) the body of a pathogenic agent; e.g., body lice. All infestations are COMMUNICABLE DISEASES. Some authors use the term also to describe invasion of the gut by parasitic worms. Not all authors restrict infestation to parasites.[8,20-22,56,188,217-219]

INFLUENCE ANALYSIS Methods to determine the ROBUSTNESS of an assessment by examining the extent to which results are affected by changes in recorded measurements and variables. The aim is to identify recorded values that made the largest contribution to the results or to find a solution that is relatively stable for the most commonly occurring values of these variables.[1,101] See also OUTLIERS; SENSITIVITY ANALYSIS.

INFODEMIOLOGY The study of the distribution of information and its determinants in an electronic medium, specifically the Internet, or in a population, with the aim to inform public health and public policies. Examples include the analysis of queries from Internet search engines to predict disease outbreaks, automated tools to measure information diffusion and knowledge translation, and tracking the effectiveness of health-marketing campaigns.[550] See also INFOVEILLANCE.

INFORMATICS The study of information and the ways to handle it, especially by means of information technology, i.e., computers and other electronic devices for rapid transfer, processing, and analysis of large amounts of data.[7]

INFORMATION Facts that have been arranged and/or transformed to provide the basis for interpretation and conversion into knowledge.

INFORMATION BIAS (Syn: measurement bias, observation bias)

1. A flaw in measuring exposure, covariate, or outcome variables that results in different quality (ACCURACY) of information between comparison groups.[1,3,5-9,42,270,276,551,797] The occurrence of information biases may not be independent of the occurrence of SELECTION BIASES. Furthermore, in clinical and epidemiological studies MISCLASS- IFICATION is often differential.

2. Bias in an estimate arising from measurement errors or MISCLASSIFICATION.

INFORMATION SYSTEM As applied in epidemiology, a combination of vital and health statistical data from multiple sources, used to derive information about the health needs, health resources, costs, use of health services, and outcomes of use by the population of a specified jurisdiction. The term may also describe the automatic release from computers of stored information in response to programmed stimuli. For example, parents can be notified when their children are due to receive booster doses of an immunizing agent against infectious disease.[67]

INFORMATION THEORY Mathematical theory dealing with the nature, effectiveness, and ACCURACY of information transfer.

INFORMED CONSENT Voluntary consent given by a subject or a responsible proxy (e.g., a parent) for participation in a study, immunization program, treatment regimen, etc., after being informed of the purpose, methods, procedures, potential benefits and potential harms, and, when relevant, the degree of uncertainty about such outcomes. The essential criteria of informed consent are that the subject has both knowledge and comprehension, that consent is freely given without duress or undue influence, and that the right of withdrawal at any time is clearly communicated to the subject.[26] Other aspects of informed consent in the context of epidemiological and biomedical research are specified in *International Ethical Guidelines for Epidemiological Studies* (Geneva: CIOMS/WHO, 2008) and *International Ethical Guidelines for Biomedical Research Involving Human Subjects* (Geneva: CIOMS/ WHO, 2002).[59,73-77,116-118,259-265] See also ETHICS.

INFOVEILLANCE The use of INFODEMIOLOGY for SURVEILLANCE.[48,160,550]

INGELFINGER RULE Rule developed by Franz Ingelfinger (1910–1980), former editor of the *New England Journal of Medicine*: "The Journal undertakes review with the understanding that neither the substance of the article nor the figures or tables have been published or will be submitted for publication during the period of review. This restriction does not apply to abstracts published in connection with scientific meetings or to news reports based on public presentations at such meetings."[552]

A revision of the rule imposed a news embargo[553] until the pertinent article is published. The rule (or modifications of it) has been adopted by many high-quality peer-reviewed academic journals. The aims of the rule are to eliminate duplicate publication and reduce uncritical acceptance of original work prior to PEER REVIEW and publication.[554]

INHERITANCE In the biological sciences, a pattern followed by the transmission from generation to generation of a given phenotype (e.g., a disease). There are several types of complex inheritance (non-Mendelian) and of Mendelian inheritance (dominant, recessive, sex-linked).[54,57] See also EPIGENETIC INHERITANCE; HEREDITY; HERITABILITY; MENDEL'S LAWS.

INHERITANCE, CULTURAL The transfer from one generation to another of values, beliefs, and customs (e.g., solidarity values, patriotic feelings, lifestyle). The process through which individuals receive, learn, and adopt norms and behaviors (e.g., on nutrition, smoking and alcohol, exercise, sleeping and dietary patterns, symptom reporting, meaning-making) from family, school, and other spheres of society.[555]

INJURY The transfer of one of the forms of physical energy (mechanical, chemical, thermal) in amounts or at rates that exceed the threshold of human tolerance. It may also result from lack of essential energy such as oxygen (e.g., drowning) or heat (e.g., hypothermia).[556] See also OCCUPATIONAL INJURY.

INOCULATION See VACCINATION.

INPUT
1. The sum total of resources and energies purposefully engaged (e.g., in a health program) in order to intervene in the spontaneous operation of a system.
2. The basic resources required in terms of manpower, money, materials, and time.

INSTANTANEOUS INCIDENCE RATE See FORCE OF MORBIDITY.

INSTITUTIONAL REVIEW BOARD (IRB) The term used in the United States to describe the standing committee in a medical school, hospital, or other health care facility that is charged with ensuring the safety and well-being of human subjects involved in research. The IRB is responsible for ethical review of research proposals. Many synonyms are used in other countries, e.g., *Ethical Review Committee, Research Ethics Board*. All research, including EPIDEMIOLOGICAL RESEARCH, that involves human subjects must be approved by an institutional review board or equivalent body.[26,59,73-77,116-118,259-265]

INSTRUMENTAL ERROR Error due to faults arising in any or in all aspects of a measuring instrument, i.e., CALIBRATION, ACCURACY, PRECISION, etc. Also applied to error arising from impure reagents, wrong dilutions, etc.

INSTRUMENT
1. A device or questionnaire used to obtain measurements.
2. An instrumental variable.

INSTRUMENTAL VARIABLE See INSTRUMENTAL VARIABLE ANALYSIS.

INSTRUMENTAL VARIABLE ANALYSIS Method that under certain assumptions allows the estimation of causal effects even in the presence of RESIDUAL CONFOUNDING of the exposure and effect. Originally used in econometrics and some social sciences. An instrumental variable, or instrument, has to meet the following conditions: (1) it is associated with the exposure, (2) it affects the outcome only through the exposure, and (3) it does not share any (uncontrolled) common cause with the outcome.[1,2,7,557] See also CONFOUNDING BIAS.

INTEGRATED DISCRIMINATION IMPROVEMENT See DISCRIMINATORY ACCURACY.

INTEGRATION
1. The action or process of integrating. To integrate: to make a new whole; to combine parts into a new system and get them to interact so that the system expresses functions unavailable to the parts. The organizing of elements to form a coherent whole or system. Integration of knowledge from different scientific disciplines yields knowledge that no discipline alone may achieve.
2. In HEALTH PROMOTION and disease PREVENTION, strategies that target several risk factors, use multiple STRATEGIES at various levels of influence, and require

INTERSECTORAL ACTION.[121] Integration entails multiplicity (more than one RISK FACTOR, level, sector, agent), and synergy resulting from multiplicity.[17]

3. In mathematics, the process of finding an antiderivative of a given function, or its value over a specified interval.

4. In medicine, the coordination within the brain of different nervous processes (e.g., sensory information from the inner ear and the eye must be integrated by the brain with other stimuli for the sense of balance and to control posture).

Integration is no less crucial to science than to the functioning of postmodern societies. Examples: quality public transportation favors integration of disabled individuals and disadvantaged groups into society; integration of racial and ethnic minorities into the educational system; integration of preventive services into clinical care.[25,33,426,548]

Synonyms, analogies, and METAPHORS are here useful as well: *integration* involves and refers to interaction, dialogue, complicity, performance, symbiosis, sharing, pooling, porousness, amalgamation, merging, coalescing, fusing, welding, blending, weaving.

INTEGRATIVE RESEARCH Research that integrates knowledge, data, methods, techniques, reasoning, and other scientific and cultural referents from multiple disciplines, approaches, and levels of analysis to generate knowledge that no discipline alone could achieve. For instance, research that integrates cultural, economic, and other "macro-level" or contextual factors with individual factors, as in MUTILEVEL ANALYSIS; analyses of the relationships among gene structure, expression, and function; research on the relationships among molecular pathways, PATHOPHYSIOLOGY, and clinical phenotypes, as in clinical pharmacology and clinical genetics; research that integrates interactions among environmental, genetic, and epigenetic processes.[1,13,26,33,80,146,202,323,339,411,548,799] Epidemiology is an inherently integrative discipline, and so are many of its subspecialities, and approaches, like CLINICAL and MOLECULAR EPIDEMIOLOGY, SOCIAL EPIDEMIOLOGY or ENVIRONMENTAL EPIDEMIOLOGY; DEVELOPMENTAL AND LIFE COURSE EPIDEMIOLOGY, for instance, attempts to integrate biological and social risk processes.[23,25] See also CLINICAL STUDY; HEALTH IMPACT ASSESSMENT; TRANSDISCIPLINARITY; REDUCTIONISM.

INTENTION-TO-TREAT ANALYSIS (ITT) A fundamental way to analyze a RANDOMIZED CONTROLLED TRIAL in which all subjects allocated to each arm of the trial are analyzed "as intended" upon randomization, whether or not they actually received the exposure allocated or completed treatment.[1,2,24,272,443-445,641,800] Failure to follow this approach defeats the main purpose and advantage of RANDOM ALLOCATION and can cause serious CONFOUNDING BIAS. This approach is virtually always required as part of the primary analysis of studies aiming to influence clinical or public-health decisions and policy formulation. It may be complemented by an explanatory analysis, in which subjects are analyzed according to the exposure they actually experienced (with adjustment for possible confounders, i.e., with an analytic approach similar to an observational cohort study), or in which some participants (e.g., subjects who complied poorly with the protocol) are excluded from analyses.[1,6,9,26,58,101,270,272,641,800] An intention-to-treat analysis does not determine whether and how to impute missing data on the outcome measure. Because of its pragmatic nature, ITT can underestimate treatment efficacy or have a low explanatory capacity; INSTRUMENTAL VARIABLE ANALYSIS and G-ESTIMATION can be used to address this bias while making use of the random allocation. See also EFFECTIVENESS; EXPLANATORY STUDY; PRAGMATIC STUDY.

INTERACTION

1. The interdependent, reciprocal, or mutual operation, action, or effect of two or more factors to produce, prevent, control, mediate, or otherwise influence the occurrence

of an event. In a broad sense, a *biological interaction* involves a biological, physical, chemical, cellular, or physiological interdependent operation of two or more factors.[14,33] See also ANTAGONISM; SYNERGISM.

2. Differences in the effect measure for one factor at different levels of another factor. See also EFFECT MODIFICATION; EFFECT MODIFIER; HETEROGENEITY.

3. The necessity for a product term in a LINEAR MODEL (Syn: statistical interaction). Based on the study substantive hypotheses, the (biological, clinical, social) nature of the interaction must guide its mathematical formulation and treatment.[1-3,5,7,8,25,37,270,798]

INTERMEDIATE VARIABLE (Syn: contingent variable, intervening (causal) variable, mediating variable, mediator) A variable that occurs in a causal pathway from a causal (independent) variable to an outcome (dependent) variable. It causes variation in the outcome variable and itself is caused to vary by the original causal variable. Such a variable will be associated with both the causal and the outcome variables.[1,24,101,791]

INTERNAL CONSISTENCY See CONSISTENCY.

INTERNAL VALIDITY See VALIDITY.

INTERNATIONAL CLASSIFICATION OF DISEASES (ICD) Short name (and acronym) for the International Statistical Classification of Diseases and Related Health Problems. The classification of specific conditions and groups of conditions determined by an internationally representative group of experts who advise the World Health Organization, which publishes the complete list in periodic revisions. Every disease entity is assigned a number. There are 21 major divisions *(chapters)* and a hierarchical arrangement of subdivisions *(rubrics)* within each in the tenth revision. Some chapters are "etiological," e.g., Infective and Parasitic Conditions; others relate to body systems, e.g., Circulatory System; and some to classes of condition, e.g., neoplasms, injury (violence). The heterogeneity of categories reflects prevailing uncertainties about causes of disease (and classification in relation to causes). The tenth revision of the manual, known as ICD-10, was endorsed by the World Health Assembly in 1990 and came into use in WHO Member States as from 1994. The eleventh revision of the classification has already started and will continue until 2015.[558] It is the latest in a series of international classifications dating back to the BERTILLON CLASSIFICATION. ICD-10 has 21 chapters:

I (A00–B99): Certain infectious and parasitic diseases

II (C00–C97): Neoplasms

III (D50–D89): Diseases of the blood and blood-forming organs and certain disorders involving the immune mechanism

IV (E00–E90): Endocrine, nutritional, and metabolic diseases

V (F00–F99): Mental and behavioral disorders

VI (G00–G99): Diseases of the nervous system

VII (H00–H59): Diseases of the eye and adnexa

VIII (H60–H95): Diseases of the ear and mastoid process

IX (I00–I99): Diseases of the circulatory system

X (J00–J99): Diseases of the respiratory system

XI (K00–K93): Diseases of the digestive system

XII (L00–L99): Diseases of the skin and subcutaneous tissue

XIII (M00–M99): Diseases of the musculoskeletal system and connective tissue

XIV (N00–N99): Diseases of the genitourinary system

XV (O00–O99): Pregnancy, childbirth, and the puerperium

XVI (P00–P96): Certain conditions originating in the perinatal period

XVII (Q00–Q99): Congenital malformations, deformations, and chromosomal abnormalities

XVIII (R00–R99): Symptoms, signs, and abnormal clinical and laboratory findings not elsewhere classified

XIX (S00–T98): Injury, poisoning, and certain other consequences of external causes

XX (V01–Y99): External causes of morbidity and mortality

XXI (Z00–Z99): Factors influencing health status and contact with health services

INTERNATIONAL CLASSIFICATION OF FUNCTIONING, DISABILITY AND HEALTH (ICF) A classification of the health components of functioning and disability. Approved by the World Health Assembly in 2001, it replaced the INTERNATIONAL CLASSIFICATION OF IMPAIRMENTS, DISABILITIES, AND HANDICAPS (ICIDH).[558] The ICF classification is structured around the following broad components: body functions and structure; activities (related to tasks and actions by an individual) and participation (involvement in a life situation); and additional information on severity and environmental factors. It complements WHO's INTERNATIONAL CLASSIFICATION OF DISEASES (ICD), which contains information on diagnosis and health condition, but not on functional status. The ICD and ICF constitute the core classifications in the WHO Family of International Classifications.

INTERNATIONAL CLASSIFICATION OF HEALTH PROBLEMS IN PRIMARY CARE (ICHPPC) See INTERNATIONAL CLASSIFICATION OF PRIMARY CARE, SECOND EDITION REVISED (ICPC-2-R).

INTERNATIONAL CLASSIFICATION OF IMPAIRMENTS, DISABILITIES, AND HANDICAPS (ICIDH) See INTERNATIONAL CLASSIFICATION OF FUNCTIONING, DISABILITY AND HEALTH (ICF).

INTERNATIONAL CLASSIFICATION OF PRIMARY CARE, SECOND EDITION REVISED (ICPC-2-R) The official classification of the World Organization of Family Doctors (WONCA).[559,560] WONCA is also known as the World Organization of Family Doctors. ICPC includes three elements of the doctor-patient encounter: the REASON FOR ENCOUNTER (RFE), the diagnosis, and the treatment or other action or intervention. It is a biaxial classification system based on chapters and components. It uses three-digit alphanumeric codes with mnemonic qualities to facilitate its day-to-day use. Chapters, each with an alpha code, form one axis; components with rubrics having a two-digit numeric code form the second axis. The components deal with symptoms and complaints, diagnoses and therapeutic interventions, administrative procedures, and diseases. ICPC includes a detailed conversion system for linking with ICD-10 codes. See also PROBLEM-ORIENTED MEDICAL RECORD.

INTERNATIONAL COMPARISONS In epidemiology and public health, comparing regions or nations of the world in terms of disease DETERMINANTS or OUTCOMES, as in tables that show the rank order of vital statistics such as INFANT MORTALITY RATES, death or incidence rates for cancer, heart disease, etc. The limits of such comparisons include the shifting tides of diagnostic fashion and the varying definitions that prevail from one nation to another. See also CROSS-CULTURAL STUDY; VALIDITY.

INTERNATIONAL FORM OF MEDICAL CERTIFICATE OF CAUSES OF DEATH In adopting the tenth revision of ICD in 1990, the World Health Assembly resolved that causes of death to be entered on the medical certificate of cause of death are all those diseases, morbid conditions, or injuries that either resulted in or contributed to death and the circumstances of the accident or violence that produced such injuries. Antecedent causes and other significant conditions are also to be recorded. See DEATH CERTIFICATE.

INTERNATIONAL HEALTH REGULATIONS (IHR) A legally binding agreement that the world has been implementing since 2007. It aims to improve global public health security by providing a new framework for the coordination of the management of events that may constitute a public health emergency of international concern, and the capacity of countries to detect, assess, notify, and respond to public health threats. Countries have to meet IHR core SURVEILLANCE and response requirements, including at airports and ports.[48]

INTERNATIONAL NOMENCLATURE OF DISEASES (IND) Since 1970, the Council for International Organizations of the Medical Sciences (CIOMS) and the WHO have collaborated in preparing an International Nomenclature of Diseases (IND). This is a complement to the ICD. The purpose of the IND is to provide a single recommended name for every disease entity. The criteria for selection are that the name should be specific, unambiguous, as self-descriptive and as simple as possible, and based on cause whenever feasible.

INTERNATIONAL STATISTICAL CLASSIFICATION OF DISEASES AND RELATED HEALTH PROBLEMS See INTERNATIONAL CLASSIFICATION OF DISEASES (ICD).

INTERPOLATE, INTERPOLATION To predict the value of variates within the range of observations; the resulting prediction.[1,78,796]

INTERPRETABILITY The degree to which a person can assign qualitative meaning (i.e., clinical or other commonly understood connotations) to an instrument's quantitative scores or change in scores. Strictly, it is not a measurement property, but an important characteristic or quality of a measurement instrument. In a wider sense, it may be a characteristic of a study design—including the analysis—that yields results with a clear (or, alternatively, obscure, low) interpretation, meaning or significance.[1-3,5,274,795] See also MEASUREMENT, TERMINOLOGY OF.

INTERPRETIVE BIAS (Syn: interpretative bias, bias of interpretation)
1. Error arising from inference and speculation. Among others, two sources of the error are (a) failure of the investigators to consider all relevant and rationally defensible interpretations coherent with the facts and to assess the scientific support of each interpretation and (b) mishandling of cases that constitute exceptions to some general conclusion.
2. Errors that can occur in interpretative and evaluative processes of scientific evidence.[99] The interpretive process is a necessary and inevitable aspect of science. Science commonly has subjective, emotional, cultural, and socioeconomic components.[561] Although unbiased interpretation of data is as important as performing rigorous experiments, evaluative processes are seldom totally objective or completely independent of scientists' convictions and organizations, theoretical apparatus, and CONTEXT. Good science inevitably embodies a certain—often, fruitful—tension between methods, results, and convictions.[201,202,562] Recognition of interpretative processes in epidemiology should not lead to a relativism or to deem all claims to knowledge equally (in)valid because of subjectivity. Views that the science enterprise is totally objective are mythical and ignore human and social elements.[38,87,99,117,135-137,248,323,335,339,467,563] See also AUXILIARY HYPOTHESIS BIAS; COGNITIVE DISSONANCE BIAS; CONFIRMATION BIAS; DATA DREDGING; DEBIASING; INVESTIGATOR BIAS; MECHANISTIC BIAS; PUBLICATION BIAS; RESCUE BIAS.

INTERSECTORAL ACTION (Syn: intersectoral collaboration) Activities and STRATEGIES involving several components of the body politic (e.g., the health sector, the education sector, the housing sector) that, working together, can enhance health conditions more effectively than when working independently of one another.[13,213,302,426,514,515] See also HEALTH IN ALL POLICIES; HEALTHY PUBLIC POLICIES.

INTERVAL The set containing all numbers between two given numbers.

INTERVAL ESTIMATE An interval within which a parameter under study is stated to lie with a particular degree of confidence, likelihood, or probability based on a statistical analysis of data.[1,7,270] See also CONFIDENCE INTERVAL; LIKELIHOOD INTERVAL; POSTERIOR INTERVAL.

INTERVAL INCIDENCE DENSITY See PERSON-TIME INCIDENCE RATE.

INTERVAL SCALE See MEASUREMENT SCALE.

INTERVENING CAUSE See INTERMEDIATE VARIABLE.

INTERVENING VARIABLE

1. Synonym for INTERMEDIATE VARIABLE.
2. A variable whose value is altered in order to block or alter the effect(s) of another factor.[1-3,101,791]

See also CAUSALITY; CAUSAL DIAGRAM.

INTERVENTION-GENERATED INEQUALITIES Unintended and unwanted variations in outcomes for individuals or population subgroups that result from any element of a health-related or social intervention.[19,248,305,424-426]

INTERVENTION INDEX An estimate of the impact of a therapeutic or preventive intervention.[564] It is the ratio of the number of persons whose risk level must change to prevent one premature death to the total number at risk. See also ABSOLUTE RISK REDUCTION; IMPACT NUMBERS; NUMBER NEEDED TO TREAT; RELATIVE RISK REDUCTION.

INTERVENTION STUDY An investigation involving intentional change in some aspect of the status of the subjects, e.g., introduction of a preventive or therapeutic regimen or an intervention designed to test a hypothesized relationship; usually an EXPERIMENT such as a RANDOMIZED CONTROLLED TRIAL.

INTERVIEWER BIAS Systematic error due to interviewers' subconscious or conscious gathering of selective data or influencing subject response.[1,7,551] See also INFORMATION BIAS.

INTERVIEW SCHEDULE The precisely designed set of questions used in an interview. See also SURVEY INSTRUMENT.

INTRACLASS CORRELATION

1. In sibship studies in genetics, the variance of genotypes as a proportion of the variance of phenotypes.
2. In surveys and group-randomized studies, the extent to which members of a group (cluster) resemble each other more than they resemble members of other groups (clusters). See DESIGN EFFECT.

"INVERSE CARE LAW" A "law" that states that "the availability of good medical care tends to vary inversely with the need for it in the population served".[19,565] Health systems are consistently inequitable, providing more and higher quality services to the well-off, who need them less, than to the poor, who are unable to obtain them. In the absence of concerted efforts to ensure that health systems reach disadvantaged groups more effectively, such inequities are likely to continue.[19,426]

INVERSE PROBABILITY WEIGHTING A method for the estimation of causal effects under the assumption of no RESIDUAL CONFOUNDING. An extension of inverse weighting methods used in survey sampling and missing data analysis. A method for adjustment for selection bias, for nonrandomly missing data, or for differences among exposure or treatment groups in the estimation of causal effects (adjustment for measured confounders).[1,2,7] In adjustment for selection bias, individuals are weighted by the inverse of their probability of selection into the study analysis. In adjustment for differences among compared populations, individuals in the study population are weighted by the inverse of their probability of having the level of exposure or treatment they actually have given their covariates, creating a pseudopopulation in which there is no confounding by the covariates used to estimate the weights.[566] When no regression models are used, inverse probability weighting and STANDARDIZATION are mathematically equivalent. See also G-ESTIMATION; MARGINAL STRUCTURAL MODELS.

INVESTIGATOR BIAS Bias on the part of the investigators of a study toward a particular research result, exposure or outcome, or the consequences of such bias.[117] Examples include bias arising from financial stakes or other CONFLICTS OF INTEREST; commitment to past hypotheses, statements, or results; moral or political leanings; or other sources of prejudicial handling in the design, conduct, analysis, or interpretation of a study or literature review. See also COGNITIVE DISSONANCE BIAS; CONFIRMATION BIAS; DATA DREDGING; INTERPRETIVE BIAS; PUBLICATION BIAS; RESCUE BIAS.

INVOLUNTARY SMOKING (Syn: passive smoking) Exposure to secondhand tobacco smoke, a mixture of exhaled mainstream smoke and sidestream smoke released from a smoldering cigarette or other smoking device (e.g., cigar, pipe, bidi) and diluted with ambient air. It involves inhaling carcinogens and other toxic components present in secondhand tobacco smoke; the latter is sometimes referred to as "ENVIRONMENTAL" TOBACCO SMOKE (ETS). It includes both smoke exhaled by smokers and smoke released directly from burning tobacco into ambient air; the latter is called SIDESTREAM SMOKE and contains higher proportions of carcinogenic substances and other toxic agents than exhaled smoke. The adjective *involuntary* is preferable to *passive*, as the latter may imply acquiescence. Involuntary smoking (exposure to secondhand or "environmental" tobacco smoke) is carcinogenic to humans (group 1 of IARC).[13,27,179]

ISLAND POPULATION A group of individuals isolated from larger groups and possessing a relatively limited gene pool; alternatively, a group that is immunologically isolated and may therefore be unduly susceptible to infection with alien pathogens.

ISODEMOGRAPHIC MAP (Syn: density-equalizing map) A type of cartogram in which the size of each area (e.g., country, state, county) is proportional to its population.

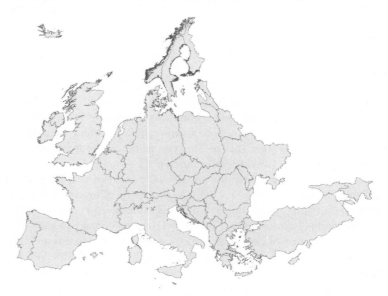

Isodemographic map. Map of Europe based on 2009 population. Source: Finnish Cancer Registry.[567] With permission.

ISOLATE (noun)

1. In genetics, a subpopulation, generally small, in which matings take place exclusively with other members of the same subpopulation.
2. In microbiology, a pure culture of an organism.

ISOLATION

1. In microbiology, the separation of an organism from others, usually by making serial cultures.
2. Separation, for the period of communicability, of infected persons or animals from others under such conditions as to prevent or limit the transmission of the infectious agent from those infected to those who are susceptible or who may spread the agent to others. The *CDC Guidelines for Isolation Precautions in Hospitals* expanded on the blood and body fluid precautions described below. *Control of Communicable Disease Manual*[188] lists seven categories of isolation:

   a. *Strict isolation:* To prevent transmission of highly contagious or virulent infections that may be spread by both air and contact. The specifications include a private room and the use of masks, gowns, and gloves for all persons entering the room. Special ventilation requirements with the room at negative pressure to surrounding areas are desirable.

   b. *Contact isolation:* For less highly transmissible or serious infections and diseases or conditions that are spread primarily by close or direct contact. A private room is indicated, but patients infected with the same pathogen may share a room. Masks are indicated for those who come close to the patient, gowns are indicated if soiling is likely, and gloves are indicated for touching infectious material.

   c. *Respiratory isolation:* To prevent transmission of infectious diseases over short distances through the air, a private room is indicated, but patients infected with the same organism may share a room. In addition to the basic requirements, masks are indicated for those who come in close contact with the patient; gowns and gloves are not indicated.

   d. *Tuberculosis isolation (AFB isolation):* For patients with pulmonary tuberculosis who have a positive sputum smear or chest x-rays that strongly suggest active tuberculosis. Specifications include use of a private room with special ventilation and closed door. Masks are used only if the patient is coughing and does not reliably and consistently cover the mouth. Gowns are used to prevent gross CONTAMINATION of clothing. Gloves are not indicated.

   e. *Enteric precautions:* For infections transmitted by direct or indirect contact with feces. Specifications include use of a private room if patient hygiene is poor. Masks are not indicated; gowns should be used if soiling is likely, and gloves are to be used for touching contaminated materials.

   f. *Drainage/secretion precautions:* To prevent infections transmitted by direct or indirect contact with purulent material or drainage from an infected body site. A private room and masking are not indicated; gowns should be used if soiling is likely and gloves used for touching contaminated materials.

   g. *Blood/body fluid precautions:* To prevent infections that are transmitted by direct or indirect contact with infected blood or body fluids. In addition to the basic requirements, a private room is indicated if patient hygiene is poor; masks are not indicated; gowns should be used if soiling of clothing with blood or body fluids is likely. Gloves should be used for touching blood or body fluids. Blood and body fluid precautions should be used consistently for all patients regardless of their blood-borne infection status ("universal blood and body fluid precautions"). These are intended to prevent parenteral, mucous membrane, and non-intact-skin exposure of health care workers to blood-borne pathogens. Protective barriers include gloves, gowns, masks, and protective eyewear.[69,188] See also QUARANTINE; UNIVERSAL PRECAUTIONS.

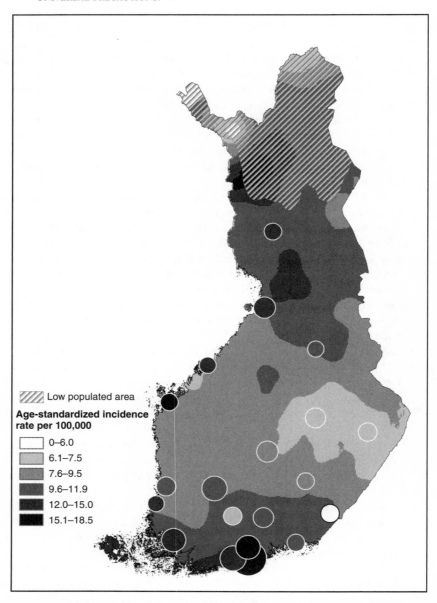

Isoline map. Regional differences in age-standardized incidence (world standard population) of lung cancer among females in Finland, 2001–2008. The rates for the 20 larger cities are shown in circles (but not with isolines) with size proportional to the number of inhabitants. Source: Finnish Cancer Registry.[567] With permission.

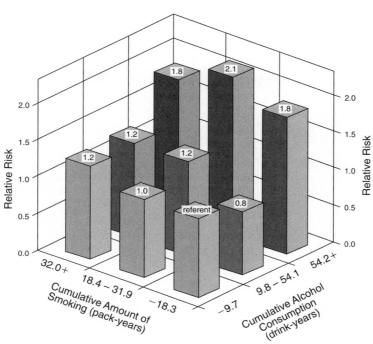

Isometric chart. Relative risks of hepatocellular carcinoma according to cumulative alcohol consumption and amount of smoking. Source: Tanaka K, et al.[568] With permission.

ISOLINE MAP (Syn: contour map, isarithmic map, isopleth map) A type of map with continuous lines connecting points of the same value.

ISOMETRIC CHART A chart or graph that portrays three dimensions on a plane surface.

IVDU Intravenous Drug User. A high-risk group for transmission of blood-borne infection (e.g., HIV, hepatitis C).

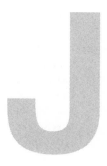

JACKKNIFE A technique for estimating the variance and the bias of an estimator. If the sample size is n, the estimator is applied to each subsample of size $n - 1$, obtained by dropping a measurement from analysis. The sum of squared differences between each of the resulting estimates and their mean, multiplied by $(n - 1)/n$, is the jackknife estimate of variance; the difference between the mean and the original estimate, multiplied by $(n - 1)$, is the jackknife estimate of bias.[7]

JAMES LIND LIBRARY A digital library created to explain and illustrate the historical development of effective therapies, and to help people understand fair tests of treatments in health care.[569]

JARMAN SCORE An index of community-wide social deprivation, used mainly by general practitioners in the United Kingdom.[570] Unlike the TOWNSEND SCORE, the Jarman score has no theoretical basis; it uses weighted values for percentages of elderly persons living alone; children aged under 5 years; single-parent families; social class V (unskilled workers); the unemployed; overcrowded dwellings; changed address in the past year; ethnic minorities. See also GINI COEFFICIENT; OVERCROWDING; TOWNSEND SCORE.

JOB EXPOSURE MATRIX (JEM) A cross-classification of jobs and occupational exposures. Some matrices are based on tasks instead of jobs. JEMs may be based on the assessment by experts of likely occupational exposures (chemical, physical, biological, and psychosocial agents) for an open or fixed list of jobs (or tasks), usually coded according to some established national or international classification system. Some JEMs also include information for different calendar time periods.[7,571]

JOB STRAIN MODELS Models to explain work-related stress based on dimensions such as job demands (e.g., psychological conflicts related to work pace or workload) and job control (or job decision latitude, defined as the combination of the worker's job decision-making authority and use of skills on the job). Jobs characterized by high "psychological workload demands" and low "decision latitude" increase risk for psychological job strain. Research in OCCUPATIONAL EPIDEMIOLOGY has shown that increased decision latitude is often preferable to reduced job demand so as to reduce mental strain. A third dimension is workplace social support (given by workmates, supervisors, employers), which may act as an effect modifier over the other two dimensions.[571,572]

JONES CRITERIA A set of clinical and laboratory findings for the diagnosis of rheumatic fever. The criteria include presence of group A hemolytic streptococcal infection; major manifestations (carditis, polyarthritis, etc.); minor manifestations (fever, arthralgia, etc.); ancillary tests (raised erythrocyte sedimentation rate, C-reactive protein, etc.).

JUSTICE

1. A morally defensible distribution of benefits and rewards in society. Equity or fairness—e.g., regarding the fair distribution in the population of benefits and risks of research, health care, or other goods. There is a diversity of views among epidemiologists worldwide with respect to the idea that health is a basic need and therefore an issue of social justice.[248] See also ETHICS; HEALTH EQUITY.

2. In law, the successful administration of the rule of law.

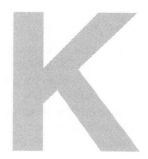

Kakwani index A measure of the progressivity or regressivity of health care payment systems. It is the difference between a CONCENTRATION INDEX for payments and the GINI COEFFICIENT for incomes, equivalent to twice the area between the payments concentration curve and the LORENZ CURVE. A positive value indicates progressivity, a negative value regressivity, and zero indicates proportionality.[573]

KAP (KNOWLEDGE, ATTITUDES, PRACTICE) SURVEY A formal survey, using face-to-face interviews, in which people are asked standardized pretested questions dealing with their knowledge of, attitudes toward, and use of contraceptive methods. Detailed reproductive histories and attitudes toward desired family size are also elicited. Analysis of responses provides much useful information on family planning and gives estimates of possible future TRENDS in population structure. The term has sometimes been used to describe other varieties of surveys of knowledge, attitudes, and practice (e.g., health promotion in general or, in particular, cigarette smoking).

Kaplan-Meier estimate (Syn: product-limit method) A nonparametric method of estimating survival probabilities from LIFE TABLES.[1,3,7,24,37,574] This combines calculated probabilities of survival and estimates to allow for CENSORED observations, which are assumed to occur randomly. The intervals are defined as ending each time an event (death, withdrawal) occurs; they may therefore be unequal.

kappa index A measure of the degree of nonrandom agreement between observers or measurements of the same categorical variable

$$\kappa \frac{P_0 - P_e}{1 - P_e}$$

where P_0 is the proportion of times the measurements agree and P_e is the proportion of times they can be expected to agree by chance alone. If the measurements agree more often than expected by chance, kappa is positive; if concordance is complete, kappa = 1; if there is no more nor less than chance concordance, kappa = 0; if the measurements disagree more than expected by chance, kappa is negative. Kappa coefficients are measures of correlation between categorical variables often used as reliability or validity coefficients.[3,7,8,24,26,37,575-577]

Kato-Katz technique A laboratory method for preparing human stool samples prior to searching and quantifying PARASITE eggs, used in epidemiological studies on schistosomiasis and other helminth diseases.

Kendall's tau See CORRELATION COEFFICIENT.

KERNEL DENSITY ESTIMATION A non-parametric method for estimating the PROBABILITY DENSITY of a random variable. A data smoothing technique through which a population distribution can be visualized without assuming anything about the exact form of that distribution. It can help in visualizing temporal and spatial distributions of disease, including clustering and spread.[1,34,37,578]

KNOWLEDGE CONSTRUCTION A production-oriented approach to the understanding of science. Analyses of how knowledge is created identify strategies that scientists employ in their work, discursive fact production, features of fact construction shared across contemporary sciences, EPISTEMIC COMMUNITIES, and social media, devices of representation, laboratory cultures, object reconfiguration in the laboratory, knowledge cultures and their "epistemic machineries" (i.e., their machineries of knowledge production), or social mechanisms of consensus formation.[135-137,323,339,579] Research on the process of knowledge production has improved understanding of science as a practical accomplishment. See also SOCIOLOGY OF SCIENTIFIC KNOWLEDGE.

KNOWLEDGE INTEGRATION The process of selecting, storing, analyzing, integrating, and disseminating information within and across disciplines. It includes knowledge management, synthesis, and translation. It aims to maximize the use of collected scientific information and accelerate translation of discoveries into individual and population health benefits.[6,9,33,58,339,485,548,580]

KOCH'S POSTULATES See HENLE-KOCH POSTULATES. See also causality; EVANS'S POSTULATES.

KRIGING A method to smooth data from spatially scattered point measurements. Used in geographic epidemiology, first used in the earth sciences.[581] It relies on analysis of the spatial variability of the data and allows representation of the variable under study as a continuous process throughout the region under study. Named for its developer, Danie G. Krige (1919 – 2013).

KURTOSIS The extent to which a unimodal DISTRIBUTION is peaked.

LANDSCAPE EPIDEMIOLOGY A branch or subspecialty of epidemiology that studies how the temporal dynamics of host, vector, and populations interact spatially within a permissive environment to enable transmission. It aims at understanding the vegetational, geologic, and other physical conditions that are necessary for or otherwise influence the maintenance and transmission of a particular pathogen or disease. GEOGRAPHICAL INFORMATION SYSTEMS are used to analyze such conditions.

LARGE-SAMPLE METHOD (Syn: asymptotic method) Any statistical method based on an approximation that becomes more accurate as sample size increases.[1] Examples include chi-square tests on a set of frequencies, and normal tests and interval estimates from frequency data.

LATE MATERNAL DEATH See MATERNAL MORTALITY.

LATENT CLASS ANALYSIS A type of statistical analysis used to group variables or observations into distinct clusters, based on the assumption that there are underlying "latent classes" within the data. Analysis can be cross-sectional or longitudinal, i.e., it can identify clusters of distinct variables at a point in time or patterns in a variable over a period of time.[1,7]

LATENT HETEROGENEITY Epidemiological data that are too heterogeneous to be described by a simple MATHEMATICAL MODEL such as the BINOMIAL DISTRIBUTION or the POISSON DISTRIBUTION; suggestive of the effect of unidentified risk factors.[1]

LATENT IMMUNIZATION See IMMUNIZATION, LATENT.

LATENT INFECTION Persistence of an infectious agent within the host without symptoms (and often without demonstrable presence in blood, tissues, or bodily secretions of the host).[56,188]

LATENCY PERIOD (Syn: latent period, latency) Two mutually incompatible definitions are commonly used in the health and life sciences:

1. The interval from initiation of the disease to clinical emergence of the disease (e.g., appearance of manifestations) or to disease detection. Thus, according to this definition, the latency period begins when the INDUCTION PERIOD ends, at the initiation of the disease. In infectious disease epidemiology, the period between exposure and the onset of infectiousness (which may be shorter or longer than the INCUBATION PERIOD).

2. The interval between initiation of exposure to the causal agent and appearance or detection of the health process; e.g., from onset of exposure to the disease-causing agent to appearance of manifestations of the disease. Thus, according to this definition, the latency period begins when the INDUCTION PERIOD begins, at the initiation of exposure to the disease-causing agent.

The two definitions agree that the latency period ends when the disease becomes clinically apparent and/or detectable; in the first definition, the induction period is followed by the latency period (there is no overlap), whereas in the second definition the latency period includes the entire induction period.[7,8] See also SOJOURN TIME.

LATIN SQUARE A statistical design for experiments that aim at removing from the experimental error the variation from two sources, which may be identified with the rows and columns of the square. In such a design, the allocation of k experimental treatments in the cells of a k by k (latin) square is such that each treatment occurs exactly once in each row and column.[7,37,283]

LAW OF LARGE NUMBERS This law, enunciated by Jacob Bernoulli (1654–1705), states that the accuracy of a sample mean is increased (or the standard error of a statistic is reduced) as the numbers studied increase. The larger the sample, the more likely it is to be representative of the "universe" population. This law is valid only with unbiased samples.[7,34]

LAY EPIDEMIOLOGY Investigations with epidemiological intent undertaken by non-epidemiologists. Individuals or groups may interpret health risks through observation and discussion of cases of illness and death in personal networks and the public arena, as well as from informal evidence arising from sources as mass media and social NETWORKS.[13,582] See also POPULAR EPIDEMIOLOGY.

LEAD TIME The time gained in treating or controlling a disease when detection is earlier than usual (e.g., in the presymptomatic stage), as when screening procedures are used for EARLY DETECTION OF DISEASE.[5-9,58]

LEAD-TIME BIAS (Syn: zero time shift) Overestimation of survival time, owing to the backward shift in the starting point for measuring survival that arises when diseases such as cancer are detected early, as by screening procedures. A systematic error arising when follow-up of groups does not begin at comparable stages in the natural history of a condition. For example, interventions for women whose breast cancer is detected by screening cannot be validly compared with interventions for women whose disease is first detected by clinical examination at a later stage of the disease.[3,5-9,24,203] See also INCEPTION COHORT; ZERO-TIME SHIFT.

LEAST SQUARES A principle of estimation, attributed to Gauss and Legendre, in which the estimates of a set of parameters in a statistical model are those quantities that minimize the sum of squared differences between the observed values of the dependent variable and the values predicted by the model.[3,7,34,37,796]

LEDERMANN FORMULA The observation by Ledermann[583] that the frequency distribution of alcohol consumption in the population of consumers may be log-normal; the curve is sharply skewed—approximately one-third of drinkers consume more than 60% of the total amount of alcohol. Among drinkers, the proportion of persons with alcoholism remains constant at around 7%–9%. The pattern of consumption of illicit drugs among users may also be log-normal. Questions have been raised, however, about the validity of some assumptions upon which the formula is based.

LEGAL EPIDEMIOLOGY A cross-disciplinary field that uses epidemiological evidence to help assess legal questions on causation and breach of duty in fields such as personal injury law, criminal law, environmental law, and insurance law.[584]

LENGTH BIAS

1. A systematic error due to selection of disproportionate numbers of long-duration cases (patients who survive longest) in one group but not in another. This can occur when prevalent rather than incident cases are included in a case-control study.

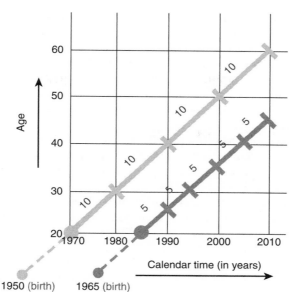

Lexis diagram.

2. Given that biologically and clinically aggressive diseases often have a shorter asymptomatic preclinical period than less aggressive diseases, a SCREENING program is more likely to detect slower progressing diseases (e.g., slow-growing tumors), which have better prognosis (e.g., survival).[3,5-9,24,203] The screening program may thus falsely appear to improve survival as compared to a cohort including a wider spectrum of disease. See also INCEPTION COHORT; LATENCY PERIOD; LEAD-TIME BIAS; SCREENING.

LENGTH OF GENERATION Time required for the replacement of a female generation by their daughters of reproductive age.

LETHALITY See FATALITY RATE.

LEVELS OF PREVENTION See PREVENTION.

LEVIN'S ATTRIBUTABLE RISK See ATTRIBUTABLE FRACTION FOR THE POPULATION.

LEXIS DIAGRAM A plot of two time dimensions: age and calendar time. Both time scales are measured in the same units (e.g., years) so that each line at 45 degrees represents the follow-up of a single individual from entry to exit from follow-up. Commonly used in the analysis of cohort data. Named after the demographer Wilhelm Lexis (1837-1914).

LIFE COURSE The natural history of human life. A term for conditions that evolve over a large part or all of the life span from infancy, or even from conception, through adolescence, adult life, and senescence. *Life cycle* has been used to describe a series of distinct, bounded life stages that are socially and/or biologically influenced. The concept of *life span* used in psychology assumes that development and aging form a continuous process from birth to death. The distinction between *life span* and *life course* is mainly a matter of scientific history.[23,312,366] See also ACCUMULATION OF RISK; DEVELOPMENTAL AND LIFE COURSE EPIDEMIOLOGY; DEVELOPMENTAL ORIGINS OF HEALTH AND DISEASE; ECOLOGICAL TRANSITION; SOCIAL EPIDEMIOLOGY.

LIFE CYCLE See LIFE COURSE.

LIFE EVENTS Aspects of the pattern of living that may be associated with or produce changes in health. The relationship of "life stress" and "emotional stress" to onset of several kinds of serious chronic disease, such as coronary heart disease and hypertension, has been the subject of epidemiological studies. The Rahe-Holmes Social Readjustment Rating Scale[585] was the first to be developed to assign ranks or ratings to significant life events such as death of a spouse or other close relative, loss of regular job, relocation, marriage, divorce, etc. Many other rating scales have since been developed.

LIFE EXPECTANCY See EXPECTATION OF LIFE.

LIFE EXPECTANCY FREE FROM DISABILITY (LEFD) An estimate of life expectancy adjusted for activity-limitation (data for which are derived from hospital discharge statistics, etc.). See also DISABILITY-ADJUSTED LIFE YEARS (DALYs); DISABILITY-FREE LIFE EXPECTANCY; QUALITY-ADJUSTED LIFE YEARS (QALYs).

LIFE EXPECTANCY WITH DISABILITY The average number of years an individual is expected to live with disability if current patterns of mortality and disability continue to apply. See DISABILITY-FREE LIFE EXPECTANCY.

LIFE SPAN See LIFE COURSE.

LIFESTYLE The set of habits and customs that is influenced by the lifelong process of socialization; examples include the use of alcohol and tobacco, dietary habits, or exercise.[1,5]

LIFESTYLE MODIFICATION The use of BEHAVIOR CHANGE INTERVENTIONS or other measures to improve LIFESTYLE. Lifestyles are modified by interventions targeting individuals, communities and populations. See also BEHAVIOR CHANGE TECHNIQUE; HEALTHY LIFESTYLE.[586]

LIFE TABLE (Syn: actuarial table) A summarizing technique used to describe the pattern of mortality and survival in populations. The survival data are time-specific and cumulative probabilities of survival of a group of individuals subject, throughout life, to the age-specific death rates in question. The life-table method can be applied to the study not only of death but also of any defined endpoint, such as the onset of disease or the occurrence of specific complication(s) of disease. The survivors to age x are denoted by the symbol l_x, the expectation of life at age x is denoted by the symbol, and the proportion alive at age x who die between age x and $x + 1$ years is denoted by the symbol nq_x. The life table method is used in public health and in assessments of treatment regimens in clinical practice, where x usually becomes time since treatment began.

The first rudimentary life tables were published in 1693 by the astronomer Edmund Halley. These made use of records of the funerals in the city of Breslau. In 1815 in England, the first actuarially correct life table was published, based on both population and death data classified by age.

Two types of life tables may be distinguished according to the reference year of the table: the current, or period, life table and the generation, or cohort, life table.

The current life table is a summary of mortality experience over a brief period (1 to 3 years), and the population data relate to the middle of that period (usually close to the date of a census). A current life table therefore represents the combined mortality experience by age of the population in a particular short period of time.

The cohort, or generation, life table describes the actual survival experience of a group, or cohort, of individuals born at about the same time. Theoretically, the mortality experience of the persons in the cohort would be observed from their moment of birth through each consecutive age in successive calendar years until all of them die.

The clinical life table describes the outcome experience of a group of individuals classified according to their exposure or treatment history; time since treatment onset, rather than age, is typically used to define the time intervals in the table.

A complete life table contains data for every single year of age, from birth to the last applicable age. An abridged life table contains data by intervals of 5 or 10 years of age.[1,3,5,8] See also EXPECTATION OF LIFE; SURVIVORSHIP STUDY.

LIFE TABLE, EXPECTATION OF LIFE FUNCTION, $\overset{o}{e}_x$ (Syn: average future lifetime) The expectation of life function is a statement of the average number of years of life remaining to persons who survive to age x.

LIFE TABLE, SURVIVORSHIP FUNCTION, l_x The survivorship function is a statement of the number of persons out of an initial population of defined size (e.g., 100,000 live births) who would survive or remain free of a defined endpoint condition to age x under the age-specific rates for the specified year. The value of l_{40}, for example, is determined by the cumulative operation of the specific death rates for all ages below 40.

LIFETIME RISK The RISK to an individual that a given health effect will occur at any time after exposure without regard for the time at which that effect occurs.

LIKELIHOOD FUNCTION A function constructed from a statistical model and a set of observed data that gives the probability of the observed data for various values of the unknown model parameters. Values for the parameters that maximize this function are called MAXIMUM LIKELIHOOD ESTIMATES of the parameters.[1,7,34,37]

LIKELIHOOD INTERVAL An interval containing all parameter values that have a value of the LIKELIHOOD FUNCTION greater than a certain proportion of the maximum; e.g., one seventh of the maximum, which roughly corresponds to a 95% confidence interval when the likelihood function has an approximately normal shape.[1,34,37]

LIKELIHOOD RATIO

1. The ratio of the values of the LIKELIHOOD FUNCTION at two different parameter values or under two different data models. Usually, one of the two values is taken to be the maximum of the function (the value of the function at the maximum-likelihood estimates). See also LIKELIHOOD-RATIO TEST.

2. The probability that a given test result would occur in a person with the target disorder divided by the probability that the same result would occur in a person without that disorder. It can be calculated for any level of a test result (for continuous diagnostic tests with many possible cutoff values) as the ratio of the probability of that test result among individuals with the target disorder to the probability of that same test result among individuals who are free of the target disorder. For a positive result, the likelihood ratio equals the ratio sensitivity/(1 − specificity). For a negative test result the likelihood ratio equals (1 − sensitivity)/specificity.[1,3,7,24]

Likelihood ratios are used to appraise screening and diagnostic tests. See also SENSITIVITY AND SPECIFICITY.

LIKELIHOOD-RATIO TEST A statistical test based on the ratio of the maximum value of the likelihood function under one statistical model to the maximum value under another statistical model; the models differ in that one includes and the other excludes one or more parameters, so that one model is a special, simpler case of the other.[1,3,7]

LIKERT SCALE An ordinal scale of responses to a question or statement ordered in a hierarchical sequence, such as from "strongly agree" through "no opinion" to "strongly disagree." Rensis Likert, a social psychologist, developed an empirical method for assigning numerical scores to such a scale.[7]

LINEAR MODEL A statistical model in which the average value of a dependent variable *y* at a given value of a factor, *x*, is assumed to be equal to $\alpha + \beta x$, where α and β are unknown constants.[1,3,7,14,37,101] See also MONOTONIC.

LINEAR MODEL, GENERALIZED A family of statistical regression models that model a response (effect, outcome) as a function of variables through a linear prediction that is specified by the link function and through an error function for the distribution of the errors. Common link functions include identity (linear models), logit (logistic regression), log (Poisson regression), and inverse (gamma regression).[1,3,7,37,244,270,796]

LINEAR REGRESSION REGRESSION analysis using linear models.

LINE GRAPH (Syn: line chart) A type of graph in which individual data points are connected by a line. The line can be displayed with or without data points. Most line graphs are used to show a TREND over time.

"LINE OF EQUALITY" See CONCENTRATION INDEX; GINI COEFFICIENT; LORENZ CURVE.

LINKAGE See GENETIC LINKAGE; RECORD LINKAGE.

LINKAGE ANALYSIS A technique used to locate a disease-causing gene by identifying genetic markers of known chromosomal location in high-risk families that are co-inherited with the TRAIT or disorder of interest.[1,5] Linkage analysis led to the discovery of genes such as the highly penetrant breast cancer genes BRCA1 and BRCA2. See also GENETIC LINKAGE.

LINKAGE DISEQUILIBRIUM A condition in which alleles at two loci or genes are found together in a population at a greater frequency than predicted simply by the product of their individual allele frequencies. Alleles at markers near disease-causing genes tend to be in linkage disequilibrium in the affected individuals.[54,57]

LIVE BIRTH WHO definition adopted by the Third World Health Assembly, 1950: "Live birth is the complete expulsion or extraction from its mother of a product of conception,

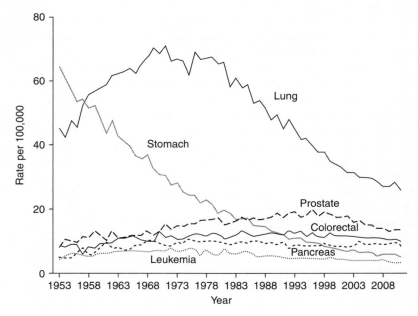

Line graph. Age-standardized mortality (world standard population) from major cancer sites among males in Finland, 1953–2011. Source: Finnish Cancer Registry. With permission.

irrespective of the duration of the pregnancy, which, after such separation, breathes or shows any other evidence of life, such as beating of the heart, pulsation of the umbilical cord, or definite movement of voluntary muscles, whether or not the umbilical cord has been cut or the placenta is attached; each product of such a birth is considered live born."

In the *Report of WHO Expert Committee on Prevention of Perinatal Mortality and Morbidity* (Technical Report Series 457, 1970), it is noted that the above definition requires the inclusion as live births of very early and patently nonviable fetuses and that accordingly it is not strictly applied. The committee suggested, therefore, that WHO should introduce a viability criterion into the definition so that very immature fetuses surviving for very short periods were excluded, even though they showed one or more of the transitory signs of life. The Conference for the Tenth Revision of the INTERNATIONAL CLASSIFICATION OF DISEASES (ICD-10) recommended that the above definitions, adopted for ICD-9, should remain unchanged.

LOCAL INDICATOR OF SPATIAL ASSOCIATION **(LISA)** Statistical measures used to identify the magnitude of spatial clustering around a particular geographical point or areal unit. Each observation gives an indication of the extent of significant spatial clustering of similar values around that observation, and the sum of LISAs for all observations is proportional to a global indicator of spatial association. Moran's I Index and Geary's C statistic are examples of LISAs.[587]

LOCUS

1. The position of a point, as defined by the coordinates on a graph.
2. The position that a gene occupies on a CHROMOSOME.

LOD SCORE The logarithm (base 10) of the odds. In genetics, the logarithm of the ratio of the probability of obtaining a set of observations assuming that two gene loci are located close to each other on a chromosome (i.e., in linkage) and, therefore, likely to be inherited together, to the probability of obtaining the same set of observations by chance. A LOD score of 3 corresponds to an odds of 1000:1 in favor of linkage between the two loci. A LOD score of 3 or higher is usually taken as an arbitrary cutoff to indicate that the two loci are linked.[57]

LOGIC The branch of philosophy and science that deals with canons of thought and criteria of validity in reasoning. Logic relies on precise definition of tangible objects, terms, and concepts; rational classification; application of fundamental principles of the underlying field of scholarship (mathematics, physics, ethics, linguistics, etc.); and minimal use of axioms and assumptions. Logic is essential but insufficient for empirical science and technology.[38,223,235] Epidemiology applies logic to arrive at conclusions about the distribution of health-related states and causal relationships, conditional on generally accepted assumptions (shared knowledge).[39,42] See also CAUSAL INFERENCE; DEDUCTIVE LOGIC; INDUCTIVE REASONING.

LOGICAL FRAMEWORK (LOGFRAME) ANALYSIS A method of project or program planning that uses a matrix of the goal, purpose, expected results, and activities on the vertical axis and the performance indicators, means of verification, and assumptions on the horizontal axis. The approach is often conducted in a group setting with facilitation, so as to promote teamwork and ownership of the plan. The matrix can be used also for project monitoring and evaluation and may be updated in response to changes in the timetable, performance, or feasibility of component activities. Logframe planning is favored by some international development agencies.

LOGIC, DEDUCTIVE See DEDUCTIVE LOGIC.

LOGIC, INDUCTIVE See INDUCTIVE REASONING.

LOGISTIC DISTRIBUTION A continuous variable Y is said to have a logistic DISTRIBUTION with mean μ and scale s if the probability $P(y)$ that Y is less than a particular value y is given by

$$P(y) = \frac{1}{1 + e^{-(y-\mu)/s}} = \mathrm{expit}\,(y - \mu)/S$$

The scale factor in this distribution is approximately 1.8 times the STANDARD DEVIATION of the distribution. This distribution resembles a normal distribution but has heavier tails; it arises in modeling various biological processes and in BAYESIAN ANALYSIS.[1,7,34,37,270]

LOGISTIC MODEL (Syn: logistic regression model) A statistical model for the probability that a binary variable Y equals 1 as a function of a covariate x, typically used when Y is an individual's disease indicator and x is the value of a risk factor or risk indicator:

$$P(Y = 1|x) = \frac{1}{1 + e^{-\alpha - \beta x}} = \mathrm{expit}\,(\alpha - \beta x)$$

where e is the (natural) exponential function and expit is the logistic function. This model has a desirable range (0 to 1), and other attractive statistical features. In this model, e^{β} is the odds ratio for the association of Y with a one-unit increase in x. In the multiple logistic model, the term βx is replaced by a linear term involving several factors, e.g., $\beta_1 x_1 + \beta_2 x_2$ if there are two factors x_1 and x_2.[1,3,7,8,24,34,37,270]

LOGISTIC REGRESSION See LOGISTIC MODEL.

LOGIT (Syn: log-odds) The natural logarithm of the ODDS.

LOGIT MODEL A linear model for the logit (natural log of the odds) of disease as a function of one or more factors X:

$$\mathrm{logit}\,(\text{disease given } X = x) = \alpha + \beta x$$

This model is mathematically equivalent to the LOGISTIC MODEL.[1]

LOG-LINEAR MODEL A statistical model that uses a LINEAR MODEL for the logarithms of frequency counts in contingency tables.[1]

LOG-NORMAL DISTRIBUTION If a variable Y is such that the natural log of Y is normally distributed, it is said to have log-normal distribution.[1,7,12,34] This is a SKEW DISTRIBUTION. See also DISTRIBUTION FUNCTION; NORMAL DISTRIBUTION.

LOG RANK TEST A test for comparing two or more sets of survival times. It is used to test the null hypothesis that there is no difference between the populations in the probability of an event (e.g., death) at any time point. The analysis is based on the times of events.[7,37,588]

LONGITUDINAL STUDY See COHORT STUDY.

LORENZ CURVE A curve developed by economist Max Lorenz (1880–1962) to describe income inequalities.[589] It shows the cumulative percentage of income, health care expenditures, and so on held by successive percentiles of the population. The percentage of individuals or households is plotted on the horizontal axis, while the percentage of income, health care expenditures, and so on is plotted on the vertical axis. A perfectly equal distribution, where each individual has the same, appears as a straight line, called the "line of perfect equality." A completely unequal DISTRIBUTION, where one person has everything, appears as a mirror L shape. This is a "line of perfect inequality." See also CONCENTRATION INDEX; GINI COEFFICIENT.

LOST TO FOLLOW-UP Subjects in a longitudinal study (COHORT STUDY, RANDOMIZED CONTROLLED TRIAL) whose status or outcome is unknown (e.g., because they could not or did not wish to attend follow-up visits). See also ATTRITION; CENSORING; DROPOUT.

LOW BIRTH WEIGHT See BIRTH WEIGHT.

"LUMPING AND SPLITTING" Derisive term describing the propensity of some researchers to arbitrarily group phenomena or to separate phenomena that hitherto had been grouped.

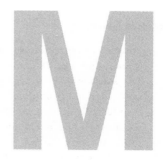

MACHINE LEARNING The ability of a program to learn from experience—i.e., to modify its execution on the basis of newly acquired information. In epidemiology and bioinformatics, examples include artificial neural NETWORKS, support vector machines, Bayesian networks, and other methods that update their procedures as new data are provided.[7]

MANHATTAN PLOT A type of scatter plot commonly used in GENOME-WIDE ASSOCIATION studies (GWAS), in which the genomic coordinates are displayed along the x axis, with the negative logarithm of the association p value for each single nucleotide polymorphism (SNP) displayed on the y axis.[87-89] The name derives from its resemblance to the Manhattan skyline.

MANN-WHITNEY TEST A test that compares two groups of ordinal scores, showing the probability that they form parts of the same distribution. It is a nonparametric equivalent of the t-test.

MANTEL-HAENSZEL ESTIMATE, MANTEL-HAENSZEL ODDS RATIO Nathan Mantel (1919 – 2002) and William Haenszel (1910 – 1998) provided an adjusted ("summary") ODDS RATIO estimate

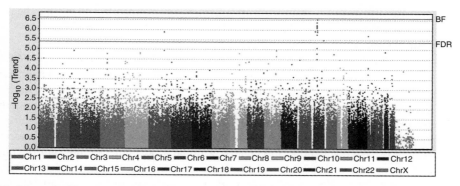

Manhattan plot. The association of SNPs with selective serotonin reuptake inhibitors (SSRIs) and serotonin–noradrenaline reuptake inhibitors (SNRIs)-induced sexual dysfunction across chromosomes. The $-\log_{10}P$ values of the Cochran–Armitage trend test were plotted across chromosomes. FDR- and Bonferroni (BF)-corrected significance levels are indicated by lines in blue and red, respectively. The association of SNPs with SSRI/SNRI-induced sexual dysfunction across chromosomes. The $-\log_{10}P$ values of the Cochran–Armitage trend test were plotted across chromosomes. FDR- and Bonferroni (BF)-corrected significance levels are indicated by lines. Source: Kurose K, et al.[590] With permission.

that may be derived from grouped and matched sets of data.[3,7,8,591] It is now known as the Mantel-Haenszel estimate, one of the few eponymous terms of modern epidemiology. The statistic may be regarded as a type of weighted average of the individual odds ratios, derived from dividing a sample into a series of strata. Ideally, the strata would be internally homogeneous with respect to confounding factors. The Mantel-Haenszel method can also be extended to the summarization of rate ratios and rate differences from follow-up studies.

MANTEL-HAENSZEL TEST (Syn: Cochran-Mantel-Haenszel test) A summary CHI-SQUARE TEST developed by Mantel and Haenszel for stratified data and used when controlling for CONFOUNDING. It is a slight modification of an earlier test by William Gemmel Cochran and a special case of certain general tests in a LOGISTIC MODEL.[1,3,24]

MANTEL'S TREND TEST A regression test of the ODDS RATIO against a numerical variable representing ordered categories of exposure. It generalizes the MANTEL-HAENSZEL TEST and can be used to analyze results of any study, including a CASE-CONTROL STUDY.

MANTOUX TEST See TUBERCULIN SKIN TEST.

MARGINAL STRUCTURAL MODELS Statistical models for the estimation of causal effects in longitudinal studies in which there are time-varying confounders affected by prior exposure.[1,2,7,101,592] They aim, for instance, to control for the effects of time-dependent confounders affected by prior treatment. They provide an alternative to G-ESTIMATION of STRUCTURAL NESTED MODELS, but cannot be used to estimate the effects of dynamic treatment regimes. They can, however, be used to estimate the effect of a nondynamic treatment regime when the data are derived from a cohort study in which the treatment regime is dynamic. Fitting of these models typically requires INVERSE PROBABILITY WEIGHTING.

MARGINALS The row and column totals of a contingency table.

MARGIN OF SAFETY An estimate of the ratio of the no-observed-effect level (NOEL) to the level accepted in regulations.[14] See also NO-OBSERVED-ADVERSE-EFFECT LEVEL.

MARKET FAILURE In economic allocation theory, the failure of a more or less idealized system of price-market institutions to sustain "desirable" activities (consumption, production). Health care markets do not merely fail to satisfy some of the standard assumptions required for competitive markets, they fail every single one of them: there is ASYMMETRY OF INFORMATION and AGENCY RELATIONSHIP, markets are incomplete, and much of health care has the character of a public good and generates EXTERNALITIES.[17,593,594]

MARKETING See SOCIAL MARKETING.

MARKOV PROCESS, MARKOV CHAIN A stochastic process such that the conditional probability distribution for the state at any future instant, given the present state, is unaffected by any additional knowledge of the past history of the system. Invented by Andrei A. Markov (1856–1922). A family of regression models for correlated data used to study event histories that include transitions between several states; Markov chains are a common way of modeling the progression of a chronic disease through various severity states; for these models, a transition matrix with the probabilities of moving from one state to another for a specific time interval is usually estimated from cohort data. Several types of Markov models (e.g., "hidden Markov models") are applied in health services research, health economics, clinical epidemiology, infectious disease epidemiology, genetic epidemiology, and systems biology.[1,7,34,37,101,595] See also MONTE-CARLO STUDY.

MASKED STUDY See BLINDED STUDY.

MASKING (Syn: blinding) Procedures intended to keep participants in a study from knowing some facts or observations that might bias or influence their actions or decisions regarding the study.[5,6,26,58]

MASS ACTION PRINCIPLE A fundamental principle of epidemic theory[385,596]: the incidence of an infectious disease one SERIAL INTERVAL in the future is dependent on the product of the current prevalence and the number of susceptibles in the population:

$$C_{t+1} = C_t \times S_t \times r$$

where

C_{t+1} = the number of new cases one serial interval in the future
C_t = the number of current cases
S_t = the number of susceptibles
r = the INFECTION TRANSMISSION PARAMETER

MATCHED CONTROLS See CONTROLS, MATCHED.

MATCHING The process of making the distribution of the matching factors to be identical across study groups.[1-3,5,7,8,38,197,269,270,280] In cohort studies, matching is used to prevent confounding due to the matching factors; if there is no source of bias other than confounding by the matching factors, adjustment for these factors may be unnecessary to remove bias. In case-control studies, matching is used to increase statistical efficiency when a subsequent procedure (e.g. stratification) is used to adjust for confounding, but it introduces selection bias; thus, adjustment for the matching factors may be necessary to remove this bias even if the factors were not confounders to begin with. Cohort matching can prevent confounding by the matched variables, but censoring or other missing data and further adjustment may necessitate control of matching variables. Case-control matching generally does not prevent confounding by the matched variables, and control of matching variables may be necessary even if those were not confounders initially. Matching on variables that are affected by the exposure and the outcome, or intermediates between the exposure and the outcome, will ordinarily produce irremediable BIAS.[280,791,795] Several kinds of matching exist:

1. *Caliper matching* is the process of matching comparison group subjects to study group subjects within a specified distance for a continuous variable (e.g., matching age to within 2 years).
2. *Frequency matching* requires that the frequency distributions of the matched variable(s) be similar in study and comparison groups.
3. *Category matching* is the process of matching study and control group subjects in prespecified categories, such as occupational groups or age groups.
4. *Individual matching* relies on identifying individual subjects for comparison, each resembling a study subject on the matched variable(s).
5. *Pair matching* is individual matching in which study and comparison subjects are paired.

MATERNAL MORTALITY Several definitions related to maternal mortality have been agreed upon by internationally representative groups under the auspices of the WHO. A *maternal death* is death of a woman while pregnant or within 42 days of termination of pregnancy, irrespective of the duration and the site of pregnancy, from any cause related to or aggravated by the pregnancy or its management but not from accidental or incidental causes.

A *late maternal death* is the death of a woman from direct or indirect obstetric causes more than 42 days but less than 1 year after termination of pregnancy.

A *pregnancy-related death* is death of a woman while pregnant or within 42 days of termination of pregnancy, irrespective of the cause of death.

Direct obstetric deaths are those resulting from obstetric complications of the pregnant state (pregnancy, labor, and the puerperium) from interventions, omissions, incorrect treatment, or a chain of events resulting from any of the above.

Indirect obstetric deaths are those resulting from previous existing disease that developed during pregnancy and not due to direct obstetric causes but aggravated by the physiological effects of pregnancy.

In order to improve the quality of maternal mortality data and provide alternative methods of collecting data on deaths during pregnancy or related to it, as well as to encourage the recording of deaths from obstetric causes occurring more than 42 days following termination of pregnancy, the 43rd World Health Assembly in 1990 adopted the recommendation that countries consider the inclusion on death certificates of questions regarding current pregnancy and pregnancy within 1 year preceding death.

MATERNAL MORTALITY RATIO The risk of dying from causes associated with childbirth. The numerator is the deaths arising during pregnancy or from puerperal causes (i.e., deaths occurring during and/or due to deliveries, complications of pregnancy, childbirth, and the puerperium). Women exposed to the risk of dying from puerperal causes are those who have been pregnant during the period. Their number being unknown, the number of live births is used as the conventional denominator for computing comparable maternal mortality rates. Thus, this indicator should be called a ratio rather than a rate because the denominator is not all pregnancies but live births. The formula is:

$$\text{Annual maternal mortality rate} = \frac{\text{number of deaths from puerperal causes in a given geographic area during a given year}}{\text{number of live births that occurred among the population of the given geographic area during the same year}} \times 1000 \ (\text{or } 100{,}000)$$

There is variation in the duration of the postpartum period in which death may occur and be certified as due to "puerperal causes," i.e., MATERNAL MORTALITY. Although WHO defines maternal mortality as death during pregnancy or within 42 days of delivery, in some areas a period as long as a year is used. Maternal deaths may be subdivided into two groups: direct obstetric deaths and indirect obstetric deaths.

MATHEMATICAL MODEL

1. A representation of a system, process, or relationship in mathematical form in which equations are used to simulate the behavior of the system or process under study. The MODEL usually consists of two parts: the mathematical structure itself (e.g., Newton's inverse square law or Gauss's "normal" law), and the particular constants or parameters associated with them (such as Newton's gravitational constant or the Gaussian standard deviation). A mathematical model is fully DETERMINISTIC if the dependent variables involved take on values not allowing for any play of CHANCE. A model is said to be stochastic, or RANDOM, if random variation is allowed to enter the picture.[1,2,7,796]

2. The set of all mathematical assumptions used to deduce or predict the behavior of a system or process.

MATRIX

1. In epidemiology and biostatistics, a display of data in columns and rows.
2. In human biology, a formative tissue.

MAXIMUM ALLOWABLE CONCENTRATION **(MAC)** See SAFETY STANDARDS.

MAXIMUM LIKELIHOOD **(ML)** ESTIMATE, MAXIMUM LIKELIHOOD ESTIMATION The ML estimates of unknown parameters in a model are the values that together maximize the probability of obtaining exactly the data that were observed. The process of finding these estimates is called ML estimation. ML is the standard method for estimating the coefficients in LOGISTIC MODELS.[1,3,7,34,37] There are many variations of ML, including conditional ML, partial ML, and marginal ML. ML and its variants are all special cases of estimating equation methods.

M-BIAS Bias in COLLIDER (C)-specific or C-adjusted exposure (E) - disease (D) associations arising from an "M pattern" within the underlying causal structure (in which all or part of the C–E association arises from shared causes A of C and E and all or part of the C–D association arises from shared causes B of C and D).[2,242] It is called "M" because of the M shape of the corresponding CAUSAL DIAGRAM, the "M diagram," in which events are temporally ordered from top (earliest) to bottom (latest), C is a COLLIDER on the "back-door" path from E to D passing through A, C and B (a back-door path from E to D is a path that begins with an arrow pointing to E; such paths are sources of CONFOUNDING). Like other collider-stratification biases and SELECTION BIASES, M-bias arises from adjustment for a variable C that numerically behaves like a classical CONFOUNDER (in that the effect estimate changes upon adjustment for C). Unlike other collider-stratification biases, M-bias attributable to C-adjustment may not be apparent from the TIME ORDER of the events, for C may be determined before E or D; hence, one may be led to adjust for C (and thus introduce bias) if one uses traditional confounder-selection criteria, even if one takes care to not adjust for variables affected by E or D.[242] See also CONFOUNDING BIAS.

McNEMAR'S TEST A form of the CHI-SQUARE TEST for matched-pairs data. It is a special case of the MANTEL-HAENSZEL TEST.[7,37]

MDR **(MULTIDRUG RESISTANT)** See DRUG RESISTANCE, MULTIPLE.

MEAN, ARITHMETIC A MEASURE OF CENTRAL TENDENCY.[37] There are two major types:

1. The sum of all the individual values in a set of measurements divided by the number of values in the set. This is an empirical quantity, usually called the group or sample mean.[7]
2. The sum (or integral) of all possible values for a variable or estimator, each weighted by the frequency or probability of the value. This is a theoretical quantity, often called the expected value of the variable or estimator. See also AVERAGE.

MEAN-DIFFERENCE PLOT (Syn: Tukey mean-difference plot) A scatter plot that shows changes in the percentiles of the distribution of a measure from samples obtained at two time points. The differences of each percentile from the earlier to the later time points are plotted on the vertical axis, and the means of the two values of each percentile are on the horizontal axis. Data are typically shown for the 2.5, 5, 10, 20, 30, 40, 50, 60, 70, 80, 90, 95, and 97.5 percentile points. Departure of the plotted points from a horizontal line indicates change of shape of the DISTRIBUTION.

MEAN, GEOMETRIC A MEASURE OF CENTRAL TENDENCY. This is calculated by adding the logarithms of the individual values, calculating their arithmetic mean, and converting back by taking the antilogarithm. Can be calculated only for positive quantities.

MEAN, HARMONIC A MEASURE OF CENTRAL TENDENCY computed by summing the reciprocals of all the individual values and dividing the resulting sum into the number of values.

MEAN SQUARED ERROR The mean (expected value) of the squared difference between an estimator and the true value of the quantity or parameter. It is equal to the sum of the squared BIAS of the estimator and the VARIANCE of the estimator. See also ACCURACY.

MEASUREMENT The procedure of applying a standard scale to a variable or to a set of values.

MEASUREMENT BIAS
1. Systematic error (BIAS) in a measurement.
2. Systematic error arising from inaccurate measurements (or classification) of subjects on study variable(s). Random errors in individual measurements typically lead to systematic errors (bias) in estimated measures of association or effect.[1-3,5-9,24,270,551] See also INFORMATION BIAS.

MEASUREMENT SCALE The range of possible values for a measurement (e.g., the set of possible responses to a question, the physically possible range for a set of body weights).[26,30]

Measurement scales can be classified according to the quantitative character of the scale:
1. DICHOTOMOUS SCALE (Syn: binary scale): One that arranges items into either of two mutually exclusive categories; e.g., Yes/No, Alive/Dead.
2. NOMINAL SCALE (Syn: polytomous scale, polytomy): Classification into unordered qualitative categories; e.g., race, religion, and country of birth. Measurements of individual attributes are purely nominal scales, as there is no inherent order to their categories.
3. ORDINAL SCALE: Classification into ordered qualitative categories, e.g., social class (I, II, III, etc.), where the values have a distinct order but their categories are qualitative in that there is no natural (numerical) distance between their possible values. See also RANKING SCALE.
4. INTERVAL SCALE: An (equal) interval involves assignment of values with a natural distance between them, so that a particular distance (interval) between two values in one region of the scale meaningfully represents the same distance between two values in another region of the scale. Examples include Celsius and Fahrenheit temperature, date of birth.
5. RATIO SCALE: A ratio is an interval scale with a true zero point, so that ratios between values are meaningfully defined. Examples are absolute (Kelvin) temperature, weight, height, blood count, and income, as in each case it is meaningful to speak of one value as being so many times greater or less than another value.

Dichotomous, nominal, and ordinal scales are sometimes called qualitative or "categorical," but the latter term has other meanings, such as *discrete* (as opposed to continuous). An example of a categorical scale that is also a ratio scale is household size (1, 2, 3,...). Interval and ratio scales are sometimes called quantitative scales. See also QUALITATIVE DATA; QUANTITATIVE DATA.

MEASUREMENT, TERMINOLOGY OF The meaning of terms used to describe the properties of measurement can be summarized as follows:

Accuracy refers to "conforming to a standard or a true value" *(OED)*. *Accuracy* may be distinguished from *precision* in this way: A measurement or statement can reflect or represent a true value without detail; e.g., a temperature reading of 37.4°C may be accurate, but it may not be precise if a thermometer that registers 37.427°C is taken as the reference. See also ACCURACY.

Precision is the quality of being sharply defined through exact detail. A faulty (inaccurate) measurement may be expressed precisely. Measurements should be both accurate and precise; the two terms are not synonymous, although precision is often considered a component of accuracy (the other being unbiasedness). See also PRECISION.

Consistency (or *reliability*) describes the property of measurements or results that conform to themselves.

Reliability A measurement is reliable when it is stable; i.e., when repetition of an experiment or measurement gives the same results. See also RELIABILITY.

Repeatability and *reproducibility* (which are synonymous and formed from their respective verbs) do not refer to a quality of measurement—rather, to the action of performing something more than once. Thus, a way of discovering whether or not a measurement is reliable is to repeat or reproduce it. The terms are used inaccurately when they are substituted for *reliability*. However, in common usage, both repeatability and reproducibility refer to the capacity of a measuring procedure to yield the same result on each occasion in a series of procedures conducted under identical conditions.

Unbiasedness If the errors in a measurement average out to zero over the long run, the measurement is said to be *unbiased.*

Validity If a measurement measures what it purports to measure, then it is said to be *valid*. The degree to which a health related-patient reported outcomes (HR-PRO) instrument measures the construct(s) it purports to measure. See also BIAS; REPEATABILITY; VALIDITY; VALIDITY, MEASUREMENT.[1-3,5-9,30,91,274]

MEASURE OF ASSOCIATION A quantity that expresses the strength or degree of association between variables. Commonly used measures of association are ratios and differences between means, proportions, risks, or rates, and correlation and regression coefficients.[1]

MEASURE OF EFFECT See EFFECT MEASURE.

MEASURES OF CENTRAL TENDENCY A general term for several values of the DISTRIBUTION of a set of values or measurements located at or near the middle of the set. The principal measures of central tendency are the MEAN (AVERAGE), MEDIAN, and MODE.

MECHANICAL TRANSMISSION Transmission of pathogens by a vector (e.g., a housefly) without biological development in or dependence on the vector. Many fecal-oral infections are spread by this means.[20,22,56,188,217-219] See also VECTOR-BORNE INFECTION.

MECHANISM In epidemiology and other health, life, and social sciences, the way in which a particular health-related event or outcome occurs, often described in terms of the agents, steps, and pathways involved. Whereas some studies focus on biological mechanisms, environmental, social, and cultural mechanisms are also relevant to epidemiology, public health, medicine, and related disciplines.

MECHANISTIC BIAS A form of INTERPRETIVE BIAS that occurs if interpretation of scientific evidence is less rigorous when basic science furnishes credibility for the putative mechanisms underlying the findings than when it does not.[99] See also BIOLOGICAL PLAUSIBILITY; COHERENCE.

MECHANISTIC EPIDEMIOLOGY Epidemiological research that focuses on MECHANISMS underlying and explaining associations between DETERMINANTS and health-related events or states. It is not a formal branch, specialty, or method of epidemiology. Loosely, a complementary opposite of "BLACK-BOX EPIDEMIOLOGY." See also APPLIED EPIDEMIOLOGY; MOLECULAR EPIDEMIOLOGY; RELEVANCE; SIGNIFICANCE.

MEDIAN A MEASURE OF CENTRAL TENDENCY. The simplest division of a set of measurements is into two parts—the lower and the upper half. The point on the scale that divides the group in this way is called the "median."

MEDIATOR (MEDIATING) VARIABLE See INTERMEDIATE VARIABLE.

MEDICAL AUDIT A health service evaluation procedure in which selected data from patients' charts are summarized in tables displaying such data as average length of stay or duration of an episode of care, the frequency of diagnostic and therapeutic procedures, and outcomes of care arranged by diagnostic category. These are often compared with predetermined norms.

MEDICAL CARE See HEALTH CARE.

MEDICAL GEOGRAPHY (Syn: geographical pathology) A branch of science concerned with the spatial variations in environmental conditions related to health and disease. It applies techniques such as mapping to health problems.[597,598] Satellite imaging and remote sensing have facilitated mapping the distribution of epidemiologically important biota, and have strengthened the integration of epidemiology, ecology, and geography in studies of medical geography and geographical medicine. Cartographic methods as CHOROPLETHIC and ISODEMOGRAPHIC MAPS provide a useful visual display of the geographical variations in the distribution of disease and health-related factors. See also GEOGRAPHICAL INFORMATION SYSTEM; GEOMATICS; SATELLITE EPIDEMIOLOGY.

MEDICAL PRACTICE VARIATIONS (MPV) Variation in the utilization of health care services that cannot be explained by variation in patient illness or patient preferences.[599] The broad literature produced in the last four decades about MPV—including clinical practice variations, unwarranted variation—shows that patients with similar diagnoses, prognoses, and demographic status receive different levels of care depending on when, where, and by whom they are treated, despite agreed and documented evidence of "best practice." MPV can occur at individual, facility, professional, and organizational levels. Wide MPV have been observed in populations with similar demographic, economic, social, and epidemiological characteristics. They appear to be largely arbitrary, and most likely reflect uncertainty about or ignorance of best professional practice.

MEDICAL RECORD A file of information relating to a transaction(s) in personal health care. In addition to facts about a patient's illness, medical records nearly always contain other information. The information in medical records includes the following:

1. Clinical, i.e., diagnosis, treatment, progress, etc.
2. Demographic, i.e., age, sex, birthplace, residence, etc.
3. Sociocultural, i.e., language, ethnic origin, religion, etc.
4. Sociological, i.e., family (next of kin), occupation, etc.
5. Economic, i.e., method of payment (fee-for-service, indigent, etc.).
6. Administrative, i.e., site of care, provider, etc.
7. "Behavioral," e.g., records of broken appointment may indicate dissatisfaction with service provided.

MEDICAL STATISTICS The branch of BIOSTATISTICS concerned with medical problems and research.

MEDICALIZATION The process by which conditions, processes, or emotional states traditionally considered nonmedical are redefined and treated as medical issues. The process of identification and labeling of a personal or social condition as a medical issue subject to medical intervention. The expansion of the influence and authority of the health

professions and industries into the domains of everyday existence.[248,292,323,337,338,363,364,470,482,600]
See also GENETIZATION; INTEGRATION; REDUCTIONISM.

MENDELIAN RANDOMIZATION

1. An approach or "strategy" of observational epidemiology that uses findings from association studies of well-characterized functional genetic variants to assess CAUSAL INFERENCES about modifiable environmental exposures. One of the INSTRUMENTAL VARIABLE approaches for making causal inferences from observational data in the face of RESIDUAL CONFOUNDING.[86,477,601] It is based on the fact that INHERITANCE of one genetic TRAIT is independent of (i.e., *randomized* with respect to) other unlinked traits. Functional variants will not be associated with other genetic variants apart from those with which they are in LINKAGE DISEQUILIBRIUM; this assumption follows from the law of independent assortment (sometimes referred to as MENDEL'S SECOND LAW), hence the term Mendelian randomization. At a population level, traits influenced by genetic variants are generally not associated with the social, behavioral, and environmental factors that confound relationships in conventional epidemiological studies. Thus genetic variants can serve as an indicator of the action of environmentally modifiable exposures. Example: studies have pointed out that the autosomal dominant condition of lactase persistence is positively associated with drinking milk; thus protective associations of lactase persistence with osteoporosis, bone mineral density, or fracture risk provide evidence that milk drinking protects against these conditions. Mendelian randomization may help to avoid CONFOUNDING, bias due to REVERSE CAUSATION or reporting tendency, and underestimation of associations due to variability in behaviors and phenotypes. Factors limiting the inferential power of Mendelian randomization include confounding of associations between genotype, intermediate phenotype, and disease through linkage disequilibrium or POPULATION STRATIFICATION; PLEIOTROPY and the multifunctionality of genes; canalization and developmental stability; and lack of suitable polymorphisms for studying modifiable exposures of interest.[477,601]

2. Originally, random assortment of genetic variants at conception, used to provide an unconfounded study design for estimating treatment effects for childhood malignancies.

MENDEL'S LAWS Derived from the pioneering genetic studies of Gregor Mendel (1822–1884). Mendel's first law states that genes are particulate units that segregate; i.e., members of the same pair of genes are never present in the same gamete, but always separate and pass to different gametes. Mendel's second law states that genes assort independently; i.e., members of different pairs of genes move to gametes independently of one another.

META-ANALYSIS A statistical analysis of results from separate studies, examining sources of differences in results among studies, and leading to a quantitative summary of the results if the results are judged sufficiently similar or consistent to support such synthesis. In the health sciences, the systematic, organized, and structured evaluation of a problem of interest, using information from a number of independent studies. A frequent application is the pooling of results from a set of randomized controlled trials, which in aggregate have more statistical precision and power to detect differences. Meta-analysis has a qualitative component (classification of studies according to predetermined characteristics capable of influencing results, such as study design, completeness and quality of data, absence of biases), and a quantitative component (extraction and analysis of the numerical information). Meta-analysis usually involves the analysis of effect estimates published by each of the participating studies. A meta-analysis is often performed on data located in a SYSTEMATIC REVIEW. Some meta-analyses re-analyze the original individual level data from each study; this type is often called POOLED ANALYSIS. The aim is to integrate the findings, if possible, and to identify overall trends or patterns in the results. Studies must be subject to critical appraisal, and various biases in the selection of subjects, detection of events, or presentation of results (e.g., PUBLICATION BIAS) must be assessed.[1,5-9,25,52,58,87,135,137,229,230,258,294,300,467,485,504] See also GRADE; WEIGHTED AVERAGE.

METABOLOME The theoretical complete set of metabolites that reflect the chemical and physiological processes occurring in a given cell, tissue, or organism.

METABOLOMICS The study of the METABOLOME. It is related to several "-omics" approaches, as genomics, proteomics, lipidomics, and transcriptomics.

METAGENOME The totality of genetic material found in and on the human body that is not human in origin. See also GENOME; EXPOSOME; HUMAN MICROBIOME.

METAPHOR A word, image, expression, concept, or symbol used as a cultural and cognitive device to convey or comprehend an idea—sometimes an abstract or complex scientific concept. In epidemiology, a classic example is the "WEB OF CAUSATION." Metaphors are important in many scientific and professional endeavors, including many epidemiology-related activities (e.g., HEALTH PROMOTION, RISK ASSESSMENT, risk communication); and, of course, in teaching epidemiology.[38,104-106,108,290,363,364,406,455,456,481,482,602,603] They may inspire or otherwise form the basis of subsequent formal developments (e.g., CAUSAL DIAGRAMS partly stem from and formalize the web-of-causation metaphor).

METHODOLOGY The scientific study of methods. Methodology should not be confused with methods. The word *methodology* is all too often used when the writer means *method*.

MIASMA THEORY An explanation for the origin of epidemics, the "miasma theory" was implied by many ancient writers and made explicit by Lancisi in *De noxiis paludum effluviis* (1717). It was based on the notion that when the air was of a "bad quality" (a state that was not precisely defined but that was supposedly due to decaying organic matter), the persons breathing that air would become ill. Malaria ("bad air") is the classic example of a disease that was long attributed to miasmata. "Miasma" was believed to pass from cases to susceptibles in those diseases considered contagious.[5,42,56]

MICROBIOME See HUMAN MICROBIOME.

MICROORGANISM (Syn: microbe) A microscopic biological entity (living) that is typically too small to be seen with the naked eye; e.g., BACTERIA.

MIGRANT STUDIES Studies taking advantage of migration to one country by those from other countries with different physical and biological environments, cultural background, and/or genetic makeup and different morbidity or mortality experience. Studies can also assess migration within-country (e.g., rural-to-urban migration). Comparisons are made between the mortality or morbidity experience of the migrant groups with that of their current country of residence and/or their country of origin. Sometimes the experiences of a number of different groups who have migrated to the same country have been compared.[5]

MILLENNIUM DEVELOPMENT GOALS (MDGs) Drawn from the actions and targets contained in the Millenium Declaration, which was adopted during the United Nations Millennium Summit in 2000. To be achieved by 2015, the eight MDGs break down into 18 quantifiable targets measured by 48 indicators. The MDGs recognize the interdependence between health, growth, poverty reduction, and sustainable development. They acknowledge that development rests on democratic governance, the rule of law, respect for human

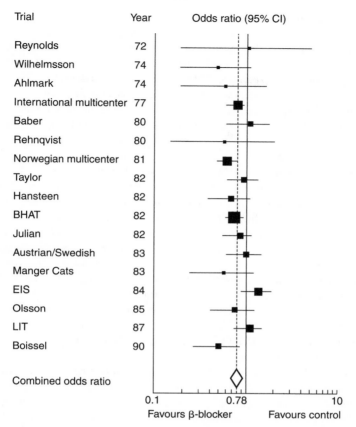

Trial	Year	Odds ratio (95% CI)
Reynolds	72	
Wilhelmsson	74	
Ahlmark	74	
International multicenter	77	
Baber	80	
Rehnqvist	80	
Norwegian multicenter	81	
Taylor	82	
Hansteen	82	
BHAT	82	
Julian	82	
Austrian/Swedish	83	
Manger Cats	83	
EIS	84	
Olsson	85	
LIT	87	
Boissel	90	
Combined odds ratio		

0.1   0.78   10

Favours β-blocker   Favours control

Meta-analysis of mortality results from 17 studies of β-blockade in secondary prevention after acute myocardial infarction. The size of the "box" in each box-and-whiskers plot is proportional to the numbers in the study, and the combined odds ratio is represented by the diamond shape in the bottom row of the diagram. Figures like this have been called meta-analysis plots, Cochrane plots, or Chalmers plots. They most often appear without an eponymous name. Source: Davey Smith G.[604]

rights, and peace and security.[605] The eight MDGs are: (1) eradicate extreme poverty and hunger; (2) achieve universal primary education; (3) promote gender equality and empower women; (4) reduce child mortality; (5) improve maternal health; (6) combat HIV/AIDS, malaria, and other diseases; (7) ensure environmental sustainability; and (8) develop a Global Partnership for Development.

MILL'S CANONS In *A System of Logic* (first edition 1843), John Stuart Mill (1806–1873) devised properties of relationships from which causal relationships may be inferred ("canons"). Four in particular are pertinent to epidemiology:[42]

Method of agreement (first canon): "If two or more instances of the phenomenon under investigation have only one circumstance in common, the circumstance in which alone all the instances agree, is the cause (or effect) of the given phenomenon."

Method of difference (second canon): "If an instance in which the phenomenon under investigation occurs, and an instance in which it does not occur, have every circumstance in common save one, that one occurring only in the former, the circumstance in which alone the two instances differ is the effect, or cause or a necessary part of the cause, of the phenomenon."

Method of residues (fourth canon): "Subduct from any phenomenon such part as is known by previous inductions to be the effect of certain antecedents, and the residue of the phenomenon is the effect of the remaining antecedents."

Method of concomitant variation (fifth canon): "Whatever phenomenon varies in any manner whether another phenomenon varies in some particular manner, is either a cause or an effect of that phenomenon, or is connected with it through some fact of causation."

See also CAUSAL CRITERIA.

MINIMALLY IMPORTANT DIFFERENCE (MID) (Syn: minimal clinically important difference) The smallest effect of a treatment that patients perceive as beneficial. In the absence of unacceptable side effects, inconvenience, or high costs, such effect may warrant treatment onset. The smallest difference or change that is important to the patient. A type of measure used in randomized trials that measure patient reported outcomes, and primary outcomes with QUALITY OF LIFE instruments, to determine the CLINICAL SIGNIFICANCE of differences observed.[606,607] See also SIGNIFICANCE, CLINICAL.

MINIMUM DATA SET (Syn: uniform basic data set) A widely agreed upon and generally accepted set of terms and definitions constituting a core of data acquired for medical records and employed for developing statistics suitable for diverse types of analyses and users. Such sets have been developed for birth and death certificates, ambulatory care, hospital care, and long-term care. See also BIRTH CERTIFICATE; DEATH CERTIFICATE; HOSPITAL DISCHARGE ABSTRACT SYSTEM.

MISCLASSIFICATION The erroneous CLASSIFICATION of an individual, a value, or an attribute into a category other than that to which it should be assigned.[1,3,5,7,8,24,25,269,270] The probability of misclassification given the true value may be the same in all study groups (nondifferential misclassification) or may vary between groups (differential misclassification; e.g., the accuracy of diagnoses in some patients depends on their alcohol consumption or educational level).[339] It is wrong to assume that nondifferential misclassification can produce only bias toward the null in measures of association or effect; other conditions must also be satisfied in order to ensure that bias is toward the null, most prominently that the misclassification must be independent of (unrelated to) the occurrence of other errors.[1] Such independence is rare in clinical and epidemiological research. See also INFORMATION BIAS; MEASUREMENT BIAS.

MISSING AT RANDOM See MISSING DATA.

MISSING COMPLETELY AT RANDOM See MISSING DATA.

MISSING DATA (Syn: incomplete data, MISSING VALUES) Lack of some information or incomplete information for some study participants. Usually (but not always) the term refers to data missing in ways deviating from the study design.[1-3,7,8,608,609] The three main types of missing data are:

1. *Missing completely at random*: there are no systematic differences between the missing values and the observed values.

2. *Missing at random*: any systematic difference between the missing values and the observed values can be explained by differences in observed data.

3. *Missing not at random*: even after the observed data are taken into account, systematic differences remain between the missing values and the observed values.

"MISSING" HERITABILITY See HERITABILITY, "MISSING."

MISSING NOT AT RANDOM See MISSING DATA.

MISSING VALUES Values that are unknown because they remained unanswered or unmeasured.

MISSION The purpose for which an organization exists. See also GOAL; OBJECTIVE; TARGET.

MITIGATION Reduction of the risk of DISASTER. Actions taken to avoid or minimize negative environmental, medical, or social impacts.[139]

MOBILITY, GEOGRAPHIC Movement of persons from one permanent place of residence (country or region) to another.

MOBILITY, SOCIAL Movement from one defined socioeconomic group to another, either upward or downward. Downward social mobility, which can be related to impaired health (e.g., alcoholism, schizophrenia, mental retardation), is sometimes referred to as "social drift."

MODE The most frequently occurring value in a set or distribution of observations. One of the MEASURES OF CENTRAL TENDENCY. See also AVERAGE.

MODEL

1. An abstract representation of the relationship between logical, analytical, or empirical components of a system.[1-3,7,12,270,796] See also MATHEMATICAL MODEL.
2. A formalized expression of a theory or the causal situation regarded as having generated observed data.
3. (Animal) model: an experimental system that uses animals because humans cannot be used for ethical or other reasons.[64]
4. A small-scale simulation, e.g., by using an "average region" with characteristics resembling those of the whole country.

In epidemiology, the use of models began with an effort to predict the onset and course of epidemics. In the second report of the Registrar-General of England and Wales (1840), William Farr developed the beginnings of a predictive model for communicable disease epidemics. He had recognized regularities in the smallpox epidemics of the 1830s. By calculating frequency curves for these past outbreaks, he estimated the deaths to be expected. See also DEMONSTRATION MODEL; MATHEMATICAL MODEL; THEORETICAL EPIDEMIOLOGY.

MODEL LIFE TABLE Simulated life table constructed for a country, used mainly when vital statistics are deficient. The model may be based on averaging of empirical data or on more sophisticated methods. The Coale-Demeny method is a range of models for life expectancies ranging from 20 to 80+ years with four variations of mortality patterns.

MODE OF INHERITANCE The manner in which a genetic TRAIT or disorder is passed from one generation to the next. Examples include autosomal dominant, autosomal recessive, X-linked dominant, X-linked recessive, multifactorial, and mitochondrial inheritance. Each mode of INHERITANCE results in a characteristic pattern of affected and unaffected family members. See also HEREDITY; HERITABILITY.

MODIFIABLE AREAL UNIT PROBLEM A phenomenon in which the results of statistical analysis may differ substantially according to the scale and pattern of the areal units used. It occurs mainly due to the arbitrary nature of the aggregation of individuals into areas, and has two interrelated components: (1) the scale effect, whereby statistical bias can occur when the information is grouped at different levels of spatial resolution; and (2) the zoning effect, whereby bias is a result of the various ways areas can be aggregated at a given scale.[610,611] See also ECOLOGICAL FALLACY.

MODIFYING FACTOR See EFFECT MODIFIER.

MOLECULAR EPIDEMIOLOGY The application of epidemiologic principles to study the molecular, biochemical, cellular and genetic mechanisms, PATHOPHYSIOLOGY, etiology and prevention of human diseases and related outcomes, as well as their early detection, treatment, or prognosis. A way of practicing INTEGRATIVE RESEARCH. Sometimes, a level of measurement (e.g., molecular, microbiological). But not a discipline with substantive research content.[53,57,612-615] From an instrumental viewpoint, the use in EPIDEMIOLOGICAL RESEARCH of the techniques of molecular and cellular biology, genetics, systems biology, and "-omics" approaches to analyze the causes and effects of certain BIOMARKERS.[91,148,434,435] The approach is used in CANCER EPIDEMIOLOGY, for instance, to identify and characterize genetic, cellular, and physiological factors and processes involved in CARCINOGENESIS.[80-82] Molecular epidemiology is making valuable contributions to biomedical, clinical, and population sciences; e.g., research on the role of gene-environment interactions in the etiology of DISEASES OF COMPLEX ETIOLOGY is generating evidence about biological mechanisms and knowledge useful for PRIMARY PREVENTION.[13,146,174,175,216,352] See also GENETIC EPIDEMIOLOGY; HuGENET.

MONITORING

1. The regular, repetitive, and intermittent conception, performance, analysis, and interpretation of measurements aimed at detecting changes in the health status of populations or in the physical or social environment. The analysis of the implementation and effects of an intervention. In principle, it is different from SURVEILLANCE, which is often a continuous process, although surveillance techniques are used in monitoring.[12,17,69,160,302] See also BENEFIT; BIOMONITORING.

2. In management, the episodic oversight of the implementation of an activity, seeking to ensure that input deliveries, work schedules, targeted outputs, and other required actions are proceeding according to plan.

MONITOR, STUDY See STUDY MONITOR.

MONOGENIC DISEASES Diseases in which a genetic variant of high PENETRANCE confers a high risk of developing the disease and may thus be thought to be the sole cause of the disease, although the penetrance and expressivity of the gene are sometimes regulated by other genes or even by lifestyle and environmental exposures (e.g., diet, access to effective medical treatment). An antonym of POLYGENIC DISEASES.

MONOTONIC (Syn: monotone) A relationship, sequence, or TREND is said to be monotonically increasing if each value is greater than or equal to the previous one and monotonically decreasing if each value is less than or equal to the previous one. Monotonic responses may be linear or nonlinear, but the slope does not change sign.[1,2,13] This justifies using high-dose testing as the standard for assessing chemical safety.[14,342] Contrast with NONMONOTONIC.

MONTE-CARLO STUDY, TRIAL Complex relationships that are difficult to solve by mathematical analysis are sometimes studied by computer experiments that simulate and analyze a sequence of events using random numbers. Such experiments are called Monte Carlo trials or studies, in reference to Monte Carlo, one of the gambling centers of the world.[7,14,37] See also MARKOV PROCESS; SIMULATION.

MORAL HAZARD In health economics, the modification of individual behaviors related to having insurance. Moral hazard refers to the effect that being insured has on behavior, increasing the probability of the event insured. Moral hazard arises because individuals or institutions do not take the full consequences and responsibilities of their actions, and therefore have a tendency to act less carefully than they otherwise would, leaving another party to hold some of the consequences of those actions. One behavioral effect of moral hazard in a market-based system is to cause premiums to rise. Premiums reflect both the inherent element of risk (the fair premium) and the additional costs generated through moral hazard. If the insurance is not compulsory, this may be sufficient to lead some insureds to withdraw from the system. In a compulsory system, it leads to a continous rising of costs, with more people being tempted to demand some services to compensate such increasing costs. The welfare effects of moral hazard ought thus to be considered in terms of its impact both on health care utilization and on the take-up of health care insurance.[17,358,616] See also ELASTICITY; MARKET FAILURE.

MORBIDITY
1. Any departure, subjective or objective, from a state of physiological or psychological well-being. In this sense *sickness, illness*, and *morbid condition* are similarly defined and synonymous (but see DISEASE).[5]
2. The WHO Expert Committee on Health Statistics noted in its Sixth report (1959) that morbidity could be measured in terms of three units:
   a. Persons who were ill.
   b. The illnesses (periods or spells of illness) that these persons experienced.
   c. The duration (days, weeks, etc.) of these illnesses.[24]

See also HEALTH INDEX; INCIDENCE RATE; NOTIFIABLE DISEASE; PREVALENCE.

MORBIDITY RATE A term, preferably avoided, used to refer to the incidence rate and sometimes (incorrectly) to the prevalence of disease.

MORBIDITY SURVEY A method for estimating the prevalence and/or incidence of disease in a population. A morbidity survey is usually designed simply to ascertain the facts as to disease distribution and not to test a hypothesis.[160] See also CROSS-SECTIONAL STUDY; HEALTH SURVEY.

MORTALITY: INCIDENCE RATIO See CANCER MORTALITY:INCIDENCE RATIO.

MORTALITY RATE See DEATH RATE.

MORTALITY STATISTICS Statistical tables compiled from the information contained in DEATH CERTIFICATES. Most administrative jurisdictions in all nations produce tables of mortality statistics. These may be published at regular intervals; they usually show numbers of deaths and/or rates by age, sex, cause, and sometimes other variables.

MOVING AVERAGES (Syn: rolling averages, running averages) A set of methods for smoothing irregularities in TREND data, such as long-term secular trends in incidence or mortality rates. Graphical display of (say, 3- or 5-year) moving averages makes it easier to discern long-term trends in rates that otherwise might be obscured by short-term fluctuations. The span over which the average is taken is sometimes called the *window width*. Within that window, the averages may be weighted by proximity to the point at which the rate is being estimated. This weighting function is sometimes called a "kernel function," and the process is then called *kernel smoothing*.[1]

MSM Men who have sex with men. In this group, high-risk practices for HIV infection may occur. See also MARGINAL STRUCTURAL MODELS.

MULTICOLLINEARITY (Syn: collinearity) In multiple regression analysis, a situation in which at least some of the regressors (independent variables) are highly correlated with each other. Such a situation can result in inaccurate or undefined estimates of the parameters in the regression model.[1,7,36,244]

MULTIDRUG-RESISTANT (MDR) See DRUG RESISTANCE, MULTIPLE.

MULTIFACTORIAL ETIOLOGY See MULTIPLE CAUSATION.

MULTILEVEL ANALYSIS (Syn: contextual analysis, hierarchical analysis) Integration of contextual, group, or macrolevel factors with individual-level factors in epidemiological analyses of health states and outcomes. The rationale is that the distribution of health and disease in populations is not explained only by characteristics of individuals.[617] Methodologies that analyze outcomes in relation to determinants simultaneously measured at different levels (e.g., individual, workplace, neighborhood, region). One aim of multilevel analyses is to explain how group- and individual-level variables interact in shaping health. Such analyses require one to select the appropriate contextual units and contextual variables, to correctly specify the model, and to account for residual correlation between individuals within contexts.[1,3,7,24,158,255,326,357,407,306]

MULTILEVEL MODEL (Syn: hierarchical model) A REGRESSION MODEL in which the coefficients of the regressors are themselves modeled as functions of properties of the regressors. For example, in a regression of colon cancer incidence in relation to food intakes, the food coefficients may be modeled as functions of their nutrient contents. In a regression of lung-cancer incidence in relation to occupation, an occupational coefficient may be modeled as a function of the chemical exposures in the occupation. The properties used to model the coefficients are called second-level or second-stage covariates. Multilevel models are equivalent to *random-coefficient models* or *mixed models* in which the second-level covariates have random coefficients.

MULTINOMIAL DISTRIBUTION The probability distribution associated with the classification of each of a sample of individuals into one of several mutually exclusive and exhaustive categories, assuming that the individual classifications are independent of one another.[7,34,37] When the number of categories is two, the DISTRIBUTION is called BINOMIAL DISTRIBUTION.

MULTIPHASE SAMPLING Method of sampling that gathers some information from a large sample and more detailed information from subsamples within this sample, either at the same time or later. Contrast to MULTISTAGE SAMPLING.

MULTIPHASIC SCREENING See SCREENING.

MULTIPLE BIAS MODELING The use of SENSITIVITY ANALYSIS techniques to assess the robustness of results to two or more biases (e.g., CONFOUNDING, MEASUREMENT ERROR, SELECTION BIAS) simultaneously.[1,2,131]

MULTIPLE CAUSATION (Syn: multifactorial etiology) The concept that a given health state or health-related process may have more than one cause. A combination of causes or alternative combinations of causes is often required to produce the health outcome. See also CAUSAL DIAGRAM; DISEASES OF COMPLEX ETIOLOGY; PLEIOTROPY; PROBABILITY OF CAUSATION; RISK FACTOR; WEB OF CAUSATION.

MULTIPLE CAUSE THEORY A theory coherent with MULTIPLE CAUSATION. By contrast, HENLE-KOCH POSTULATES do not admit multiple causes of a single disorder, nor do they contemplate causal relations not susceptible to experimentation. Early in the twentieth century, German scientists raised questions about the limitation of such postulates and paved the way for new ideas on multifactorial causality.[618] Consensus about MULTIPLE CAUSATION coalesced a half-century later, when chronic noninfectious disease had become a leading public health concern.[163-169] Thereafter, the theory permeated epidemiology up to the present time.[25,39,101,128,206,207,326,406,407,557,566,592]

MULTIPLE COMPARISON PROBLEMS Problems that arise from the fact that the greater the number of conventional statistical tests of SIGNIFICANCE conducted on a data set, the greater the probability that at least one or more tests will falsely reject the NULL HYPOTHESIS solely because of the play of chance. Adjustment of the ALPHA LEVEL in this situation is a debatable option; it has been strongly criticized because it will dramatically raise the false-negative rate (rate of TYPE-II ERROR, failure to reject a false null).[1,24,26,53,91] See also *P* VALUE; RELEVANCE.

MULTIPLE COMPARISON TECHNIQUES Statistical procedures to adjust for differences in probability levels in setting up simultaneous confidence limits involving several distributions or sets of data or in comparing the means of several groups.[37] *Tukey's method* is the most conservative; this uses the difference between the largest and smallest means as a measure of their dispersion; the q statistic, based on the α level (acceptable rate of TYPE I ERROR), and the number of groups are used as multipliers of the standard deviation. The *Bonferroni correction* adjusts the α error level to compensate for multiple comparisons between three or more groups or two or more response variables.

Such conventional multiple comparisons techniques are problematic because they raise the false-negative rate (rate of TYPE II ERROR, failure to reject a false null), often to the point that it may become impossible to detect any true effects. Modern techniques that attempt to address both Type I and Type II errors have been developed, especially under the topic of EMPIRICAL-BAYES METHODS and SHRINKAGE ESTIMATION.

MULTIPLE DRUG RESISTANCE See DRUG RESISTANCE, MULTIPLE.

MULTIPLE LOGISTIC MODEL A LOGISTIC MODEL with multiple regressors.[3]

MULTIPLE OF THE MEDIAN (MoM) A measurement of a positive quantity expressed in units of the median. MoM is sometimes used to report the results of medical screening tests, particularly where the results of the individual tests are highly variable. The method is not much affected by variation in measurement errors; however, it is affected by the DISTRIBUTION of results used to determine the median, and there is no correction for the spread of the data. For these reasons the Z SCORE is usually considered preferable.

MULTIPLE REGRESSION TECHNIQUES Techniques for REGRESSION ANALYSIS that allow the inclusion of multiple regressors (independent variables).[1,3,7,11,36,110,244]

MULTIPLE RISK Where more than one RISK FACTOR for the development of a disease or other outcome is present and their combined presence results in an increased RISK, we speak of "multiple risk." The increased risk may be due to the additive effects of the risks associated with the separate risk factors, or to SYNERGISM. See also MULTIPLE CAUSATION.

MULTIPLICATIVE MODEL A model in which the joint effect of two or more factors is the product of their individual effects.[1,3,8,270] For instance, if factor X multiplies risk by the amount x in the absence of factor Y, and factor Y multiplies risk by the amount y in the absence of factor X, then the multiplicative risk model states that the two factors X and Y together will multiply the risk by $x \times y$. See also ADDITIVE MODEL.

MULTIPLY ROBUST ESTIMATOR An estimator for an effect which, when multiple statistical models are specified, is CONSISTENT for the effect of interest whenever one of multiple (three or more) non-nested sets of models is correctly specified.[101,619,620] See also DOUBLY ROBUST ESTIMATOR.

MULTISTAGE MODELS Conceptual and mathematical models—mainly for carcinogenesis—based on theory and preclinical, clinical, and epidemiological evidence suggesting that a CARCINOGEN may affect one or more stages in the development of cancer.[78-82] At least five fundamental models of carcinogenesis have been proposed.[78] Model 1 is centered around mutations, the chemical environment, radiation and viruses. Model 2 focuses on genomic dysregulation, genome instability, and familiality. Model 3 is based on non-genotoxic mechanisms, clonal expansion, and epigenetics. Model 4 encompasses the previous three, based on the concept of a "Darwinian" (somatic) cell selection. Model 5 is based on "tissue organization." The five models have been formalized mathematically, partly overlap, and differ in considering that biological changes in the epithelium alone lead to malignancy, or that changes in stroma/extracellular matrix are also necessary. See also ARMITAGE-DOLL MODEL.

MULTISTAGE SAMPLING Selection, random or otherwise, of entities (such as geographical regions, schools, workplaces) followed by random sampling of persons within each sampled group. The method has advantages such as convenience and FEASIBILITY, but it complicates analysis. Contrast to MULTIPHASE SAMPLING.

MULTIVARIATE ANALYSIS A set of techniques used when the variation in several variables has to be studied simultaneously. In statistics, any analytical method that allows the simultaneous study of two or more DEPENDENT VARIABLES (regressands).[1,3,7,34,36,37,244,269,270]

MUTAGEN A microbiological, physical, or chemical agent that raises the frequency of mutations above the spontaneous rate. Any substance that can cause genetic mutations. Mutagens cause mutations in different ways.[57,78,80-82,183-186,245,316-321,409-417]

MUTATION Any change in a DNA sequence. In a clinical sense, any such change that disrupts the information contained in DNA and leads to disease. Many types of mutations and mechanisms leading to mutations exist. Change in the genetic material not caused by genetic segregation or recombination that is transmitted to daughter cells and to succeeding generations provided that it is not a dominant lethal factor.

MUTUALISM The interaction of two organisms that results in a fitness advantage for both organisms. See also COMMENSAL; HUMAN MICROBIOME; METAGENOME; PARASITE.

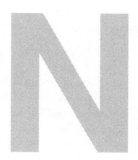

NARRATIVE REVIEW See SYSTEMATIC REVIEW.

NATURAL EXPERIMENT Naturally occurring circumstances in which subsets of the population have different levels of exposure to a hypothesized causal factor in a situation resembling an actual EXPERIMENT.[5,26] The presence of persons in a particular group is typically nonrandom; yet for a natural experiment, it suffices that their presence is independent of (unrelated to) potential confounders. See also EXPERIMENTAL EPIDEMIOLOGY; OBSERVATIONAL STUDY.

Investigation by John Snow (1813–1858) of the distribution of cholera cases in London in relation to the sources of water supply is an excellent example of a natural experiment. It would have been unethical for Snow to allocate subjects to groups exposed to a lethal infection; but tracing the source of their drinking water, using what is now sometimes called SHOE-LEATHER EPIDEMIOLOGY, gave him the opportunity to make crucially important observations. "To turn this grand experiment to account, all that was required was to learn the supply of water to each individual house where a fatal attack of cholera might occur... I resolved to spare no exertion which might be necessary to ascertain the exact effect of the water supply on the progress of the epidemic, in the places where all the circumstances were so happily adapted for the inquiry... I had no reason to doubt the correctness of the conclusions I had drawn from the great number of facts already in my possession, but I felt that the circumstances of the cholera-poisoning passing down the sewers into a great river, and being distributed through miles of pipes, and yet producing its specific effects was a fact of so startling a nature, and of so vast importance to the community, that it could not be too rigidly examined or established on too firm a basis."[69,621]

NATURAL FOCUS OF INFECTION (Syn: natural nidality of disease). A focus existing outside a human population (e.g., in domestic or wild animals) often transmitted by a vector; humans can be infected if they enter such a biotype.[56,69] A concept developed by zoologist, parasitologist, and epidemiologist Yevgeny Pavlovsky (1884–1965).

NATURAL HISTORY OF DISEASE The course of a disease from pathological onset or inception to resolution. Many diseases have certain relatively well-defined stages that, taken all together, are referred to as the "natural history of the disease" in question. These stages are as follows:

1. Stages of pathological onset. They are constantly being changed in many diseases; "onset," in particular, tends to be redefined in increasingly smaller microbiological (e.g., molecular and genetic) terms.

2. Presymptomatic stage: from initiation of disease to the first appearance of symptoms and/or signs.
3. Clinically manifest disease, which may progress inexorably to a fatal termination, be subject to remissions and relapses, or regress spontaneously, leading to recovery.

The nature and borders of these broad stages varies vastly across diseases. Some diseases have precursors. For example, elevated serum cholesterol is among the precursors of coronary heart disease. Precursor lesions may long precede the stage of pathological onset, but many alterations will be reversible or of unknown prognostic SIGNIFICANCE. An intense search is presently taking place for genetic, biochemical, or peptidomic "precursors" or "markers" of many diseases; a common aim is to market tests for EARLY DETECTION, which should be able to alter the natural history of the disease if they are promptly followed by effective interventions (e.g., surgical treatment). Studies on precursor and prognostic factors must integrate evidence on the putative biochemical or molecular markers with clinical, anatomopathological, and pathophysiological reasoning.

Often it is more a model or framework than a reality: the presentation and course of human disease tends to vary a lot in different individuals and contexts. The term *natural* should not be taken as a synonym of *biological*, since the course of disease in humans is not influenced only by biological and health care processes but also by social and cultural interactions (e.g., by cultural beliefs and norms on health care seeking, attributions of meaning to symptoms, economic barriers to treatment).[5-9,58,332] The term has also been used to mean "descriptive epidemiology of disease." See also CLINICAL STUDY; EARLY CLINICAL DETECTION; INCUBATION PERIOD; INDUCTION PERIOD; LATENCY PERIOD; SCREENING; SICKNESS "CAREER."

NATURAL HISTORY STUDY A study, generally longitudinal, designed to yield information about the natural course of a disease or condition. See also INCEPTION COHORT.

NATURAL RATE OF INCREASE (DECREASE) See GROWTH RATE OF POPULATION.

NEAREST NEIGHBOR METHOD

1. In statistics, a regression method in which the prediction at a given combination of regressor values is estimated only from the nearest neighbors to that combination, where "nearest" is defined in terms of a multivariate distance criterion.[1]
2. A means of analyzing the spatial patterns of a free-living population. A term originating from VETERINARY EPIDEMIOLOGY. Random sampling points are located throughout an area and the distance from each point to the nearest individual is measured; alternatively, individuals are selected at random and, from each of these, the distance to the nearest neighbor is measured.

NECESSARY CAUSE A factor whose presence is required for the occurrence of the effect.[1-3,5,8,39,42,84,101,206-210,406,407,433,798] See also ASSOCIATION; CAUSALITY; COMPONENT CAUSES; DISEASES OF COMPLEX ETIOLOGY; HILL'S CONSIDERATIONS FOR CAUSATION; INTEGRATION; SUFFICIENT CAUSE.

NEEDLE STICK Puncture of the skin by a needle that may have been contaminated by contact with an infected patient or fluid. See also SHARPS.

NEED(S) In health economics, the minimum amount of resources required to exhaust an individual's or a specified population's capacity to benefit from an intervention.[116] Sociologists allude to *perceived need*, meaning the beliefs or perceptions of health care providers or users about their requirements. Physicians speak of *professionally defined needs*, meaning undiagnosed and/or untreated conditions ranging from dangers to the public health, such as the risk of TB posed by persons who are excreting tubercle bacilli in sputum, to mild myopia in persons who would benefit from wearing corrective lenses.[28,622]

NEEDS ASSESSMENT A systematic procedure for determining the nature and extent of problems experienced by a specified population that affect their health either directly or indirectly. It uses epidemiological, sociodemographic, and qualitative methods to describe health problems and their environmental, social, economic, and behavioral DETERMINANTS. The aim is to identify unmet health care needs and make recommendations about ways to address these needs, whether they are explicit health problems such as untreated diseases or "problems waiting to happen," such as inadequate housing, ignorance due to low literacy levels, domestic violence, lack of ACCESS to long-term care, etc. Needs assessment is a routine or an ad hoc activity in many local public health departments.[28,43,38,303,304,623-625]

NEGATIVE CONTROLS See CONTROLS, NEGATIVE.

NEGATIVE PREDICTIVE VALUE See PREDICTIVE VALUE, NEGATIVE.

NEGATIVE STUDY Often taken to mean a study that fails to find evidence for an effect.[626] It is a somewhat confusing term because it also suggests a "negative effect," which in turn may mean a preventive or a deleterious effect.[58] See also CONFOUNDING, NEGATIVE; FALSE NEGATIVE; NULL STUDY; PUBLICATION BIAS.

NEGATIVE TRANSITION See DISEASE TRANSITION.

NEONATAL MORTALITY RATE

1. In VITAL STATISTICS, the number of deaths in infants under 28 days of age in a given period, usually a year, per 1000 live births in that period.[627] See also MATERNAL MORTALITY RATIO.

2. In obstetrical and perinatal research, the term *neonatal mortality rate* is often used to denote the cumulative mortality rate of live-born infants within 28 days of age. See DEATH RATE.

NESTED CASE-CONTROL STUDY A type of CASE-CONTROL STUDY in which cases and controls are drawn from the population in a fully enumerated COHORT. Typically, some data on some variables are already available about both cases and controls; thus concerns about differential (biased) MISCLASSIFICATION of these variables can be reduced (e.g., environmental or nutritional exposures may be analyzed in blood from cases and controls collected and stored years before disease onset). With nested DENSITY SAMPLING, controls are selected from subjects who remain at risk of developing the outcome of interest at the time of occurrence of each case that arises in the cohort.[1,3,149,197,269,270,795] With nested CUMULATIVE SAMPLING, controls are instead selected only from subjects who do not experience the outcome throughout the entire study period.

NESTED DESIGN A study design that is applied to a population already identified in an existing population or study; an example is a nested case-control study, in which cases and controls are drawn from a fully enumerated cohort, which may already be under investigation in a cohort study.[1-3,795]

NET MIGRATION The numerical difference between immigration and emigration.

NET MIGRATION RATE The net effect of immigration and emigration on an area's population, expressed as an increase or decrease per 1000 population of the area in a given year.

NET RECLASSIFICATION INDEX See DISCRIMINATORY ACCURACY.

NET REPRODUCTION RATE (NRR) The average number of female children born per woman in a cohort subject to a given set of age-specific fertility rates, a given set of age-specific mortality rates, and a given sex ratio at birth. This rate measures replacement fertility under given conditions of fertility and mortality: it is the ratio of daughters to mothers assuming continuation of the specified conditions of fertility and mortality. It is a measure of population growth from one generation to another under constant conditions. This rate is similar to the gross reproduction rate but takes into account that some women will die before completing their childbearing years. An NRR of 1.00 means that each generation of mothers is having exactly enough daughters to replace itself in the population. See also GROSS REPRODUCTION RATE; REPLACEMENT-LEVEL FERTILITY.

NET REPRODUCTIVE RATE (R) (Syn: case reproduction rate) In infectious disease epidemiology, the average number of secondary cases that will occur in a mixed host population of susceptibles and nonsusceptibles when one infected individual is introduced. Its relationship to the BASIC REPRODUCTIVE RATE (R_0) is given by

$$R = R_0 x$$

where x is the proportion of the host population that is susceptible.

NETWORK A dynamically interconnected group or system. The interpersonal and social connections among individuals, groups, organizations, companies, or institutions. Physical and social networks are involved in many *processes* of relevance for epidemiology, such as the spread of communicable diseases and healthy and toxic habits (exercising, consumption, leisure and cultural habits, smoking, alcohol use), information sharing and social networking, food webs, (un)employment and work relationships, urban pollution, world trade, or global warming. Some of the most important natural systems and social phenomena of relevance to public health and medicine have a networked structure.[17,27,28,160,628] This makes the absence of the concept in most epidemiologic and medical textbooks remarkable.[399] See also ACQUAINTANCE NETWORK; SENTINEL SURVEILLANCE.

NIDUS A focus of infection. The term can be used to describe any heterogeneity in the distribution of a disease, but it is usually applied to a small area in which conditions favor occurrence and spread of a COMMUNICABLE DISEASE. Also, the site of origin of a pathological process.

NNT See NUMBER NEEDED TO TREAT.

NNH See NUMBER NEEDED TO HARM.

NNS See NUMBER NEEDED TO SCREEN.

NOCEBO An unpleasant or adverse effect attributable to administration of a PLACEBO.

NODE See CAUSAL DIAGRAM.

N-OF-ONE STUDY (Syn: single-patient trial) A variation of a randomized controlled CROSSOVER CLINICAL TRIAL, in which a sequence of alternative treatments is randomly allocated to only one patient. Changes in signs and symptoms (or other reversible outcomes) experienced by the patient are compared, with the aim of deciding on the optimal regimen for the patient.[6,26,37,58,629-631]

NOISE (IN DATA) This term is used when extraneous uncontrolled variables and/or errors influence the distribution of measurements made in a study, thus rendering difficult or impossible the determination of relationships between variables under scrutiny.

NOMENCLATURE A list of all approved terms for describing and recording observations.

NOMINAL SCALE See MEASUREMENT SCALE.

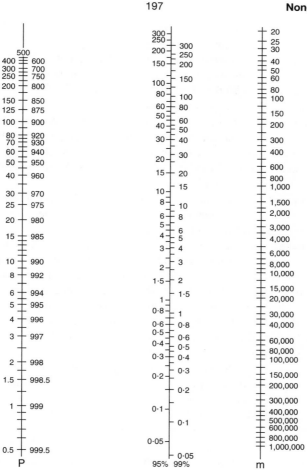

Nomogram of confidence limits to a rate. Source: Rosenbaum R.[632]

NOMOGRAM A form of line chart showing scales for the variables involved in a particular formula in such a way that corresponding values for each variable lie on a straight line intersecting all the scales.

NON-COMMUNICABLE DISEASE (Syn: non-transmissible disease) A disease for which evidence is lacking that transmission from individual to individual is possible by CONTAGION, a VECTOR, biological HEREDITY or INHERITANCE.[20,22,163-169,633,634]

NONCONCURRENT STUDY See HISTORICAL COHORT STUDY.

NON-CONTAGIOUS EVENTS. Events for which the occurrence in one individual does not increase the risk of the event in other individuals. This definition does not exclude the possibility that the event in one individual may decrease risk in other individuals. Both possibilities are however excluded by INDEPENDENCE. See also CONTAGIOUS.

NONDIFFERENTIAL MISCLASSIFICATION See MISCLASSIFICATION.

NONEXPERIMENTAL STUDY See OBSERVATIONAL STUDY.

NONGENOTOXIC CARCINOGENS Carcinogens that do not cause direct damage to the DNA. Nongenotoxic processes and mechanisms include induction of inflammation, immunosuppression, formation of reactive oxygen species (ROS), activation of receptors such as the arylhydrocarbon receptor (AhR) or estrogen receptor (ER), and EPIGENETIC silencing. Together, GENOTOXIC and nongenotoxic mechanisms can alter signal-transduction pathways, finally resulting in hypermutability, genomic instability, loss of proliferation control, and resistance to apoptosis—features characteristic of cancer cells. At early stages of tumorigenesis the nongenotoxic effects are reversible and may require continuous presence of the compound. Long-term exposure to low doses of GENOTOXIC carcinogens also contributes to nongenotoxic alterations. Some nongenotoxic environmental CARCINOGENS weaken cell-cycle checkpoint functions, thus leading to genetic instability or to heritable alterations of the genome.[13,14,78,80-82,178,415,416,635] See also CARCINOGENESIS; MUTAGEN.

NON-INFERIORITY TRIAL A trial designed to test that a treatment is not inferior to a comparison treatment; i.e., that one treatment is "not worse than" or is "at least as good as" another treatment.[73,76,77] See also SUPERIORITY TRIAL.

NON-INFERIORITY MARGIN The acceptable amount for which the experimental therapy may be worse than the control therapy and still be noninferior to the control therapy. Typically, the non-inferiority margin is based on a systematic review of the effect of the control therapy, so that the experimental therapy would be regarded as beneficial and/or efficacious should the effect of the experimental therapy be greater than the difference in the effect of the control therapy and the non-inferiority margin.[73,76]

NONMALEFICENCE The ethical principle of causing no harm.[59,73-77,116-118,259-265] See also PRECAUTIONARY PRINCIPLE.

NONMONOTONIC A nonmonotonic relationship between an exposure and an outcome or effect is a nonlinear relationship in which the slope of the curve changes sign from positive to negative or vice versa at one or more points along the range of doses examined.[1,2] Such curves and TRENDS often have a U- or inverted U-shape, and are thus referred to as biphasic. Abundant examples of biological and social mechanisms responsible for nonmonotonicity exist in the biological, clinical, epidemiological, and economic literature. Natural hormones and endocrine-disrupting chemicals frequently show nonmonotonic relationships and low-dose effects. When nonmonotonic DOSE-RESPONSE curves occur, the effects of low doses cannot be predicted by the effects observed at high doses.[12-14,342] Contrast with MONOTONIC.

NONPARAMETRIC METHODS See DISTRIBUTION-FREE METHOD.

NONPARAMETRIC TEST See DISTRIBUTION-FREE METHOD.

NONPARTICIPANTS (Syn: nonresponders) Members of a study sample or population who do not take part in the study for whatever reason, or members of a target population who do not participate in an activity. Differences between participants and nonparticipants have been demonstrated repeatedly in studies of many kinds, and this is often a source of BIAS.

NO-OBSERVED-ADVERSE-EFFECT LEVEL (NOAEL) The highest dose at which no adverse health effects are detected in an animal population. A NOAEL-SF is a no-observed-effects level with an added safety factor for human exposures; it is used in setting human safety standards. In practice, the safety factor added is commonly two or more orders of magnitude (i.e., a hundredfold or a thousandfold greater than the NOAEL).[14]

NORM

1. What is usual; e.g., the range into which blood pressure values usually fall in a population group, the dietary or infant feeding practices that are usual in a given culture, or the way that a given illness is usually treated in a given health care system.

2. What is desirable; e.g., the range of blood pressures that a given authority regards as being indicative of present good health or as predisposing to future good health, the dietary or infant feeding practices that are valued in a given culture, or the health care procedures or facilities for health care that a given authority regards as desirable. In the latter sense, norms may be used as criteria in evaluating health care in order to determine the degree of conformity with what is desirable (e.g., the average length of stay of patients in hospital). Behavior that is considered culturally desirable and appropriate and therefore expected from members that belong to the community.

NORMAL

1. Within the usual range of variation in a given population or group. Frequently occurring in a given population or group. In this sense, "normal" is frequently defined as "within a range extending from two standard deviations below the mean to two standard deviations above the mean," or "between specified percentiles of the distribution" (e.g., the 10th and 90th percentiles).[1-3,5-9,37,38]
2. Indicative or predictive of good health or conducive to good health. For a diagnostic or screening test, a "normal" result is one in a range within which the probability of a specific disease is low. See also NORMAL LIMITS.
3. (Of a distribution) Gaussian distribution or NORMAL DISTRIBUTION.[7]

NORMAL DISTRIBUTION (Syn: Gaussian distribution) The continuous frequency distribution of infinite range whose PROBABILITY DENSITY is given by the equation

$$f(x) = \frac{1}{(2\pi\sigma^2)^{1/2}} e^{-(x-\mu)^2/2\sigma^2}$$

where x is the abscissa, $f(x)$ is the ordinate, μ is the mean, $e \approx 2.718$ is the base of the natural logarithm, and σ the standard deviation. All possible values of the variable are displayed on the horizontal axis. The relative frequency (relative probability) of each value is displayed on the vertical axis, producing the graph of the normal distribution. The properties of a normal distribution include the following:

1. It is a continuous, symmetrical distribution; both tails extend to infinity.
2. The arithmetic mean, mode, and median are identical.
3. Its shape is completely determined by the mean and standard deviation.
4. In common situations found in epidemiology, it is the approximate distribution for sums and means of variables provided that there are enough variables being summed or averaged, no one variable dominates the sum or average, and the variables are not too highly correlated among themselves. Then this is so even if the component variables are not themselves normal. An example is the mean of independent binary variables; the individual variables are far from normal, but the DISTRIBUTION of their mean gets close to normal even if there are as few as five of them. This property is sometimes called the *central limit* property.[7,12,34,37]

NORMAL LIMITS The limits of the "normal" range of a test or measurement, in the sense of being indicative of or conducive to good health. One way to determine normal limits is to compare the values obtained when the measurements are made in two groups, one that is healthy and has been found to remain healthy and another that is ill or subsequently found to become ill. The result may be two overlapping distributions. Outside the area where the distributions overlap, a given value clearly identifies the presence or absence of disease or some other manifestation of poor health. If a value falls into the area of overlap, the individual may belong either to the normal or the abnormal group. The choice of the normal limits depends upon the relative importance attached to the identification of individuals as healthy or unhealthy. See also FALSE NEGATIVE; FALSE POSITIVE; SENSITIVITY AND SPECIFICITY.

NORMATIVE Pertaining to the normal, usual, accepted standards or values. See also NORM.

NOSOCOMIAL Relating to a hospital. Arising while a patient is in a hospital or as a result of being in a hospital. Denoting a new disorder (unrelated to the patient's primary condition) associated with being in a hospital.[69]

NOSOCOMIAL INFECTION (Syn: hospital-acquired infection) An infection originating in a medical facility; e.g., occurring in a patient in a hospital or other health care facility in whom the infection was not present or incubating at the time of admission.[56,69,188,196,217-219] Includes infections acquired in the hospital but appearing after discharge; it also includes such infections among staff. See also HOSPITAL EPIDEMIOLOGY.

NOSOGRAPHY, NOSOLOGY Classification of ill persons into groups, whatever the criteria for their CLASSIFICATION, and agreement as to the boundaries of the groups. The assignment of names to each disease entity in the group results in a nomenclature of disease entities, or nosography.[636]

NOTIFIABLE DISEASE A disease that, by statutory requirements, must be reported to the public health authority in the pertinent jurisdiction when the diagnosis is made. A disease deemed of sufficient importance to the public health to require that its occurrence be reported to health authorities.

The reporting to public health authorities of COMMUNICABLE DISEASES is, unfortunately, very incomplete. The reasons for this include diagnostic inexactitude; the desire of patients and physicians to conceal the occurrence of conditions carrying a social stigma (e.g., sexually transmitted diseases) and the indifference of physicians to the usefulness of information about such diseases as hepatitis, influenza, and measles. Yet notifications are extremely important. They provide the starting point for investigations into the failure of preventive measures, such as immunizations, for tracing sources of infection, finding common vehicles of infection, describing the geographic CLUSTERING of infection, and various other purposes, depending upon the particular disease.[28,56,188,196,217-219]

N.S. Abbreviation, usually written lower case (n.s.), for *not statistically significant*. See also SIGNIFICANCE.

NULL HYPOTHESIS The statistical hypothesis that one variable has no association with another variable or set of variables, or that two or more population distributions do not differ from one another. In statistical terms, the null hypothesis states that the differences observed in a study or test occurred as a result of the operation of chance alone.[3,7,26] A CAUSAL NULL HYPOTHESIS states that one variable has no EFFECT on another. See also TEST HYPOTHESIS.

NULL STUDY A study that fails to find evidence for an association or effect (e.g., coffee drinking does not increase or decrease the risk of pancreatic cancer). The term is more precise than the often used synonym NEGATIVE STUDY. A study is not null simply because it fails to reach STATISTICAL SIGNIFICANCE; it may in fact provide evidence for an association or an effect (evidence against the NULL HYPOTHESIS) by exhibiting an association, but fail to reach conventional levels of statistical significance because it is too small (underpowered) for the observed association to reach statistical significance.[1,3,91,270]

NUMBER NEEDED TO HARM (NNH) (Syn: Number Needed to be treated to Harm one person)

1. The number of persons needed to be treated, on average, to produce one more adverse event (e.g., occurrence of a disease, complication, adverse reaction, relapse) than would have occurred without the treatment. Average number of persons who need to receive the treatment for one of them to experience an adverse effect. It is a clinically oriented way of expressing the RISK of one intervention over another and takes the absolute risk of the event into account. It is used to summarize results of studies and to assist in clinical decision-making.

2. The reciprocal of the ABSOLUTE RISK INCREASE. Let ARC be the absolute risk of events in the control group and ART the absolute risk of events in the treatment group; then the absolute risk increase (ARI) = ART – ARC and NNH = 1 / ARI. It may also be calculated as 100 divided by the ARI to express it as a percentage.[9,10,58] Example: the occurrence of adverse outcomes in a clinical trial was 10% (0.10) in the treated group and 4% (0.04) in the placebo group; hence, the ARI was 0.06 and 1 / 0.06 = 16.7; i.e., on average, about 17 patients have to be treated in order to increase the number having an adverse outcome by 1.

Definitions 1 and 2 look equivalent but are not unless the treatment acts independently of other background factors leading to the harm. See also ABSOLUTE RISK REDUCTION; NUMBER NEEDED TO TREAT; RELATIVE RISK REDUCTION.

NUMBER NEEDED TO SCREEN (NNS) The average number of persons who must undergo a SCREENING test and the ensuing diagnostic and therapeutic procedures in order to prevent one case of the disease of interest:

$$NNS = NNT / PrC$$

where NNT is the NUMBER NEEDED TO TREAT and PrC is the prevalence of carriers of the variant of interest in the population screened. When the NNT is to be used to compute the NNS, computation of the NNT is based, as usual, on the reciprocal of the ABSOLUTE RISK REDUCTION (ARR) (i.e., NNT = 1 / ARR); yet in GENETIC SCREENING, the ARR is the lifetime risk of the disease among carriers of the genetic variant of interest minus the risk of the disease achieved once the carriers are identified, diagnosed, and treated with the available means. A reasonable (low) NNS is attained only by screening for highly penetrant genetic variants in high-risk families, not for such mutations in the general population or for low-penetrant polymorphisms.[478] See also GENETIC PENETRANCE; MONOGENIC DISEASES; POLYGENIC DISEASES; SCREENING.

NUMBER NEEDED TO TREAT (NNT) (Syn: Number Needed to be Treated)

1. The number of persons needed to be treated, on average, to prevent one more event (e.g., occurrence of a disease to be prevented, complication, adverse reaction, relapse). It is a clinically meaningful way of expressing the benefit of an intervention over another; it takes the absolute risk of the event into account. It is used to summarize results of studies and to assist in clinical decision-making.[2,7,9,26,58,637,638]

2. The reciprocal of the ABSOLUTE RISK REDUCTION. Let ARC be the absolute risk of events in the control group and ART the absolute risk of events in the treatment group; then the absolute risk reduction (ARR) = ARC – ART and the NNT = 1 / ARR. It may also be calculated as 100 divided by the ARR expressed as a percentage. Example: the occurrence of adverse outcomes in a clinical trial was 10% (0.10) in the placebo group and 4% (0.04) in the treated group; hence, the ARR was 0.06 and 1 / 0.06 = 16.7 (i.e., on average, about 17 patients have to be treated in order

to prevent one of them from having an adverse outcome or to reduce the number having an adverse outcome by 1). The ARR is higher and the NNT lower in groups with higher absolute risks.[9,10,58]

Definitions 1 and 2 seem equivalent but are not so unless the treatment acts independently of other background factors leading to the harm. See also MEASURE OF ASSOCIATION; NUMBER NEEDED TO HARM; RELATIVE RISK REDUCTION.

NUMERATOR The upper portion of a ratio.[1,7,34,37,106-108] See also DENOMINATOR.

NUMERICAL TAXONOMY The construction of homogeneous groupings or taxa using numerical methods.

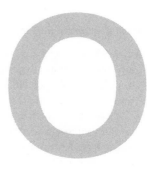

OBESITY See BODY MASS INDEX.

OBJECTIVE

1. (n.) The precisely stated end to which efforts are directed, specifying the population outcome, variable(s) to be measured, etc.[17] See also GOAL; TARGET.

2. (adj.) Free of prejudice, bias, favoritism, special interest; e.g., an objective perspective or method. Some authors believe that such perspectives do not exist in reality and that at best an objective view is simply an ideal to strive for.[1-3,38]

OBSERVATIONAL EPIDEMIOLOGY The use of epidemiological reasoning, knowledge, and methods in studies that are nonexperimental. Epidemiological studies and programs (e.g., SURVEILLANCE) in which main conditions (e.g., exposures) are not under the direct control of the researcher.[1-3,12,48,83,160,270]

OBSERVATIONAL STUDY (Syn: nonexperimental study) A study that does not involve any intervention (experimental or otherwise) on the part of the investigator.[1-3,6,9,25,26,39-42,197,239,269,270,272,795] A study with RANDOM ALLOCATION of treatments or other exposures is inherently experimental or nonobservational. Observations are not just a haphazard collection of facts; in their own way, observational studies must apply the same rigor as experiments, and vice versa.[201,276] Many important preclinical, clinical, and epidemiological studies (and studies in other branches of science) are completely observational or have strong observational components.[101] Dismissive attitudes toward observational research have a weak scientific basis. In the health, life, and social sciences—and in other sciences as well—there has long been a fruitful dialectic tension between observation and experiment; facts and reasons; actions, explanations, mechanisms.[1,3,6,9,26,38-42,64,83,101,201-203,639-641,798,800] Often, observational and experimental studies on the apparently same issue actually answer *different questions*; for example, a randomized clinical trial will compare women allocated to hormone replacement therapy (HRT) and women allocated to another therapy or a placebo, and perform an INTENTION-TO-TREAT ANALYSIS, whereas an observational study will compare rather different women (than those included in a RCT) who were actually exposed to HRT and women exposed to other therapies or none; characteristics of subjects, context, exposures, timing, confounders, and interactions are just six of the many reasons that usually make different designs answer different questions. Also, different designs have different strengths and weaknesses to help make decisions and CAUSAL INFERENCES. Some observational studies may be analyzed as experiments; and some experiments, as observational studies.[2,641,800] See also CASE REPORTS; CLINICAL STUDY.

OBSERVATIONAL EPIDEMIOLOGICAL STUDY Epidemiological study that does not involve any intervention (experimental or otherwise) on the part of the investigator; e.g., a population study in which changes in health status are studied in relation to changes in other characteristics. Most analytical epidemiological designs (notably, CASE-CONTROL and COHORT STUDIES) are properly called observational because investigators observe without intervening other than to record, classify, count, and analyze results.[1-3,197,795]

OBSERVER BIAS Systematic difference between a true value and the value actually observed due to OBSERVER VARIATION.[3,6,26] See also INFORMATION BIAS; INTERVIEWER BIAS.

OBSERVER VARIATION (ERROR) Variation (or error) due to failure of the observer to measure or to identify a phenomenon accurately. All observations are subject to variation. Discrepancies between repeated observations by the same observer and between different observers are to be expected; these can be diminished but probably never absolutely eliminated.

Variation may arise from several sources. The observer may miss an abnormality or think that one has been found where none is present; a measurement or a test may give incorrect results due to faulty technique or incorrect reading and recording of the results; or the observer may misinterpret the information. Two varieties of observer variation are *interobserver variation* (the amount observers vary from one another when reporting on the same material) and *intraobserver variation* (the amount one observer varies between observations in reporting more than once on the same material).

OCCAM'S RAZOR (Syn: Ockham's razor) The philosophical principle of scientific parsimony (parsimony in the sense of unwillingness to use unnecessary resources, frugality, austerity). An ancient principle often attributed to the philosopher and Franciscan friar William of Ockham (c.1285–c.1349), who said: *Entia non sunt multiplicanda praeter necessitatem* (i.e., assumptions to explain a phenomenon must not be multiplied beyond necessity). In *The Grammar of Science* (1892), Karl Pearson called this the most important canon in the whole field of logical thought. The maxim does not contradict the conclusion that multiple causes may operate in a system. The number of possible causes implicated depends upon the frame of reference and scope of the inquiry. The principle is also important in MULTIVARIATE ANALYSIS (i.e., models should not be complicated beyond necessity).[1,36,101,268-270] Nonetheless, its primacy in statistics has been challenged by modern computing developments, in which highly complex models, augmented by computer-intensive fitting and validation methods (such as CROSS-VALIDATION, SHRINKAGE, and the bootstrap), may outperform parsimonious methods. See also OVERFITTING.

OCCUPATIONAL DISEASE A disease or health disorder related to exposure to WORKING CONDITIONS, in which the relationship to specific causative processes at work has been reasonably established, and causal factors can be identified, measured, and hopefully controlled.[267,571,572,642] See also OCCUPATIONAL INJURY; WORK-RELATED DISEASE.

OCCUPATIONAL EPIDEMIOLOGY The study of the distribution of workplace exposures, EMPLOYMENT CONDITIONS, and WORKING CONDITIONS (including psychosocial, chemical, and physical processes), and of their effects on health states and outcomes in defined populations. The application of epidemiological knowledge to labor force.[571,572,643] See also OCCUPATIONAL INJURY; OCCUPATIONAL DISEASE; WORK-RELATED DISEASE.

OCCUPATIONAL HEALTH The specialized practice of medicine, public health, and other professions (e.g., industrial hygienist, ergonomist, safety technician, occupational psychologist) in an occupational setting or with a focus on the working conditions as determinants of health. It aims to promote health as well as to prevent occupationally related diseases and injuries and the impairments arising therefrom—and, when work-related injury or illness occurs, to treat these conditions, and/or to promote return to work. It combines preventive, therapeutic, and rehabilitation services.[644] Bernadino Ramazzini (1633–1714) is regarded as "the father of occupational medicine," having published *De Morbis Artifi cum* (On the Diseases of Workers) in 1700.

OCCUPATIONAL INJURY Any damage inflicted to the body by energy transfer during work with a short time between exposure and the health event, usually less than 48 hours. Acute symptoms of disease due to deleterious WORKING CONDITIONS. The term mostly refers to traumatic injuries, although conditions such as stroke are considered occupational INJURIES in some worker's compensation schedules.[13,267,358,571,643,644] See also OCCUPATIONAL DISEASES; WORK-RELATED DISEASES.

OCCURRENCE In epidemiology, a general term describing the frequency of a disease or other event or attribute in a population; it does not distinguish between INCIDENCE and PREVALENCE. The term is also used to allude to processes that lead to disease or that influence the incidence of health outcomes.[1]

ODA See OFFICIAL DEVELOPMENT ASSISTANCE.

ODDS The ratio of the probability of occurrence of an event to that of nonoccurrence, or the ratio of the probability that something is one way to the probability that it is another way. If 60% of smokers develop a chronic cough and 40% do not, the odds among smokers in favor of developing a cough are 60 to 40, or 1.5; this may be contrasted with the probability or risk that smokers will develop a cough, which is 60 over 100 or 0.6. The natural logarithm of the odds is often called the LOGIT.[1,3,5,7,270]

ODDS RATIO (Syn: cross-product ratio, relative odds) The ratio of two odds. The term *odds* is defined differently according to the situation under discussion. Consider the following notation for the distribution of a binary exposure and a disease in a population or a sample:

	Exposed	Unexposed
Disease	*a*	*b*
No disease	*c*	*d*

The odds ratio (cross-product ratio) is *ad/bc*.

The *exposure-odds ratio* for a set of case-control or cross-sectional data is the ratio of the odds in favor of exposure among the cases *(a/b)* to the odds in favor of exposure among noncases *(c/d)*. This reduces to *ad/bc*. In a case-control study with incident cases, unbiased subject selection, and a "rare" (uncommon) disease, *ad/bc* is an approximate estimate of the RISK RATIO; the accuracy of this approximation is proportional to the RISK of the disease. With incident cases, unbiased subject selection, and DENSITY SAMPLING of controls, *ad/bc* is an estimate of the ratio of the PERSON-TIME INCIDENCE RATES in the exposed and unexposed (no rarity assumption is required for this).

The *disease-odds ratio* for a cohort or cross-sectional study is the ratio of the odds in favor of disease among the exposed *(a/c)* to the odds in favor of disease among the unexposed *(b/d)*. This reduces to *ad/bc* and hence is equal to the exposure-odds ratio for the cohort or cross section.

The *prevalence-odds ratio* refers to an odds ratio derived cross-sectionally, as, for example, an odds ratio derived from studies of prevalent (rather than incident) cases.

The *risk-odds ratio* is the ratio of the odds in favor of getting disease if exposed to the odds in favor of getting disease if not exposed. The odds ratio derived from a cohort study is an estimate of this ratio.[1,3,5,7,197] See also CASE-CONTROL STUDY; LOGISTIC MODEL; RARE-DISEASE ASSUMPTION.

ONCOGENE A gene that can cause neoplastic transformation of a cell; oncogenes are slightly transformed equivalents of normal genes.

ONE-SIDED TEST A statistical test based on the assumption that only one direction of departure from the TEST HYPOTHESIS is of interest. Sometimes called a "one-tailed test," although that term has other meanings.[1] See also TWO-SIDED TEST.

ONTOLOGY The study of what is the form and nature of reality and what can be known about it.[420] The set of things whose existence is acknowledged by a particular theory or system of thought; it is in this sense that some experts speak of the ontology of a theory. The natural sciences embody implicit ontological schemes that cannot be wholly justified on purely empirical grounds and can engender theoretical perplexities.[223] See also EPISTEMOLOGY.

OPEN-ENDED QUESTION A question that allows respondents to answer in their own words rather than according to a predetermined set of possible responses, i.e., a closed-ended question. Open-ended questions can be difficult to code and classify for statistical analysis.

OPEN POPULATION A study population that is allowed to gain and lose members over time. Similar to DYNAMIC POPULATION except that gains and losses may occur but need not occur. Contrast to FIXED COHORT, in which entry (gain in membership) cannot occur after a defining event or starting point.[1]

OPERATIONAL DEFINITION A definition embodying criteria used to identify and classify individual members of a set or concept to facilitate classification and counting.

OPERATIONAL RESEARCH The systematic study, by observation and experiment, of the working of a system (e.g., health services), with a view to improvement.

OPERATIONS RESEARCH
1. The fitting of models to data or the designing of models
2. Synonym for OPERATIONAL RESEARCH

OPPORTUNISTIC INFECTION Infection with organism(s) that are normally innocuous (e.g., COMMENSALS in the human) but become pathogenic when the body's immunological defenses are compromised, as in the ACQUIRED IMMUNODEFICIENCY SYNDROME (AIDS).[56]

OPPORTUNITY COST The benefit foregone, or value of opportunities lost, by engaging resources in a service; usually quantified by considering the benefit that would accrue by investing the same resources in the best alternative manner. The concept of opportunity cost derives from the notion of scarcity of resources.[17]

ORDINAL SCALE See MEASUREMENT SCALE.

ORDINATE The distance of a point, P, from the horizontal or x axis of a graph, measured along the vertical or y axis. See also ABSCISSA; AXIS; GRAPH.

OUTBREAK An epidemic limited to localized increase in the incidence of a disease, e.g., in a village, town, or closed institution; *upsurge* is sometimes used as a euphemism for outbreak.[5,24,56,188]

OUTCOME RESEARCH Research on outcomes of interventions. This is a large part of the work of clinical epidemiologists and epidemiologists involved in health services research.[17,24,26,58,202,270,499]

OUTCOMES All the possible results that may stem from exposure to a causal factor or from preventive or therapeutic interventions. All identified changes in health status arising as a consequence of the handling of a health problem.[2,3,5,6,17,26,38,255] See also CAUSALITY; CAUSATION OF DISEASE, FACTORS IN; DEPENDENT VARIABLE; RISK FACTOR.

OUTLIERS Observations with values differing widely from the rest of the data. This may suggest that an error was committed in their measurement or recording, or that the values come from a population different from that giving rise to the bulk of the observations. Yet, the values may be valid and precise.[1,7,37] See also MEASUREMENT, TERMINOLOGY OF.

OUTPUT The immediate result of professional or institutional health care activities, usually expressed as units of service (e.g., patient hospital days, outpatient visits, laboratory tests performed).

OVERADJUSTMENT Statistical adjustment by an excessive number of variables or parameters, uninformed by substantive knowledge (e.g., lacking coherence with biological, clinical, epidemiological, or social knowledge). It can obscure a true effect or create an apparent effect when none exists.[1,3,270] See also CAUSAL DIAGRAM; CONFOUNDING BIAS; CONFOUNDING, NEGATIVE; OVERMATCHING.

OVERCROWDING This sociodemographic term is variously defined. The UK Office of Population Censuses and Surveys (OPCS) uses an *index of overcrowding*, defined as the number of persons in private households living at a density greater than one person per room as a proportion of all persons in private households.

OVERFITTING Fitting a statistical model with a large number of parameters relative to the amount of data available and the fitting method used. It contradicts the principle of scientific parsimony, or OCCAM'S RAZOR. Chance error produced when large numbers of potential predictors are used to discriminate among a small number of outcome events and discrimination cannot be reproduced in a different sample. Genomic-based diagnostic research has been seen to be particularly prone to this type of error.[91,434] Statistical methods such as CROSS-VALIDATION, EMPIRICAL-BAYES METHODS, and SHRINKAGE can be used to address this problem without oversimplifying the model. See also CROSS VALIDATION; DATA DREDGING.

OVERMATCHING An undesirable result from matching COMPARISON GROUPS too closely or on too many variables.[1,3,5,7,38,280,791] Several varieties can be distinguished:

1. The MATCHING procedure partially or completely obscures evidence of a true causal association between the independent and dependent variables. Overmatching may occur if the matching variable is involved in—or is closely connected with—the mechanism whereby the independent variable affects the dependent variable. The matching variable may be an intermediate cause in the causal chain under study, or it may be strongly affected by such an intermediate cause or a consequence of it.

2. The matching procedure uses one or more unnecessary matching variables (e.g., variables that have no causal effect or influence on the dependent variable) and hence cannot confound the relationship between the independent and dependent variables but reduces PRECISION.

3. The matching process is unduly elaborate, involving the use of numerous matching variables and/or insisting on very close similarity with respect to specific matching variables. This leads to difficulty in finding suitable controls. See also MATCHING.

OVERVIEW See META-ANALYSIS; SYSTEMATIC REVIEW.

OVERWEIGHT See BODY MASS INDEX.

OVERWINTERING See VECTOR-BORNE INFECTION.

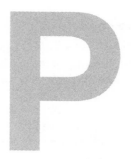

P See *P* VALUE.

PAIRED SAMPLES In a CLINICAL TRIAL, pairs of subject patients may be studied. One member of each pair receives the experimental regimen, and the other receives a suitably designated control regimen. Pairing should be based on a prognostic variable, such as age.

Pairing may similarly be used in a CASE-CONTROL STUDY or in a COHORT STUDY.[3,197] See also MATCHING.

PANDEMIC An EPIDEMIC occurring over a very wide area, crossing international boundaries, and usually affecting a large number of people. Only some pandemics cause severe disease in some individuals or at a population level. Characteristics of an infectious agent influencing the causation of a pandemic include: the agent must be able to infect humans, to cause disease in humans, and to spread easily from human to human.[69,116,645-647]

PANEL STUDY A combination of cross-sectional and cohort methods in which the investigator conducts a series of cross-sectional studies of the same individuals or study sample. This method of study permits changes in one variable to be related to changes in other variables.

PARADIGM A broad intellectual framework or set of assumptions used to analyze a scientific issue or a field of scientific inquiry. Loosely, a pattern of thought or conceptualization — an overall way of regarding phenomena within which scientists normally work. In the particular sense used by Thomas Kuhn, paradigms are governing concepts of cause in a given science during a given period. Paradigms reflect causal concepts operative in current or so-called normal science. In Kuhn's influential view (one not accepted by all philosophers of science), such paradigms can be displaced only by scientific revolutions.[648] The causal theories of disease governing the thought of successive eras reflect different paradigms (e.g., miasma, germs, MULTIPLE CAUSATION). The inductive methods of Aristotle in the fourth century B.C. and of Bacon in the seventeenth century were rejected by David Hume in the eighteenth century and again by Karl Popper in the twentieth. However, they have been given modern forms in the machine-learning, artificial intelligence, and Bayesian literature. A paradigm may dictate what form of explanation will be found acceptable or well supported, but a science may change paradigms.[40,101,438] See also DEDUCTIVE LOGIC; HYPOTHETICO-DEDUCTIVE METHOD; INDUCTIVE REASONING.

PARAMETER In statistics and epidemiology, a measurable characteristic of a population that is often estimated by a statistic, e.g., mean, standard deviation, regression coefficients.

In mathematics, a quantity in a formula or model that determines the characteristics or behavior of the population or system under study.

PARAMETRIC TEST A statistical test that depends upon assumptions about the distribution of the data that are represented by explicit PARAMETERS in a model (e.g., that errors are normally distributed or that outcomes follow a linear model). All statistical tests require assumptions about the underlying data generating mechanism (e.g., that it was random in some known way), but parametric methods make assumptions beyond those used in DISTRIBUTION-FREE METHODS.[7,34,37]

PARAMUTATION In EPIGENETICS, an interaction between two alleles of a single locus, resulting in a heritable change of one allele that is induced by the other allele. Paramutation violates MENDEL'S FIRST LAW, which states that in the process of the formation of the gametes (egg or sperm) the allelic pairs separate, one going to each gamete, and that each gene remains completely uninfluenced by the other. In paramutation, an allele in one generation heritably affects the other allele in future generations, even if the allele causing the change is itself not transmitted. Paramutation can result in a single allele of a gene controlling a spectrum of phenotypes. See also EPIGENETIC INHERITANCE; HERITABILITY.

PARASITE Loosely, a foreign entity that lives at the expense of a host. An animal or vegetable organism that lives on or in another and derives its nourishment therefrom. Strictly, a eukaryote whose vital cycle is only possible in close association with a host. An *obligate parasite* is one that cannot lead an independent nonparasitic existence. A *facultative parasite* is one that is capable of either parasitic or independent existence. An *ectoparasite* lives on the surface of its host, while an *endoparasite* lives within. Strictly, parasites are involved in INFESTATIONS.[20-22,56,188,217-219] See also COMMENSAL; COMMUNICABLE DISEASE; INFECTION; MUTUALISM; PATHOGEN.

PARASITE COUNT See WORM COUNT.

PARASITE DENSITY The collective degree of parasite load (or of parasitemia) in a population. Calculated by the geometric mean or the weighted average of the individual parasite counts (e.g., by using a frequency distribution based on a geometric progression).

PARASITEMIA Presence of parasites in the blood. The term can also be used to express the quantity of parasites in the blood (e.g., "a parasitemia of 2%").

PARATENIC HOST (Syn: transport host) A second, third, or subsequent intermediate host of a parasite, in which the parasite does not undergo any development or replication but remains, usually encysted, until the paratenic host is ingested by the definitive host of the PARASITE.

PARITY The status of a woman with regard to having borne viable children. The number of full-term children previously borne by a woman, excluding miscarriages and abortions in early pregnancy but including STILLBIRTHS.

PARTICIPANT Person upon whom research is conducted. The term *research participant* is suggested in preference to *research subject* on the grounds that *subject* may be demeaning, but this can be ambiguous, because members of research teams are also called participants. *Volunteer* may be an alternative, but this too can be misleading, because not all persons upon whom research is conducted are volunteers. The term *research subject* is less ambiguous. The most suitable term differs according to the setting and should be selected for both clarity and for acceptability in that setting.

PARTICIPANT OBSERVATION A method used in the social sciences in which the research worker (observer) is (or pretends to be) a member of the group being studied. Epidemiologists distrust the method on the grounds that objectivity of the observations may be compromised.

PARTICULARIZATION A method of analysis opposite to generalization or abstraction. It focuses on the specificity of a number of facts and illustrates an issue through the use of example.

PASSAGE The transfer of microorganisms from human to animal host(s) either directly or via laboratory culture; in the laboratory, this procedure is used to check for conformity with the HENLE-KOCH POSTULATES.

PASSENGER VARIABLE A variable that varies systematically with the dependent (outcome) variable under study without having a direct causal relation to it.[50] A third (explanatory) variable, the common cause of both the dependent and the passenger variable, "explains," or accounts for, their association.

PASSIVE SMOKING See INVOLUNTARY SMOKING; ENVIRONMENTAL TOBACCO SMOKE.

PASTEURIZATION The process of heat-treating milk or other perishable foodstuffs to kill pathogens. Developed by and named for bacteriologist Louis Pasteur (1822–1895).

PATH ANALYSIS A mode of analysis involving assumptions about the direction of causal relationships between linked sequences and configurations of variables. This permits the analyst to construct, fit, and test the appropriateness of alternative models (often represented as a PATH DIAGRAM) of the causal relations that may exist within the array of variables included in the finite system studied.[7]

PATH DIAGRAM The original term for what has commonly come to be called a CAUSAL DIAGRAM.

PATHOGEN Any organism, agent, factor, or process capable of causing disease (literally, causing a pathological process). Traditionally, biological pathogens include INFECTIOUS AGENTS, PARASITES, and genetic variants.

PATHOGENESIS The mechanisms by which a risk factor or other etiological agent contributes to cause a disease or disorder. The etiology of some diseases includes causes that initiate or promote pathogenesis; control of such causes favors PRIMARY PREVENTION of the disease.

PATHOGENICITY The property of an organism that determines the extent to which overt disease is produced in an infected population, or the power of an organism to produce disease. Also used to describe comparable properties of toxic chemicals. Pathogenicity of infectious agents is measured by the ratio of the number of persons developing clinical illness to the number exposed to infection. See also VIRULENCE.

PATHOPHYSIOLOGY

1. In epidemiology and medicine, the altered physiological processes that contribute to cause a disease or disorder, through which a disease develops, or that are otherwise associated with the clinical condition of interest. The integration of knowledge on human physiology and pathophysiology is essential in APPLIED EPIDEMIOLOGY and EPIDEMIOLOGICAL RESEARCH (e.g., to control EPIDEMICS, to conduct ETIOLOGICAL STUDIES and INTEGRATIVE RESEARCH, in MOLECULAR EPIDEMIOLOGY, to avoid the pitfalls of REDUCTIONISM and GENETIZATION when studying DISEASES OF COMPLEX ETIOLOGY).[6,26,58,201,202,323,649] A compelling reminder of such need is the number of human genes (c. 30,000): much lower than expected, and with only small differences among the genomes of humans, the mouse, fruit fly, worm, or other primates; current understanding of the genome does not explain the complexity of human physiology, pathophysiology, and behavior, nor why and how most human diseases occur.[53,91] See also PATHOGENESIS.

2. The discipline that studies such processes.

PATIENT-REPORTED OUTCOMES, PERSON-REPORTED OUTCOMES A measure of a patient's health status or condition that comes directly from the patient; in principle, without interpretation of her response by a health professional. Measures of QUALITY OF LIFE outcomes. Like other such measures, their assessments may include subtle effects, symptoms, and side effects of treatments.[499,650,651] Non-biological assessments of health status (traditionally, an essential qualitative part of the practice of clinical medicine, but rarely of quantitative clinical and epidemiological research) have helped assess a wider, more relevant spectrum of beneficial and adverse effects of therapies.[202] See also HEALY; MINIMALLY IMPORTANT DIFFERENCE; QUALITY OF LIFE; UTILITY; SYMPTOMATOLOGY.

PEARSON'S CHI-SQUARE See CHI-SQUARE TEST.

PEARSON'S PRODUCT MOMENT CORRELATION See CORRELATION COEFFICIENT.

PEDIGREE A diagram showing the ancestral relationships and transmission of genetic TRAITS over several generations of a family. See also FAMILY HISTORY.

PEER REVIEW A process of evaluation of scientific or professional work by experts in the same field (reviewers) to assess whether the work meets the necessary methodological and ethical standards before it is accepted or published. The critical assessment of manuscripts submitted to journals by experts who are not part of the editorial staff.[138,266] The term may also refer to review of clinical performance in a medical AUDIT.

PENALIZED ESTIMATION See SHRINKAGE ESTIMATION.

PENETRANCE See GENETIC PENETRANCE.

PERCEIVED NEED A felt need. It usually refers to the need for health care felt by the person or community concerned; it may not be perceived by health professionals or political authorities.

PERCENTAGE A PROPORTION in which the denominator is 100; e.g., 0.98 equals a percentage of 98. It is a dimensionless quantity ranging from 0 to 100. It is often denoted using the percent sign, "%." See also RATE; RATIO.

PERCENTILE The set of divisions that produce exactly 100 equal parts in a series of continuous values, such as children's heights or weights. Thus, a child above the 90th percentile has a greater value for height or weight than over 90% of all in the series. See also QUANTILE.

PERFORMANCE BIAS

1. Systematic differences in the care provided to members of the different study groups other than the intervention under investigation. For instance, patients who know they are in the control group may be more likely to use other forms of care, patients who know they are in the intervention group may be more likely to experience PLACEBO EFFECTS, and health care providers may treat patients differently according to what group they are in. See also BLINDED STUDY; DETECTION BIAS; PERFORMANCE BIAS.

2. Bias that may arise when the intervention actually received by study subjects differed substantially from the intervention that was intended or planned.

PERINATAL MORTALITY Literally, mortality around the time of birth. Perinatal mortality includes STILLBIRTHS and first week deaths. Conventionally, the time is limited to the period between 28 weeks gestation (when fetuses weigh on average 1000 g) and early neonatal deaths (occurring in the first seven days of life). In most high-income countries, the perinatal mortality rate is defined as:

$$\text{Perinatal mortality rate} = \frac{\text{Fetal deaths and early neonatal deaths}}{\text{Total births}} \times 1000$$

An alternative, more recent definition includes fetal deaths with a gestational age of 22 weeks (or 500 g) or more, rather than 28 weeks or more. However, in low- and middle-income countries exact ascertainment of gestational age is often impossible, and there is a preference for defining cutoffs based on BIRTH WEIGHT instead of gestational ages. As a consequence, there is considerable inconsistency across countries (and probably within some countries) regarding the definition and measurement of perinatal mortality, with different countries adopting alternative definitions. The main reasons for inconsistencies include: (a) whether the lower limit should be set at 500 g (or 22 weeks' gestation) or 1000 g (or 28 weeks' gestation); (b) whether the upper limit should be extended to the first 28 days instead of the first 7 days; (c) whether the denominator should include stillbirths (in which case the indicator would be the perinatal mortality rate) or only live births, given that the latter tend to be more reliably reported (in which case the indicator would be the perinatal mortality ratio); and (d) whether live born infants weighing less the 1000 g should be included in the denominator of the early neonatal component, because of underreporting and of the difficulties in establishing signs of life in very small newborns.

Because of these difficulties, the WHO recommends that countries should present, solely for international comparisons, "standard perinatal statistics" in which both the numerator and denominator of all rates are restricted to fetuses and infants weighing 1000 g or more, or, where BIRTH WEIGHT is unavailable, the corresponding gestational age (28 weeks) or body length (25 cm crown–heel).[652]

$$\text{Perinatal mortality rate, weight specific} = \frac{\begin{array}{c}\text{Fetal deaths weighing 1000 g and over,}\\ \text{plus early neonatal deaths of infants}\\ \text{weighing 1000 g and over at birth}\end{array}}{\text{Total births weighing 1000 g and over}} \times 1000$$

PERIODICITY A repeating pattern of a phenomenon or an event, especially the repetition of comparable values; e.g., seasonal fluctuation in numbers of cases of respiratory infections.

PERIODIC (MEDICAL) EXAMINATIONS Assessment of health status conducted at predetermined intervals (e.g., annually or at specified milestones in life, such as infancy, school entry, preemployment, or preretirement). This form of medical examination generally follows a formal protocol, employing a set of structured questions and/or a predetermined set of laboratory tests.

PERIOD OF COMMUNICABILITY See COMMUNICABLE PERIOD.

PERIOD PREVALENCE See PREVALENCE.

PERMISSIBLE EXPOSURE LIMIT (PEL) An occupational health standard to safeguard workers against dangerous substances in the workplace. See SAFETY STANDARDS.

PERSONAL HEALTH CARE Those services to individuals that are performed on a one-to-one basis by a health care worker for the purpose of maintaining or restoring health.

PERSONAL MONITORING DEVICE An instrument attached to a person to measure the exposure of that person to hazardous substance(s).

PERSON-TIME A measurement combining persons and time as the denominator in incidence and mortality rates when, for varying periods, individual subjects are at risk of developing disease or dying. It is the sum of the periods of time at risk for each of the subjects. The most widely used measure is person-years. With this approach, each subject contributes only as many years of observation to the population at risk as the period over which that subject has been observed to be at risk of the disease; a subject observed over 1 year contributes 1 person-year, a subject observed over a 10-year period contributes 10 person-years. This method can be used to measure incidence rate over extended and variable time periods.[1-3,5,24,270] See also CONTEXT.

PERSON-TIME INCIDENCE RATE (Syn: interval incidence density) A measure of the incidence rate of an event (e.g., a disease or death) in a population at risk, given by

$$\frac{\text{Number of events occurring during the interval}}{\text{Number of person-time units at risk observed during the interval}}$$

Although widely used, a problem with this measure is that it treats equally events among persons with short and long follow-up. This problem can be addressed by stratifying on follow-up time and computing the rates within the resulting time intervals, as in LIFE TABLES.[1] See also HAZARD RATE; INCIDENCE RATE; LIFE TABLE.

PERSON-TO-PERSON SPREAD OF DISEASE See TRANSMISSION OF INFECTION.

PERSON-YEARS See PERSON-TIME.

PERSPECTIVE PLOT Diagrammatic representation of the relationship among three variables, one each on the horizontal and vertical axes and the third represented by a series of lines drawn so as to convey an illusion of three dimensions. See also CONTOUR PLOT.

PHARMACOEPIDEMIOLOGY (Syn: drug epidemiology) The study of the distribution and determinants of drug-related events in populations and the application of this study to efficacious treatment. The application of epidemiological knowledge, methods, and reasoning to describe, explain, control, and predict the uses and effects (beneficial and adverse) of drugs, vaccines, and related biological products in human populations. The public health foundation of pharmacoepidemiology is that drugs and vaccines are among the factors that influence the distribution of health states in human populations.

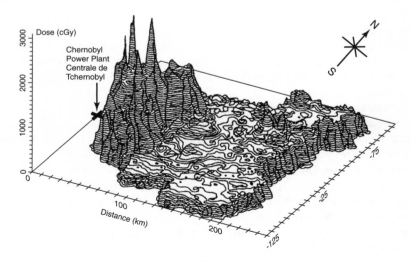

Perspective plot. Average distribution of thyroid doses of radioactive iodine, Ukraine, 1986. Source: Buzunov VA, et al.[653] With permission.

Its core lies at the intersection of two subspecialties: clinical pharmacology and CLINICAL EPIDEMIOLOGY. Pharmacoepidemiology also aids pharmacology, public health, and other health sciences by increasing knowledge about the occurrence and causes of diseases, the distribution of health states, and the functioning of the health care system.[272,654,655,797]

PHARMACOVIGILANCE See POSTMARKETING SURVEILLANCE.

PHASE I, PHASE II, PHASE III TRIAL See CLINICAL TRIAL.

PHENOTYPE The observable properties, characteristics, or form of an organism or person produced by the GENOTYPE in synergy or interaction with the environment. All aspects of a living organism other than its genetic constitution. See also GENETIC PENETRANCE.

PHYSICIAN (Syn: medical practitioner, doctor) Professional person qualified by education and authorized by law to practice medicine.

PIE CHART A circular diagram divided into segments, each representing a category or subset of data. The amount for each category is proportional to the angle subtended at the center of the circle and hence to the area of the sector. When several pie charts are used to describe several populations, the area of each circle is proportional to the size of the population it represents.[102-108,505]

PILOT INVESTIGATION, STUDY A small-scale test of the methods and procedures to be used on a larger scale if the pilot study demonstrates that these methods and procedures can work.[3]

PLAs Persons living with AIDS.

PLACEBO A medication or procedure that is inert (i.e., one having no pharmacological effect) but intended to give patients the perception that they are receiving treatment or assistance for their complaint. From Latin *placebo*, "I shall please."[5,6,24,26,38]

PLACEBO EFFECT The beneficial effect resulting solely from the administration of a treatment, no matter whether strictly a placebo, an active drug, or another therapeutic procedure. Hence, placebo effects accompany also the prescription of efficacious drugs. They may be due to a variety of factors and occur through different mechanisms, including an empathic relationship between the prescribing professional and the patient, and the patient's expectation of an effect. The very accomplishments of EVIDENCE-BASED MEDICINE, attained through scientific research, have augmented its placebo effects and metaphoric power.[6,335] See also HALO EFFECT; NOCEBO.

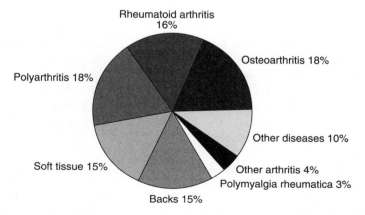

Pie chart. Percentage distribution of new outpatients in a rheumatic diseases clinic. Source: Silman AJ, et al.[656] Copyright held by editors.

PLASTICITY The potential for change in the intrinsic characteristics of a cell, tissue, system, or whole organism in response to environmental stimuli. The ability of a genotype to produce more than one alternative form of structure, physiological state, or behavior in response to environmental conditions. It is a quality of organisms as they develop, and diminishes with increasing age or after a critical developmental period. Within the limits imposed by genetic and mechanical constraints, each person has a range of options for her LIFE COURSE and final body form and function.[23,32,161,316,799] See also DEVELOPMENTAL ORIGINS OF HEALTH AND DISEASE; EPIGENETICS; PROGRAMMING; SENSITIVE PERIOD.

PLAUSIBILITY See BIOLOGICAL PLAUSIBILITY; COHERENCE; HILL'S CONSIDERATIONS FOR CAUSATION.

PLEIOTROPY The influence of a single gene or variant on multiple distinct phenotypic traits (disease endpoints or quantitative traits). Thus, a mutation in a pleiotropic gene may have an effect on some or all traits simultaneously. There is evidence of pleiotropic effects in human complex diseases, with each individual gene mutation affecting multiple diseases.[657] It is a common property of genes and SNPs associated with disease TRAITS. It has implications for genetic testing as a mutation that predisposes a person to one disease also affects her probability of developing other diseases.

PLHIV See PLWHA.

PLOT, BOX AND WHISKER See BOX-AND-WHISKERS PLOT.

PLOT, CAT AND WHISKER See BOX-AND-WHISKERS PLOT.

PLOT, FOREST See FOREST PLOT.

PLOT, FUNNEL See FUNNEL PLOT.

PLOT, MANHATTAN See MANHATTAN PLOT.

PLWHA People Living With HIV/AIDS. Also abbreviated as PLHIV.

POINT SOURCE EPIDEMIC See EPIDEMIC, COMMON SOURCE.

POISSON DISTRIBUTION A DISTRIBUTION FUNCTION used to describe the occurrence of rare events or the sampling distribution of isolated counts in a continuum of time or space (e.g., cases of an uncommon disease). The number of events X has a Poisson distribution with parameter λ (lambda) if the probability of observing k events ($k = 0, 1,...$) is equal to

$$Pr(X = k) = \frac{e^{-\lambda}\lambda^k}{k!}$$

where e is the base of natural logarithm, 2.7183.... The mean and variance of the distribution are both equal to λ. This DISTRIBUTION is used in modeling PERSON-TIME INCIDENCE RATES and caseloads.[1,3,7,8,34,37]

POLICY A guide to action to change what would otherwise occur; a decision about amounts and allocations of resources; a statement of commitment to certain areas of concern; the distribution of the amount shows the priorities of decision makers. *Public policy* is policy at any level of government.[13,14,17,24,38,83,248,252,267,290,302,426,515,522] See also BENEFIT; HEALTHY PUBLIC POLICIES.

POLICY BRIEF A decision-making tool for policy makers based on a summary of the scientific evidence. It facilitates the transfer of knowledge from researchers to decision makers and thus the process of EVIDENCE-INFORMED HEALTH POLICYMAKING.[658] Policy briefs are recommended by the Evidenced Informed Policy Network (EVIPNet) of the World Health Organization.[659]

POLYGENIC TRAIT A TRAIT whose phenotype is influenced by more than one gene. Many polygenic traits are also influenced by the environment and are therefore called multifactorial. See also GENETIC PENETRANCE; PLEIOTROPY.

POLITICAL EPIDEMIOLOGY The scientific study of political factors, processes, and conditions affecting the health of human populations.[352] The effects on health of the institutions derived from political power.[660] Even before Rudolf Virchow (1821–1902) proposed medicine as a political science, many epidemiologists studied the effects on individual and population health of politically modifiable processes as democracy, political rights, and civil liberties.[661] *Political economy* is the discipline that examines the relationships of individuals to society, economic production, and the activities of the state. *Political economy of health* is a theoretical framework used to study HEALTH INEQUALITIES; it proposes that health disparities and inequalities are caused by social structures and institutions, which create, enforce, and perpetuate poverty and privilege. *Political ecology* is the study of the political and economic principles controlling the relations of human beings to one another and to the environment.[19,31,214,248,252,267,279,307,357,358,426,662-665]

POLLUTANT (Syn: contaminant) Any undesirable solid, liquid, or gaseous matter in a solid, liquid, or gaseous environmental medium.

POLLUTION Any undesirable modification of air, water, or food by substances that are toxic or may have adverse effects on health or that are offensive even if not necessarily harmful to health.[13,33] See also CONTAMINATION.

POLYGENIC DISEASES Diseases in which multiple gene variants or genetic alterations jointly influence the risk of developing the disease, often through complex processes in which environmental and EPIGENETIC factors also intervene.[799] An antonym of MONOGENIC DISEASES. See also DISEASES OF COMPLEX ETIOLOGY; PLEIOTROPY.

POLYGENIC INHERITANCE The transmission of a phenotypic TRAIT whose expression depends on the effect of multiple genes.

POLYMORPHISM, GENETIC The occurrence in a population of two or more genotypes. The existence of two or more genetic variants. A genome segment or locus in which alternate forms (alleles) are present. In population genetics, variation is polymorphic if all alleles are found at frequencies >1%. Genetic polymorphims can have opposite relations with different diseases; e.g., people with the NAT2-slow genotype are thought to have an increased risk of bladder cancer if exposed to aromatic amines (which are deactivated by acetylation) but a decreased risk of colon cancer if exposed to heterocyclic amines (activated by acetylation).[57,415,416,479-485,666]

POLYTOMOUS Divided or involving division into multiple parts.

POLYTOMOUS VARIABLE A categorical variable with three or more categories. See also MEASUREMENT SCALE.

PONDERAL INDEX The anthropometric index of body mass. Defined as height divided by the cube root of the body weight. The BODY MASS INDEX is generally regarded as a better index of body mass because it appears better correlated with tissue composition (percent body fat).

POOLED ANALYSIS (Syn: meta-analysis of individual data) A type of META-ANALYSIS in which investigators have access to and analyze the original individual level data from each one of the participating studies. It minimizes some methodological problems of traditional meta-analysis because it allows the use of similar inclusion criteria, variable definitions, and statistical methods across studies. It also minimizes publication bias, as data from unpublished studies may be included.[26,229,230,467]

POPULAR EPIDEMIOLOGY The process by which regular citizens gather scientific information and knowledge to understand and change the EPIDEMIOLOGY of various health states.[13,26,667] Based on different needs, goals, and methods, lay people and professionals may have conflicting perspectives on how to investigate and interpret evidence on POPULATION HEALTH, including differences in definitions of data quality, levels of SIGNIFICANCE, and relations between evidence and policy. See also LAY EPIDEMIOLOGY.

POPULATION

1. All the inhabitants of a given country or area considered together; the number of inhabitants of a given country or area.
2. In sampling, the whole collection of units (the "UNIVERSE") from which a sample may be drawn; not necessarily a population of persons—the units may be institutions, records, or events. The sample is intended to give results that are representative of the whole population; it may deviate from that goal owing to random and systematic errors.[1,3,5,24] See also GENERAL POPULATION.

POPULATION ATTRIBUTABLE RISK This term was sometimes used as a synonym for ATTRIBUTABLE FRACTION FOR THE POPULATION. It was also used for the difference of the population rate or risk of disease and the rate or risk in the unexposed.[668,669]

POPULATION ATTRIBUTABLE RISK PERCENT This is the ATTRIBUTABLE FRACTION FOR THE POPULATION expressed as a percentage.

POPULATION-BASED Based on a defined POPULATION (e.g., a study, a project); as opposed to based on a hospital, or by contrast with programs or studies with no population reference, frame, or base. Pertaining to a general population defined by geopolitical boundaries; this population is the denominator and/or the sampling frame.[1,7,211,270] See also CASE SERIES; EARLY CLINICAL DETECTION; SCREENING: STUDY BASE.

POPULATION DYNAMICS Changes in the structure of a population; loosely used as a synonym for DEMOGRAPHY.

POPULATION GENETICS Study of the genetic composition of populations. The main aim is to estimate gene frequencies and detect selective factors in the environment that influence these frequencies.

POPULATION HEALTH

1. The health of the population measured by health status indicators; it is influenced by physical, biological, social, and economic factors in the environment, by personal health behavior, and by access to and effectiveness of health care services.
2. The prevailing or aspired level of health in the population of a specified country or region or in a defined subset of that population. The distinction between *population health* and PUBLIC HEALTH is that population health describes the condition whereas public health includes the policies, programs, practices, procedures, institutions, and disciplines required to achieve the desired state of population health. The term also sometimes means the disciplines involved in studying the determinants and dynamics of a population's health status.[17,24,28,164,165,211,212,366,515,670]

POPULATION IMPACT NUMBER See IMPACT NUMBERS.

POPULATION MEDICINE See COMMUNITY MEDICINE.

POPULATION MOMENTUM In a growing population, the phenomenon of continuing population growth beyond the time when replacement-level fertility has been achieved because of the increasing size of childbearing and younger age cohorts resulting from higher fertility and/or falling mortality in preceding years.

POPULATION PREVENTIVE STRATEGY See STRATEGY, "POPULATION."

POPULATION PYRAMID A graphic presentation of the age and sex composition of the population. The population pyramid is constructed by computing the percentage distribution of a population simultaneously cross-classified by sex and age. The percentage that each female age group is of the total is plotted on the right and the corresponding percentages for males are plotted on the left. Sometimes the pyramid is constructed using absolute numbers, rather than proportions, in each age and sex group. A population pyramid is intended to provide a quick overall comprehension of age and sex structure in the population. A population whose pyramid has a broad base and narrow apex may be identified as a high-fertility population. Changing shape over time reflects the changing composition of the population associated with changes in fertility and mortality at each age. Since the figure is two-dimensional, the word *pyramid* is incorrectly used, but the more accurate word *profile* has never caught on.

POPULATION, SOURCE (Syn: base population) The group from which a study group is selected.

POPULATION STRATIFICATION A type of CONFOUNDING that occurs when there are systematic differences in allele frequencies between subpopulations with a different ancestry. For instance, when the risk of disease varies between two ethnic groups, then any factor—whether genetic or environmental—that also varies between the groups will appear to be related to the disease. Population stratification can be a problem for ASSOCIATION STUDIES, such as case-control studies and GWAS, where the association found could be due to the underlying structure of the population and not to a disease-associated locus.[53,87-89]

POPULATION, STUDY (Syn: study group, study sample) The group selected for investigation.

POPULATION, TARGET See TARGET POPULATION.

POPULATION THINKING By contrast to INDIVIDUAL THINKING, a reasoning and mode of reasoning that dynamically integrates fluxes in human populations, sociogeographic spaces, and time. It observes, analyzes, and predicts the experiences of a whole group of people defined in a specific way (e.g., geophysically, socially, clinically, biologically).[42,211,426] Population thinking is important—perhaps indispensable—for GROUP COMPARISONS. See also CLINICAL STUDY; PREVENTION PARADOX; STRATEGY, "POPULATION."

POSITIVE PREDICTIVE VALUE See PREDICTIVE VALUE, POSITIVE.

POSITIVE TRANSITION See DISEASE TRANSITION.

POSITIVITY (Syn: experimental treatment assignment assumption) The assumption that each exposure or treatment level of interest occurs with non-zero probability at all values of confounding variables that can occur in the target population. A necessary assumption for CAUSAL INFERENCE in observational studies. To meet the assumption, exposed and unexposed participants must be present at every combination of the values of the observed confounder(s) in the population under study. Positivity is present by design in randomized controlled trials. In observational studies, violations of positivity can happen because participants at one or more levels of the confounder cannot receive or are not observed at 1 or more levels of the exposure; i.e., theoretical violations of the positivity assumption occur when there is zero probability of some exposure or treatment level for at least one combination of confounder values. Practical violations occur in finite samples when by chance zero observations with a given treatment or exposure level occur in some confounder strata. Such violations can be problematic, particularly when using INVERSE PROBABILITY WEIGHTING estimators. Weaker positivity assumptions are also possible in some cases.[2,671,672]

Causal inference with observed positivity violations requires at least interpolation between—and possibly extrapolation beyond—the data, with the hazards either may entail. This is especially so when precise inferences are needed. For example, it may be safe to extrapolate that the rate of fatal overdose from prescribing 50 mg/day of diazepam would be higher than the rates observed at lower doses, even if no dose higher than 30 mg/day was observed; on the other hand, it would be dangerous to infer that the risk is below an acceptable threshold even if that risk was below the threshold at the lower, observed doses.

POSTERIOR ODDS The odds calculated after reference to results of a study. See BAYES' THEOREM.

POSTERIOR PROBABILITY The probability calculated after reference to results of a study. See BAYES' THEOREM.

POST HOC ANALYSIS An analysis of the data that is undertaken after essential parts of the study protocol or planning are finished, to look at patterns or associations that were not sought out when the study was designed. See also DATA DREDGING.

POSTMARKETING SURVEILLANCE Studies conducted after a drug or vaccine has been licensed for marketing and public use. Designed to provide information on the actual uses and effects of the product under common conditions of living, especially on the occurrence of side effects and adverse reactions unlikely to be detected with the lower numbers of subjects that take part in premarketing studies (e.g., in phase III clinical trials). It uses epidemiological and nonepidemiological designs. The latter include voluntary reporting systems of adverse events by health professionals. Postmarketing epidemiological studies may be observational and experimental.[48,49,272,654] See also CLINICAL TRIAL.

POSTNEONATAL MORTALITY RATE The number of infant deaths between 28 days and 1 year of age in a given year per 1000 live births in that year. It is an important rate to monitor in developing countries, where older infants frequently die of infections and malnutrition.[315,627]

POTENCY The strength of a particular drug, toxin, or hazard; the ratio of the dose of a standard amount required to elicit a specific response to the dose of the test agent that elicits the same response.

POTENTIAL OUTCOME The outcome of a person, group, or other unit of study under a possibly hypothetical sequence of events.[271] For example, it may be hypothesized that a person will survive at least 5 more years by accepting a treatment but not survive by declining the treatment. Under this model for the person's potential outcomes, survival is a hypothesized outcome under treatment. If the person declines treatment and then dies, we will not know if indeed the hypothetical model is correct because we will not observe what her outcome would have been had the treatment been accepted. If treatment is declined, treatment becomes a counterfactual and any further reasoning about the person's outcome under treatment will thus require COUNTERFACTUAL LOGIC. Some authors prefer the term "potential outcomes" over "COUNTERFACTUAL OUTCOMES" to emphasize that, depending on the treatment that is received, one of the outcomes can be potentially observed.[1,2,101]

POTENTIAL YEARS OF LIFE LOST (PYLL) A measure of the relative impact of various diseases and lethal forces on society. PYLL highlights the loss to society as a result of youthful or early deaths. The figure for PYLL due to a particular cause is the sum, over all persons dying from that cause, of the additional years that these persons would have lived had they reached a specified age.[5,24] The concept derives from Petty's *Political Arithmetic* (1687) and is elaborated upon in Dublin and Lotka's *Money Value of a Man* (1930).

POVERTY A condition of absolute or relative deprivation of material and cultural resources. Absolute poverty refers to the condition in which the basic resources necessary to sustain

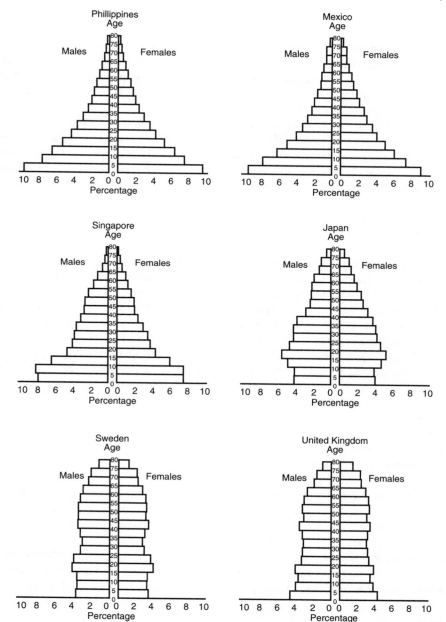

Population pyramids. Age pyramids for populations of six countries, 1965. Source: Basch PF.[673]

life are lacking; relative poverty is the lack of resources in comparison with other members of a given society.[649,662,674] See also ABSOLUTE POVERTY LEVEL; RELATIVE POVERTY LEVEL.

POWER, STATISTICAL Roughly, the ability of a study to demonstrate an association or effect if one exists. The probability that the TEST HYPOTHESIS will be rejected if it is false; it is equal to $1 - \beta$, where β is the probability of TYPE II ERROR (failing to reject a false NULL HYPOTHESIS). The statistical power of a study is influenced by factors as the frequency of the condition under study, the magnitude of the effect, the study design, and sample size.[1-3,7,37,270]

PRAGMATIC STUDY, PRAGMATIC TRIAL (Syn: effectiveness trial, management trial) A study (including randomized clinical trials) whose aim is to determine the effects of an intervention under the usual conditions in which it will be applied. By contrast with an EXPLANATORY STUDY, the focus is on guiding decisions (e.g., about health care).[6,9,24,110,232,443-445] See also EFFECTIVENESS; INTENTION-TO-TREAT ANALYSIS.

PRECAUTIONARY PRINCIPLE The "better safe than sorry" approach to assessing and managing health risks, such as those associated with environmental hazards. Where there is strong evidence that a relevant risk exists, prudence and ethical norms warrant that action be taken to reduce or eliminate the risk, even if the evidence is not conclusive.[13,267] Similar in some ways the medical maxim *primum non nocere* ("first do no harm") and the ethical principle of NONMALEFICENCE.[17,59,73-77,116,213,360] See also COSTS OF INACTION.

PRECIPITATING FACTORS See CAUSATION OF DISEASE, FACTORS IN.

PRECISION
1. Relative lack of random error. Contrast with INTERNAL VALIDITY, the relative lack of BIAS, or systematic, nonrandom error. As a principle, in etiological research internal validity must take precedence over precision. However, a slightly biased, highly precise estimate may be preferable to an unbiased but highly imprecise estimate.[1-3,37]
2. In statistics, one measure of precision is the inverse of the variance of a measurement or estimate. A measure of imprecision is the standard error of measurement — the standard deviation of a series of replicate determinations of the same quantity.
3. The quality of being sharply defined or stated. One measure of precision is the number of distinguishable alternatives from which a measurement was selected, sometimes indicated by the number of significant digits in the measurement. Precision does not imply ACCURACY. See also MEASUREMENT, TERMINOLOGY OF.

PRECURSOR A condition or state preceding pathological onset of a disease; sometimes detectable by SCREENING. See also RISK MARKER.

PREDICTIVE ACCURACY See DISCRIMINATORY ACCURACY.

PREDICTIVE CAPACITY See DISCRIMINATORY ACCURACY.

PREDICTIVE VALIDITY See VALIDITY, MEASUREMENT.

PREDICTIVE VALUE (of a screening test or of a diagnostic test) The probability of the disease given the results of the test. Predictive values of a test are determined by the SENSITIVITY and SPECIFICITY of the test and by the PREVALENCE of the condition for which the test is used.[1,5-9,37,58,796] See also SCREENING.

PREDICTIVE VALUE, NEGATIVE (Syn: predictive value of a negative test) The probability that a person with a negative test result is a true negative (e.g., does not have the disease).[6,58]

PREDICTIVE VALUE, POSITIVE (Syn: predictive value of a positive test) The probability that a person with a positive test result is a true positive (e.g., does have the disease).[6,58]

PREDISPOSING FACTORS See CAUSATION OF DISEASE, FACTORS IN.

PREGNANCY-RELATED DEATH See MATERNAL MORTALITY.

PREMUNITION A state of resistance in a host harboring a parasite to superinfection by a PARASITE of the same species. The state is dependent on the continued survival of parasites in the body and disappears after their elimination; it may be complete or partial. A term used mainly in the epidemiology of parasitic diseases, especially malaria.[56]

PREPATENT PERIOD In parasitology, the period equivalent to the incubation period of microbial infections; the corresponding phase may be biologically different from microbial multiplication when the invading organism is a multicellular parasite that undergoes developmental stages in the host.

PRESCRIPTIVE SCREENING See SCREENING.

PRESENTEEISM The practice of being present at one's place of work for more hours than required, especially as a manifestation of job insecurity. The situation in which workers go to work despite being sick. It can be a source of inequalities and of decreased productivity.[358,675,676] See also ABSENTEEISM; SICKNESS ABSENCE.

PRESPECIFIED FALSIFICATION HYPOTHESIS A claim, distinct from the one that is being tested, that researchers believe is highly unlikely to be causally related to the intervention in question. It may provide a safeguard when observational data are used to study rare events.[677]

PRESUMPTIVE TREATMENT Treatment of clinically suspected cases without, or prior to, results from confirmatory laboratory tests.

PREVALENCE A measure of disease occurrence; in fact, a measure of the OCCURRENCE of any type of health condition, exposure, or other factor related to health (e.g., prevalence of depression, of smoking): the total number of individuals who have the condition (e.g., disease, exposure, attribute) at a particular time (or during a particular period) divided by the population at risk of having the condition at that time or midway through the period. When used without qualification, the term usually refers to the proportion of individuals in a population who have the condition at a specified point in time (point prevalence).[1,3,8,24,269,270,678] It is a proportion, not a rate. Types of prevalence include:

Point prevalence The proportion of individuals with the condition at a specified point in time.

Period prevalence The proportion of individuals with the condition at any time during a specified time period or interval. Examples include:

Annual prevalence The proportion of individuals with the condition at any time during a year. It includes cases of the disease arising before but extending into or through the year as well as those having their inception during the year. Only occasionally used.

Lifetime prevalence The proportion of individuals who have had the condition for at least part of their lives at any time during their LIFE COURSE.

One-year prevalence The proportion of individuals with the condition at any time during a calendar year. It includes cases arising before and during the year.

PREVALENCE POOL The diseased subset of a population.[1]

PREVALENCE STUDY See CROSS-SECTIONAL STUDY.

PREVENTABLE FRACTION FOR THE POPULATION In a situation in which exposure to a given factor is believed to protect against a disease or other outcome, the preventable fraction for the population is the proportion of the disease in the population that would be prevented if the whole population were exposed to the factor. This measure must be interpreted with great caution, as part or all of the apparent protective effect may be due to other factors associated with the apparent protective factor.

In a study of a total population, the preventable fraction for the population of the incidence rate is computed as

$$\left(I_p - I_e\right)/I_p,$$

where I_p is the incidence rate of the disease or other outcome in the population and I_e is what the incidence rate would be if everyone were exposed.

The same approach may be applied to other measures of disease frequency; e.g., the preventable fraction of the caseload is

$$\left(A_p - A_e\right)/A_p,$$

where A_p is the caseload in the population and A_e is what the caseload would be if everyone were exposed.[1] See also ATTRIBUTABLE FRACTION.

PREVENTED FRACTION FOR THE POPULATION In a situation in which exposure to a given factor is believed to protect against a disease or other outcome, the prevented fraction for the population is the proportion of the hypothetical total load of disease in the population that has been prevented by exposure to the factor. This measure must also be interpreted with great caution, as part or all of the apparent protective effect may be due to other factors associated with the apparent protective factor.

In a study of a total population, the prevented fraction of the incidence rate is computed as

$$\left(I_u - I_p\right)/I_u, \text{ or } P_e\left(1 - I_p/I_u\right)$$

where I_p is the rate of the disease in the population, I_u is what the rate would be if everyone were not exposed, and P_e is the prevalence of exposure. See also ATTRIBUTABLE FRACTION.

PREVENTION Actions that prevent disease occurrence. Actions aimed at eradicating, eliminating, or minimizing the impact of disease and disability, or if none of these is feasible, retarding the progress of disease and disability.

The concept is best defined in the context of *levels* of prevention, traditionally called primary, secondary, and tertiary prevention.[24] Other levels (primordial prevention, quaternary prevention) are also used. There is significant conceptual and practical overlapping among levels—largely, depending on the type of disease (e.g., on the NATURAL HISTORY OF THE DISEASE). Effective prevention STRATEGIES often interact and operate across levels.

1. PRIMORDIAL PREVENTION: conditions, actions, and measures that minimize hazards to health and that hence inhibit the emergence and establishment of processes and factors (environmental, economic, social, behavioral, cultural) known to increase the risk of DISEASE.[213,678] Primordial prevention is accomplished through many public and private HEALTHY PUBLIC POLICIES and INTERSECTORAL ACTION. It may be seen as a form of primary prevention.

2. PRIMARY PREVENTION aims to reduce the incidence of disease by personal and communal efforts, such as decreasing environmental risks, enhancing nutritional status, immunizing against communicable diseases, or improving water supplies.[3,5,13,24,28,67,84,121,211,214,366,426] It is a core task of PUBLIC HEALTH, including HEALTH PROMOTION. See also COSTS OF INACTION.

3. SECONDARY PREVENTION aims to reduce the prevalence of disease by shortening its duration. If the disease has no cure, it may increase survival and QUALITY OF LIFE; it will also increase the prevalence of the disease. It seldom prevents disease occurrence; it does so only when EARLY DETECTION of a precursor lesion leads to complete removal of all such lesions. It is a set of measures available to individuals and communities for the early detection and prompt intervention to control disease and minimize disability; e.g., by the use of SCREENING programs. It is a core task of PREVENTIVE

MEDICINE. Both EARLY CLINICAL DETECTION and population-based SCREENING usually aim at achieving secondary prevention. in certain diseases, these activities may also contribute to tertiary prevention.[5]

4. TERTIARY PREVENTION: measures aimed at softening the impact of long-term disease and disability by eliminating or reducing impairment, disability, and handicap; minimizing suffering; and maximizing potential years or useful life. It is mainly a task of rehabilitation.

5. QUATERNARY PREVENTION: procedures and policies that identify individuals and groups at risk of overdiagnosis or overmedication, and that decrease excessive medical and sanitary intervention.[679] Actions that prevent IATROGENESIS and "DISEASE MONGERING."

PREVENTION, CLARK'S LEVELS OF See PREVENTION.

PREVENTION LEVEL See PREVENTION.

PREVENTION PARADOX As formulated by Geoffrey Rose (1926–1993), a preventive measure that brings large benefits to the community but may offer little to each participating person.[211,426] For example, to prevent one death due to a motor vehicle accident, many hundreds of people must wear seat belts. Conversely, an intervention that brings much benefit to an individual may have a small impact in the population. See also STRATEGY.

PREVENTIVE MEDICINE The application of preventive measures by clinical practitioners. A specialized field of medical practice composed of distinct disciplines that utilize skills focusing on the health of defined populations in order to promote and maintain health and well-being and prevent disease, disability, and premature death.

In addition to the knowledge of basic and clinical sciences and the skills common to all physicians, the distinctive aspects of preventive medicine include knowledge of and competence in biostatistics; epidemiology; administration, including planning, organization, management, financing, and evaluation of health programs; environmental health; application of social and behavioral factors in health and disease; and the application of primary, secondary, and tertiary prevention measures within clinical medicine. See also HEALTH EDUCATION; HEALTH PROMOTION; STRATEGY.

PRIMARY CASE The individual who introduces the disease into the family or group under study. Not necessarily the first diagnosed case in a family or group. See also INDEX CASE.

PRIMARY CARE EPIDEMIOLOGY The application of epidemiological principles and methods to the study and control of problems arising in primary care. It includes studies at the interface between primary care and the general population, as well as on the interfaces between primary, secondary, and tertiary care. Much work involves the determinants and outcomes of consultations in primary care. Here, DETERMINANTS include also the nature of symptoms, signs, or illnesses occurring in the community and factors influencing decisions to consult or not to consult. OUTCOMES include—in addition to all other conventional outcomes—the duration, severity, and impact of illnesses and symptom complexes.[17,24,680]

PRIMARY HEALTH CARE

1. Health care that begins at the time of first encounter between a patient and a provider of health care. It often is primary *medical* care.[681]

2. Primary health care is essential health care made accessible at a cost the country and the community can afford, with methods that are practical, scientifically sound, and socially acceptable.[17,432,682] Everyone in the community should have access to it. Related sectors should also be involved in it in addition to the health sector. At the very least it should include education of the community on the health problems

prevalent and on methods of preventing health problems from arising or of controlling them; the promotion of adequate supplies of food and of proper nutrition; safe water and basic sanitation; maternal and child health care, including family planning; the prevention and control of locally endemic diseases; immunization against the main infectious diseases; appropriate treatment of common diseases and injuries; and the provision of essential drugs. See also COMMUNITY-ORIENTED PRIMARY HEALTH CARE.

PRIMORDIAL PREVENTION See PREVENTION.

PRINCIPAL COMPONENT ANALYSIS A statistical method to simplify the description of a set of interrelated variables. Its general objectives are data reduction and interpretation; there is no separation into dependent and independent variables; the original set of correlated variables is transformed into a smaller set of uncorrelated variables called the principal components. Often used as the first step in a factor analysis.

PRION An infectious protein, to which several neurological diseases once attributed to a slow virus diseases are now attributed, including Creutzfeldt-Jakob disease and kuru in humans, bovine spongiform encephalopathy in cattle, and scrapie in sheep. Unlike viruses and bacteria, prions do not contain DNA or RNA. The word was coined in 1982 by neurologist Stanley B. Prusiner (b. 1942), from *pro*teinaceous *in*fectious particles, reversing the order of the vowels. He received the Nobel Prize in 1997.

PRIOR ODDS The odds of the event (e.g., disease) before knowing the symptoms; the odds given a hypothesis before a study is analyzed.[1,37] See BAYES' THEOREM.

PRIOR PROBABILITY Probability of the disease before seeing diagnostic test results; probability of a hypothesis calculated or estimated from past data, theory, and judgment, before a study is analyzed.[1,7,37,101] See BAYES' THEOREM.

PRISMA Preferred Reporting Items for Systematic Reviews and Meta-Analyses. An evidence-based approach to reporting SYSTEMATIC REVIEWS and META-ANALYSES utilizing a 27-item checklist and four-phase flow diagram. It is an update and expansion of the Quality of Reporting of Meta-Analyses (QUOROM) statement.[229,230,423,683,684] See also CONSORT; EQUATOR; QUOROM; STARD; STREGA; STROBE.

PRIVACY The state of being undisturbed or free from public attention. The rules, regulations, and laws governing privacy and access to health-related information vary and change frequently. Privacy and CONFIDENTIALITY are protected by public interest groups and in some nations by privacy commissioners; the safeguards can affect EPIDEMIOLOGICAL RESEARCH requiring access to personal, private information. The concepts are increasingly important in situations where epidemiologists require access to data in medical and other records.[264] See also INFORMED CONSENT.

PROBABILITY

1. Frequency probability: the limit of the relative frequency of an event in a sequence of N random trials as N approaches infinity, i.e., the limit of

$$\frac{\text{Number of occurrences of the event}}{N}$$

2. Subjective probability: a measure, ranging from zero to 1, of the degree of belief in a hypothesis or statement.

Other definitions of probability exist (e.g., logical probability) but are rarely found in epidemiology, statistics, and clinical research. All probabilities obey the laws given by the axioms that:

a. All probabilities are 0 or greater: for any event or statement A, $Pr(A) \geq 0$.
b. The probability of anything certain to happen is 1; i.e., If A is certain, $Pr(A) = 1$.
c. If two events or statements A and B, cannot both be true at once (they are mutually exclusive), then the probability of their disjunction (A or B) is the sum of their separate probabilities: $Pr(A \text{ or } B) = Pr(A) + Pr(B)$.[1,3,7,34,37,38]

PROBABILITY DENSITY For a continuous variable, the function that gives the rate at which its PROBABILITY DISTRIBUTION is increasing. Not to be confused with FREQUENCY DISTRIBUTION.

PROBABILITY DISTRIBUTION For a discrete random variable, the function that gives the probabilities that the variable equals each of a sequence of possible values. Examples include the binomial and Poisson DISTRIBUTIONS. For a continuous random variable, the function that gives the probability that the variable is less than or equal to any given value; but the term is often used synonymously with the probability density function.[1,34,37,38]

PROBABILITY OF CAUSATION For a given case, the probability that exposure played a role in disease occurrence.[1,2,101] It should not be equated with the ATTRIBUTABLE FRACTION: the probability of causation can be much greater than that fraction, and the two measures are of different nature. To illustrate, suppose 100 patients given an incorrect treatment each lived 8 years but would have lived 10 years each had they not received the incorrect treatment. Then the probability of causation of death by the incorrect treatment is 100%. After 10 years of follow-up, the total PERSON-TIME at risk of death was $100(8) = 800$; but if the incorrect treatment had not been given, it would have been $100(10) = 1000$. Therefore the death rate over the 10 years was $100/800 = 0.125$/year, but it would have been only $100/1000$ had the incorrect treatment not been given. Thus the attributable fraction for the death rate was $(0.125 - 0.100)/0.125 = 0.20$ or 20%, which is far less than the probability of causation. In realistic examples the difference is less dramatic, but it still may be huge. See also ETIOLOGIC FRACTION.

PROBABILITY SAMPLE (Syn: random sample) See SAMPLE.

PROBABILITY THEORY The branch of mathematics dealing with the purely logical properties of probability. Its theorems underlie most statistical methods.

PROBAND The individual through whom a family with a genetic disorder is ascertained. In males he is called a *propositus*, and in females, a *proposita*. The INDEX CASE in a genetic study.

PROBIT The inverse of the NORMAL DISTRIBUTION FUNCTION. Used in exploratory statistical graphics and some regression modeling of binary response variables.[37]

PROBLEM-ORIENTED MEDICAL RECORD (POMR) A medical record in which the patient's history, physical findings, laboratory results, etc., are organized to give a cumulative record of problems (e.g., hemoptysis, rather than disease, such as pneumonia). The record includes subjective, objective, and significant negative information; discussions and conclusions; and diagnostic and treatment plans with respect to each problem. This type of record, which was developed by Lawrence Weed,[685] contrasts with the traditional medical record, which is less formally organized, usually recording all information from each source (history, physical, and laboratory findings) together without regard to the problems the information describes.

Since the problems may not be described in terms of conventional disease labels, their classification and counting for epidemiological purposes are sometimes difficult. The INTERNATIONAL CLASSIFICATION OF HEALTH PROBLEMS IN PRIMARY CARE (ICHPPC) is an attempt to overcome this difficulty.

PROCARCINOGEN The precursor of an active carcinogen. The procarcinogen itself is not usually carcinogenic but is converted to the active carcinogen after it has been metabolized by "xenobiotic metabolizing enzymes" such as cytochrome P450, dependent monooxygenases, glutathione S-transferases, sulfotransferases, and others. To elicit detrimental effects, the great majority of human chemical carcinogens require metabolic activation.[14,78,80-82,178,415,416,666] See also CARCINOGEN; MUTAGEN.

PRODUCT LIMIT METHOD See KAPLAN-MEIER ESTIMATE.

PROFESSIONAL ACTIVITY STUDY (PAS) The HOSPITAL DISCHARGE ABSTRACT SYSTEM, which covers many acute short-stay hospitals in the United States. It provides regularly published statistical tables arranged according to hospital service, diagnostic category, etc., giving details on diagnostic and therapeutic procedures, length of stay, and outcome.

PROFILE PLOT (Syn: barycentric coordinates) A graphical method of data presentation used when several categories add to 100%; it permits the categories to be plotted on a plane surface using coordinates running inward at right angles from each side of an equilateral polyhedron.

PROFILE, TRIAL See CONSORT.

PROGRAM
1. A (formal) set of procedures to conduct an activity, e.g., control of malaria.
2. An ordered list of instructions directing a computer to carry out a desired sequence of operations. The objective is normally the solution of a problem.

PROGRAM EVALUATION AND REVIEW TECHNIQUES (PERT) A work-scheduling method that uses ALGORITHMS and also enunciates general principles of procedure for allocating resources. It calls for the listing of specific tasks to be completed and the resources—personnel, equipment, supplies, and other items—that will be needed, along with their costs; a time chart indicating when each component task is to begin and end; an enumeration of interim accomplishment levels during that period; and a specification of times for interim review of the progress of the plan.

PROGRAMMING As defined by Alan Lucas,[686] the process whereby a stimulus or insult at a SENSITIVE PERIOD of development has lasting effects on the structure or function of the body. It is not recommended to describe the DEVELOPMENTAL ORIGINS OF HEALTH AND DISEASE.

PROGRAM REVIEW An evaluative study of a specific health program operating in a specific setting that is performed to provide a basis for decisions concerning the operation of the program.

PROGRAM TRIAL An experimental or quasi-experimental evaluative study of a (health) program.

PROLECTIVE Pertaining to data collected by planning in advance. A research study may use data collected for the study purposes or RETROLECTIVE data. Two of many terms coined by Alvan R. Feinstein (1925–2001),[224,687] aiming to be more precise than the common terms *prospective* and *retrospective*. Rarely used. See also DIRECTIONALITY.

PROPENSITY SCORE The conditional probability of being exposed or treated given a certain set of measured covariates. It can be estimated using (for example) regression methods. When comparing outcomes of different exposure or treatment groups, the estimated propensity score can be used to adjust for differences in the covariate distributions among the compared groups. This propensity adjustment can be done through matching, stratification, or regression adjustment for the score, or by a combination of these methods, and it can be used along with other covariate adjustments.[1,2,7,24,26,101,688,797]

PROPERTIES OF A CAUSE As described by David Hume in 1739, they are ASSOCIATION (cause and effect occur together), TIME ORDER (causes precede effects), and CONNECTION or DIRECTION.[42,84] When discussing CAUSALITY in the health and life sciences it is often essential that scientists clarify what properties they believe a cause should have.[101] See also CAUSAL CRITERIA; CAUSES IN PUBLIC HEALTH SCIENCES; COHERENCE, EPIDEMIOLOGICAL.

PROPHYLAXIS The preventive management of disease in individuals and populations. See also CHEMOPROPHYLAXIS.

PROPORTION A type of RATIO in which the numerator is included in the denominator. The ratio of a part to the whole, expressed as a "decimal fraction" (e.g., 0.2), as a "common fraction" (1/5), or as a PERCENTAGE (20%). By definition, a proportion *(p)* must be in the range (decimal) $0.0 \leq p \leq 1.0$. Since numerator and denominator have the same dimension, any dimensional contents cancel out, and a proportion is a dimensionless quantity. Where numerator and denominator are based on counts rather than measurements, the originals are also dimensionless, although proportions can be used for measured quantities (e.g., the skin area of the lower limb is x percent of the total skin area) as well as for counts (e.g., 15% of the population died). A PREVALENCE is a count-based proportion. The nondimensionality of a proportion, and its range limitations, do not necessarily apply to other kinds of ratios, of which "proportion" is a subset.[1,7] See also RATE; RATIO.

PROPORTIONAL HAZARDS MODEL (Syn: Cox model) A statistical model in SURVIVAL ANALYSIS proposed by Paul Sheehe in 1962 and more fully developed by D. R. Cox in 1972. It asserts that the effect of the study factors on the HAZARD RATE in the study population is multiplicative and does not change over time. For example, the model for the two factors x_1 and x_2 asserts that the rate at time t $\lambda(t)$, is given by

$$e^{\beta_1 x_1 + \beta_2 x_2} \lambda_0(t)$$

where $\lambda_0(t)$ is the rate when $x_1 = x_2 = 0$, and e is the base of the natural logarithm.[1,3,7,8,11,37]

PROPORTIONAL MORTALITY-ODDS RATIO The odds of deaths from a specified condition in a defined population divided by the odds of deaths expected from this condition in a STANDARD POPULATION, usually expressed either on an age-sex-specific basis or sex-specific after age adjustment. Often preferred to the proportional mortality ratio on the grounds that it tends to better approximate the ratio of mortality rates in the two populations.

PROPORTIONAL MORTALITY RATIO The proportion of observed deaths from a specified condition in a defined population divided by the proportion of deaths expected from this condition in a STANDARD POPULATION, usually expressed either on an age-sex-specific basis or sex-specific after age adjustment. Unlike the STANDARDIZED MORTALITY RATIO, it does not require data on the age composition of the population but only on the deaths. The acronym PMR is preferably avoided because the same initial letters can stand for perinatal mortality rate.[1,7,8]

PROPOSITUS See PROBAND.

PROSPECTIVE STUDY See COHORT STUDY.

PROTEOME The entire network or set of proteins expressed by the genome and epigenome within distinct cells and tissues in the body.

PROTOCOL The plan, or set of steps, to be followed in a study or investigation or in an intervention program.[3,6,26] See also ALGORITHM, CLINICAL.

PROTOPATHIC BIAS A type of BIAS that can occur if the first symptoms of the outcome of interest are the reasons for using the treatment under study.[224] See also CONFOUNDING BY INDICATION.

PROTOZOA (singular: protozoan) A group of unicellular or acellular, usually microscopic, eukaryotic organisms which vary greatly in size, morphology, nutritional requirements, and life cycle. It includes some plant-like forms and animal species that are free-living, COMMENSAL, mutualistic, and parasitic, and some important disease-causing organisms.

PROXIMAL DETERMINANT See DETERMINANT, PROXIMAL.

PSEUDO-LONGITUDINAL STUDY If a population is randomly sampled, for example annually, it is possible to identify a sequence of subsamples with age ranges increasing in step with the dates of the samples. The sequence of subsamples resembles a regularly measured cohort except that it consists of a different sample at each sampling occasion, which may overlap little if at all.

PSYCHOSOCIAL EPIDEMIOLOGY See SOCIAL EPIDEMIOLOGY.

PUBLICATION BIAS

1. The result of the tendency of authors to submit, organizations to encourage, reviewers to approve, and editors to publish articles containing "positive" findings (e.g., a gene-disease association), especially "new" results, in contrast to findings or reports that do not report statistically significant or "positive" results.

2. A tendency of authors to preferentially include in their study reports findings that conform to their preconceived notions, or outcomes preferred by their institution, sponsor, or EPISTEMIC COMMUNITY.

Publication bias distorts available scientific evidence on a wide range of issues. It can be a particularly important source of bias in META-ANALYSIS. Efforts are underway to promote that all clinical trials be registered and all results reported.[1,3,6,9,26,58,64,87,91,117,135-137,226,294,300,467,504,626] See also DATA DREDGING; KNOWLEDGE CONSTRUCTION; INTERPRETIVE BIAS; SCIENTIFIC MISCONDUCT; SUPPRESSION BIAS.

PUBLIC HEALTH Like most sculptures, symphonies, and other works of art, certain important things in life have several dimensions. The definition of public health has four dimensions. Public health is:

1. The health of a whole society. It can be measured and assessed through quantitative and qualitative indicators and analytic processes.

2. The specific policies, services, programs and other essential efforts agreed (ideally, and often, democratically), organized, structured, financed, monitored, and evaluated by society to collectively protect, promote, and restore the people's health and its determinants.

3. The institutions, public and private organizations — including private and public companies —, and other citizens organizations, that plan, develop, fund, and implement such efforts, and which are thus an integral part of local, national, regional, and global public health systems.

4. The scientific disciplines and professions, knowledge, methods, art, and craft essential to positively influence HEALTH DETERMINANTS, and thus prevent disease and disability, prolong life, and promote HEALTH through the organized and collective efforts of society.

Public health takes care daily of what we breathe, drink, and eat, how we work, move, and live together. Economic, environmental, social, educational, occupational, medical, and other policies intertwined with public health change with changing social values and networks, policies and technologies; yet, the goals—diverse as they are in democratic societies—remain the same: to reduce the amount of health-related suffering, disease, disability, and premature death in the population. Public health is a SYSTEM of professions and scientific disciplines, social organizations and institutions, values, and actions.[1,2,5,6,13,14,17,19,28,33,38-42, 67,72,83,85,96,113-117,123,128,140,150,158,160,161,164,183,186,188,213-215,248-250,254,267,279,285-287,302-320,357-360,366,382,436-439,522,678]

PUBLIC HEALTH IMPACT ASSESSMENT See HEALTH IMPACT ASSESSMENT.

PUBLIC HEALTH MEDICINE The practice of public health by physicians. See also SOCIAL MEDICINE.

PUBLIC HEALTH SIGNIFICANCE See SIGNIFICANCE, PUBLIC HEALTH.

PURIFIED PROTEIN DERIVATIVE SKIN TEST (PPD) See TUBERCULIN SKIN TEST.

P **VALUE** (Syn: probability value, observed significance level) The probability that a test statistic would be as extreme as observed or more extreme if the TEST HYPOTHESIS were true. The letter *P* stands for this probability. The *P* value is a continuous measure of the compatibility between the data and the test hypothesis, given the statistical model used to compute the test, with $P = 1$ representing maximum compatibility and $P = 0$ representing complete incompatibility. When the tested hypothesis is a null hypothesis, the *P* value is usually close to the probability that the difference observed or greater could have occurred by chance alone given the null hypothesis is true. In most health and social science research, a study result whose *P* value is less than 5% ($P < 0.05$) is considered sufficiently unlikely to have occurred by chance to justify the designation "statistically significant," but the use of such cutoffs has been criticized extensively for degrading the information contained in the precise value of *P*. A *P* value is said to be *calibrated* or *valid* if it has a uniform DISTRIBUTION between 0 and 1 when the test hypothesis is correct (i.e., if it has equal probability of lying anywhere between 0 and 1). It is said to be *powerful* to the extent that its distribution shifts toward 0, away from 1 when the test hypothesis is false.[1] See also SIGNIFICANCE, STATISTICAL.

QALYs See QUALITY-ADJUSTED LIFE YEARS.

Q–Q PLOT A probability plot for comparing two probability distributions by plotting their quantiles against each other ("Q" stands for quantile). If the two distributions are similar, the points in the Q–Q plot will approximately lie on the line y = x. If the distributions are linearly related, the points in the Q–Q plot will approximately lie on a line, but not necessarily on the line y = x. Commonly used in genetic epidemiology to assess data quality.[54]

QUADAS-2 Quality Assessment of studies of Diagnostic Accuracy included in Systematic reviews. An evidence-based quality assessment tool to be used in SYSTEMATIC REVIEWS of diagnostic accuracy studies. The checklist includes items that cover patient spectrum, reference standard, DISEASE PROGRESSION BIAS, verification bias, review bias, clinical review bias, incorporation bias, test execution, study withdrawals, and indeterminate results. It is presented together with guidelines for scoring each of the items included in the tool.[340,423,689] See also CONSORT; EQUATOR; PRISMA; QUOROM; STARD; STROBE; TREND.

QUALITATIVE DATA

1. Observations or information characterized by measurement on a categorical scale, i.e., a dichotomous or nominal scale, or, if the categories are ordered, an ordinal scale. Examples are sex, hair color, death or survival, and nationality. See also MEASUREMENT SCALE.

2. Systematic nonnumerical observations by sociologists, anthropologists, etc., using approved methods such as participant observation or key informants. Qualitative data can enrich understanding of complex problems and help to explain why things happen.

QUALITATIVE RESEARCH Any type of research that employs nonnumeric information to explore individual or group characteristics, producing findings not arrived at by statistical procedures or other quantitative means. Examples include clinical case studies, narrative studies of behavior, ethnography, and organizational or social studies.[229,690]

QUALITY-ADJUSTED LIFE EXPECTANCY (QALE) A model for clinical decision-making in which estimates of impairment or disability are included in the calculation of life expectancy.

QUALITY-ADJUSTED LIFE YEARS (QALYs) An adjustment of life expectancy that reduces the overall life expectancy by amounts that reflect the existence of chronic conditions causing impairment, disability, and/or handicap as assessed from health survey data, hospital discharge data, etc.[163-169] In practice, numerical weights representing severity of residual disability are established by the judgment of patients and health professionals.

Procedures for calculating QALYs, like those for calculating DALYs, begin with chronological age and multiply this by a "utility-weight" for the health state. A variety of techniques have been used, including STANDARD GAMBLE and TIME TRADE-OFF. See also DISABILITY-ADJUSTED LIFE YEARS.

QUALITY ASSURANCE System of procedures, checks, audits, and corrective actions to ensure that all research, testing, MONITORING, sampling, analysis, and other technical and reporting activities are of the highest achievable quality. The term is used in health services with the same meaning.[17]

QUALITY CONTROL The supervision and control of all operations involved in a process, usually involving sampling and inspection, in order to detect and correct systematic or excessively random variations in quality.[3,7,26]

QUALITY OF CARE A level of performance or accomplishment that characterizes the health care provided. Measures of the quality of care depend upon value judgments, but there are ingredients and determinants of quality that can be measured objectively. Such factors were classified by Donabedian[517] into measures of structure (e.g., manpower, facilities), process (e.g., diagnostic and therapeutic procedures), and outcome (e.g., case fatality rates, disability rates, and levels of patient satisfaction with the service).[17,232,432] See also HEALTH SERVICES RESEARCH.

QUALITY OF LIFE

1. The degree to which persons perceive themselves able to function physically, emotionally, mentally, and socially. Contrast HEALTH STATUS, which is an objective measurement. In a general sense, that which makes life worth living.[17,38,227,651]

2. In a more "quantitative" sense, an estimate of remaining life free of impairment, disability, or handicap, as used in the expression QUALITY-ADJUSTED LIFE YEARS. Somewhere between these is an estimate of the utility of life; for instance, in clinical decision analysis, the utility of life that is impaired by a disabling degree of angina pectoris may be compared with that of a life that may be shorter in duration but free of disabling pain as a result of applying therapeutic procedures. Such trade-offs are part of clinical decision analysis.[202] See also MINIMALLY IMPORTANT DIFFERENCE; PATIENT-REPORTED OUTCOMES; UTILITY.

QUANGO A quasi-autonomous nongovernmental organization (NGO). Originally, slang. A semipublic body partly or wholly supported by government funds and with some members appointed by the government but otherwise having the characteristics of an NGO.

QUANTAL EFFECT (Syn: all-or-none effect) An effect that can be expressed only in binary form, e.g., as "occurring" or "not occurring."[449]

QUANTILE The p'th quantile of a PROBABILITY DISTRIBUTION is the point x at which the probability (proportion of the distribution) falling below x is p. Quantiles are divisions of a DISTRIBUTION into equal, ordered subgroups. Deciles are tenths; quartiles, quarters; quintiles, fifths; terciles, thirds; and centiles, hundredths.[7] See also PERCENTILE.

QUANTITATIVE DATA Data in numerical quantities, such as continuous measurements or counts or binary variables. QUALITATIVE DATA can be coded to create quantitative data. See also MEASUREMENT SCALE.

QUARANTINE

1. Restriction of the activities of well persons or animals who have been exposed to a case of COMMUNICABLE DISEASE during its period of communicability (i.e., contacts) to prevent disease transmission during the incubation period if infection should occur.

a. *Absolute* or *complete quarantine*: The limitation of freedom of movement of those exposed to a communicable disease for a period of time not longer than the longest usual incubation period of that disease in such manner as to prevent effective contact with those not so exposed.

b. *Modified quarantine*: A selective, partial limitation of freedom of movement of contacts, commonly on the basis of known or presumed differences in susceptibility and related to the danger of disease transmission. It may be designed to meet particular situations. Examples are exclusion of children from school, exemption of immune persons from provisions applicable to susceptible persons, or restriction of military populations to the post or to quarters. It includes personal SURVEILLANCE, the practice of close medical or other supervision of contacts in order to permit prompt recognition of infection or illness but without restricting movements; and segregation, the separation of some part of a group of persons or domestic animals from the others for special consideration, control, or observation — for example, removal of susceptible children to homes of immune persons or establishment of a sanitary boundary to protect uninfected from infected portions of a population.[48,69,160,188]

2. The word *quarantine* comes from the Italian *quaranta*, meaning forty, and refers to the 40 days arbitrarily (or empirically) believed to be an adequate isolation period, perhaps based on the biblical 40 days. The clinical distinction between ISOLATION and quarantine is that isolation is the procedure for persons already sick, whereas quarantine is often applied to (apparently) healthy contacts. This has legal and ethical implications if apparently healthy persons must submit to restrictions upon their freedom to move at large in society.

QUASI-EXPERIMENT A situation in which the investigator lacks full control over the allocation and/or timing of intervention but nonetheless conducts the study as if it were an experiment, allocating subjects to groups. Inability to allocate subjects randomly is a common situation that may be best described as a quasi-experiment.[1,7,24] See also NATURAL EXPERIMENT.

QUESTIONNAIRE A predetermined set of questions used to collect data—clinical data, social status, occupational group, etc.[26,551] This term is often applied to a self-completed survey instrument, as contrasted with an INTERVIEW SCHEDULE.

QUETELET'S INDEX See BODY MASS INDEX.

QUEUEING THEORY A mathematical discipline featuring models that analyze the flow of people through a service or their use of resources and that attempts to optimize utilization.

"QUICK AND DIRTY" METHOD A colloquial expression to refer to a method that yields a result rapidly but not necessarily with scientific rigor or validity. RAPID EPIDEMIOLOGICAL ASSESSMENT has value and is not necessarily unreliable.

QUOROM Quality of Reporting of Meta-analyses. A consensus checklist and a flow diagram to improve the quality of reports of META-ANALYSES of randomized clinical trials.[276,294,691] The checklist describes ways to present the sections of a report of a meta-analysis. The flow diagram provides information about the numbers of trials identified, included, and excluded. It has been revised and replaced by the PRISMA statement to encompass both meta-analyses and SYSTEMATIC REVIEWS.[423] See also CONSORT; EQUATOR; QUADAS-2; STARD; STROBE; STREGA; TREND.

QUOTA SAMPLING A method by which the proportions in the sample in various subgroups (according to criteria such as age, sex, and social status of the individuals to be selected) are chosen to agree with the corresponding proportions in the population. The resulting sample may not be representative of characteristics that have not been taken into account.

QUOTIENT The result of the division of a numerator by a denominator.

Q-VALUE The minimum level at which the FALSE DISCOVERY RATE (FDR) is considered significant. Also known as an FDR level, the q-value is an arbitrary cutoff that can be thought of as the proportion of expected false discoveries. For example, if out of 100,000 tests, 1000 discoveries (rejected null hypotheses) were made, then a q-value of 0.05 would indicate the expectation that 50 out of 1000 discoveries were FALSE POSITIVES.

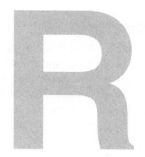

RACE
1. By historical and common usage, the group (*subspecies* in traditional scientific use) a person belongs to as a result of a mix of physical features such as skin color and hair texture, which reflect ancestry and geographical origins; as identified by others or as self-identified. The importance of social factors in the creation and perpetuation of racial categories has led to broadening of the concept to include a common social and political heritage, making its use similar to ETHNICITY.[430]
2. In biology, a category used in the classification of organisms or groups of individuals within a species that are geographically, ecologically, physiologically, or genetically distinct from other members of the species.[692]

Biological classification of human races is difficult — and sometimes meaningless — because of significant genetic and environmental overlaps among population groups. Concepts of race often reflect social and ideological conventions.[279,693] Socioeconomic, cultural, and behavioral differences are often more important than racial differences in influencing health status. However, race may be a useful concept in PUBLIC HEALTH because some exposures and diseases are correlated with biological and physical aspects of race; this may relate to gene-environment interactions or to specific gene variants, which may be associated with environmental exposures of prior generations. Useful insights into human biology and genetics have come from analysis by racial group of census data and national health surveys.[5,375] See also ETHNIC GROUP.

RADIX The size of the hypothetical BIRTH COHORT in a life table, commonly 1000 or 100,000.

RAHE-HOLMES SOCIAL READJUSTMENT RATING SCALE See LIFE EVENTS.

RANDOM (Syn: aleatory, stochastic) Governed by CHANCE; not completely determined by measurable factors.[2,34,37,38,101]

RANDOM ALLOCATION (Syn: randomization) Allocation of individuals to groups in a CLINICAL TRIAL (e.g., intervention and control) by chance. It makes the trial a RANDOMIZED CONTROLLED TRIAL.[1,3,5,6,24,58,101,270,272,641,800] If there is no effect of the intervention, it makes differences between the intervention and control groups random. Within the limits of chance variation (e.g., if the number of subjects is large), it yields groups similar at the start of an investigation and does so for both known and unknown variables (i.e., for measured and unmeasured determinants of the outcomes). No other methodological procedure can accomplish this. Yet, the "benefits of randomization" do not last forever: for explanatory purposes (e.g., to assess mechanisms), the randomized trial may need to be analyzed as an observational cohort study if post-randomization events affect differently the different study groups.[272,641,800] Randomization enables statistical procedures to account for uncertainty about unmeasured baseline differences via standard errors, *P* values, and confidence intervals. It also ensures that personal judgment and views of the investigator do not influence allocation. Random allocation follows a strictly predetermined plan, devised with the aid of a computer program. Nonrandom methods (e.g., allocation by alternation, date of birth, case record, day of the week, presenting or enrollment order), sometimes called "pseudorandomization," are not reliable in producing similar groups, prone to breakdown of ALLOCATION CONCEALMENT, and thus usually unacceptable as valid allocation methods.[37] See also BLOCKED RANDOMIZATION; CONFOUNDING BIAS; EXPLANATORY STUDY; POSITIVITY; STRATIFIED RANDOMIZATION.

RANDOM-DIGIT DIALING A method for sampling people in telephone surveys in which telephone numbers are randomly dialed.

RANDOMIZATION See RANDOM ALLOCATION.

RANDOMIZATION, MENDELIAN See MENDELIAN RANDOMIZATION.

RANDOMIZED CONTROLLED TRIAL (RCT) A clinical-epidemiological experiment in which subjects are randomly allocated into groups, usually called *test* and *control* groups, to receive or not to receive a preventive or a therapeutic procedure or intervention. The results are assessed by comparison of rates of disease, death, recovery, or other appropriate outcome in the study groups. RCTs are generally regarded as the most scientifically rigorous method of hypothesis testing available in epidemiology and medicine. Nonetheless, they may suffer lack of GENERALIZABILITY due, for example, to the non-REPRESENTATIVENESS of patients who are ethically and practically eligible, chosen, or consent to participate.[1,2,5,6,24,26,37,58,73-77,91,101,110,227,270,272,641,800] A few authors refer to this design as "randomized control trial." See also CLINICAL TRIAL; COMMUNITY TRIAL; EXPERIMENTAL EPIDEMIOLOGY.

RANDOM SAMPLE A sample that is arrived at by selecting sample units such that each possible unit has a fixed and known or equal probability of selection. See also SAMPLE; SAMPLING.

RANDOM SAMPLING VARIATION See SAMPLING VARIATION.

RANDOM VARIABLE

1. A variable whose distribution incorporates some element of chance, randomness, or unpredictability.
2. A variable that has or may be assigned a (possibly unknown) PROBABILITY DISTRIBUTION.[2,7]

RANDOM WALK The path traversed by a particle that moves in steps, each step being determined by chance in regard to direction, magnitude, or both. The theory of random walks has many applications (e.g., to sequential sampling and to the migration of insects, including disease vectors).

RANGE OF DISTRIBUTION The difference between the largest and smallest values in a DISTRIBUTION.

RANK (v.) To arrange in a meaningful order or sequence (e.g., numerical order, degree of severity).

RANKING SCALE (Syn: ordinal scale) A scale that arrays the members of a group from high to low according to the magnitude of the observations, assigns numbers to the ranks, and neglects distances between members of the array. See also MEASUREMENT SCALE.

RAPID EPIDEMIOLOGICAL ASSESSMENT Methods that can be used to yield results as rapidly and efficiently as available resources permit; e.g., to assess health problems and evaluate health programs in developing countries or to delineate the health impact of a PUBLIC HEALTH emergency, such as a disaster or an epidemic with unusual features.[28,694] See also DISASTER EPIDEMIOLOGY; TRIAGE.

RARE-DISEASE ASSUMPTION (Syn: rarity assumption) Reliance on the use of approximations, based on the assumption that the disease being studied is rare in the studied population. This assumption must be met for (1) prevalence to be approximately equal to the incidence rate multiplied by the average duration of disease (i.e., for the validity of the approximation $P = I \times D$); (2) the incidence proportion to be approximately equal to the incidence rate multiplied by the length of the follow-up period (i.e., for $IP = IR \times T$); and (3) for the odds ratio to be approximately equal to the INCIDENCE RATE RATIO or the RISK RATIO (i.e., $OR \approx IRR$ or $OR \approx RR$) in some but not other case-control studies, depending on the method used to select controls. When DENSITY SAMPLING is used to select controls, $OR = IRR$ regardless of the rarity or frequency of the disease. Decisions about "rarity" are rather arbitrary; the odds ratio will usually be within p% of the risk ratio if the risk does not exceed p% in any group being compared (e.g., if the risk is always below 5%, the odds ratio will generally be within 5% of the risk ratio and even closer to the rate ratio).[1,2,24,197]

RATE A measure of the frequency of occurrence of a phenomenon. In epidemiology, demography, and vital statistics, a rate is an expression of the frequency with which an event occurs in a defined population, usually in a specified period of time. The components of a rate are the numerator, the denominator, the specified time in which events occur, and usually a multiplier, a power of 10, that converts the rate from an awkward fraction or decimal to a whole number.

In vital statistics,

$$\text{Rate} = \frac{\text{Number of events in specified period}}{\text{Average population during the period}} \times 10^n$$

In epidemiology, the denominator is usually PERSON-TIME. Physical units other than time may be used for constructing rates; e.g., in accident epidemiology, deaths per passenger-mile is a more meaningful way of comparing modes of transportation.

Other uses of *rate* in epidemiology include: (1) As a wrong synonym for ratio, it refers to proportions as rates, as in the terms *cumulative incidence rate* or *survival rate*. PROPORTION and RATIO are not synonyms for rate. (2) In other situations, rate refers only to ratios representing relative changes (actual or potential) in two quantities. (3) Sometimes rate is further restricted to refer only to ratios representing changes over time. In this sense, the term *prevalence rate* is to be avoided, because PREVALENCE cannot (and does not need to) be expressed as a change in time; of course, different prevalence estimates may vary, change, and be compared. In contrast, the force of mortality and the force of morbidity (hazard rate) are proper rates, for they can be expressed as the number of cases developing per unit time divided by the total size of the population at risk.[1-3,5,197] See also HAZARD RATE.

RATE DIFFERENCE (RD) The difference between two rates; for example, the difference in incidence rate between a population group exposed to a causal factor and a population group not exposed to the factor:

$$RD = I_e - I_u$$

where I = incidence rate among exposed and I_u = incidence rate among unexposed. In comparisons of exposed and unexposed groups, the term *excess rate* may be used as a synonym for *rate difference*.[1]

RATE-ODDS RATIO See ODDS RATIO.

RATE RATIO The ratio of two rates; e.g., the rate in an exposed population divided by the rate in an unexposed population:

$$Rate\ Ratio = \frac{I_e}{I_u}$$

where I_e is the incidence rate among the exposed and I_u is the incidence rate among the unexposed.[1] See also RELATIVE RISK.

RATIO The value obtained by dividing one quantity by another. RATES and PROPORTIONS (including RISK) are ratios, though not synonyms.[1] The numerator of a proportion is included in the population defined by the denominator, whereas in other types of ratios numerator and denominator are distinct quantities, neither being included in the other. The dimensionality of a ratio is obtained through algebraic cancellation, summation, etc., of the dimensionalities of its numerator and denominator terms. Both counted and measured values may be included in the numerator and in the denominator. There are no general restrictions on the dimensionalities or ranges of ratios, but there are in some types of ratios (e.g., proportion, prevalence). Ratios are sometimes expressed as percentages (e.g., standardized mortality ratio). In these cases, the value may exceed 100. See also MATERNAL MORTALITY RATIO; SEX RATIO.

RATIO SCALE See MEASUREMENT SCALE.

RAW DATA The entire set of information that has been collected in a study before any cleaning, editing, or statistical analysis begins.

REASON FOR ENCOUNTER (RFE) The statement of reason(s) why a person enters the health care system, representing that person's demand for care. The terms recorded by the health care provider clarify the reason for encounter without interpreting it in the form of a diagnosis.[560]

RECALL BIAS Systematic error due to differences in ACCURACY or completeness of recall to memory of past events or experiences.[1,3,6,9,26,551] For example, a mother whose child has died of leukemia may be more likely than the mother of a healthy living child to remember details of such past experiences as use of x-ray services when the child was in utero. A type of INFORMATION or MEASUREMENT BIAS.

RECEIVER OPERATING CHARACTERISTIC (ROC) CURVE (Syn: relative operating characteristic curve) A graphic means for assessing the ability of a screening or diagnostic test to discriminate between persons with and without the target disorder. For an ordinal or continuous diagnostic test, the ROC curve depicts the plot of all pairs of SENSITIVITY and 1-SPECIFICITY (false-positive probability) over all possible or chosen cutoff values.[6,9,24,26,58,796] The term *receiver operating characteristic* comes from psychometry, where the characteristic operating response of a receiver-individual to faint stimuli or nonstimuli was recorded, and it was first used in studies of radar during World War II. See also DISCRIMINATORY ACCURACY.

RECESSIVE In genetics, a gene that is phenotypically manifest only when present in the homozygous state.[57,349,549]

RECOMMENDATIONS See GUIDELINES.

RECORD LINKAGE A method for bringing together the information contained in two or more records—e.g., in different sets of medical charts, in birth and death certificates—and a procedure to ensure that each individual is counted only once. The procedure incorporates a unique identifying system such as a personal identification number and/or birth name(s) of the individual's mother.[696]

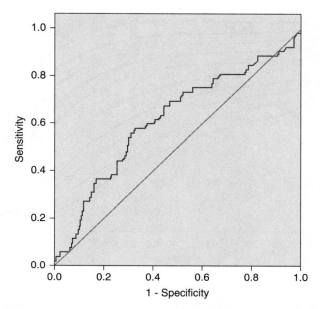

ROC curve. Performance of the Gail model to assess the individual risk of breast cancer in a screening setting. The ROC curve is barely over the diagonal ("line of no-discrimination"); i.e., regardless of the cutoff point used, the model performs only slightly better than random guessing in discriminating women with and without breast cancer. Source: Buron A, et al.[695] With permission.

Record linkage makes it possible to relate significant health events that are remote from one another in time and place, or to bring together records of different individuals (e.g., members of a family).

PRIVACY and CONFIDENTIALITY must both be respected in record linkage studies. "Each person in the world creates a Book of Life. This Book starts with birth and ends with death. Its pages are made of the records of the principal events in Life. Record linkage is the name given to the process of assembling the pages of this Book into a volume." [7,8,697] See also LIFE COURSE.

RECRUDESCENCE Reactivation of infection. See also RELAPSE.

RECTANGULARIZATION OF MORTALITY The shape of survival curves as life expectancy increases: higher proportions of all who are born survive to old age and the graph becomes more "rectangular" in shape. Empirical observations in several countries have failed to demonstrate it, and the opposite was found in the United States, where the range of age at death was widening because of the impact of HIV disease and violence. See also COMPRESSION OF MORTALITY.

RECURRENCE The second episode of a disease occurring after a first episode was considered cured. For instance, in tuberculosis, molecular techniques have shown that some recurrences are due to reinfection by a different strain rather than relapse with the same strain that had caused the first episode.[217-219,698] Thus REINFECTION and RELAPSE are two different causes of disease recurrence.

RECURRENCE RISK Risk of a second episode (and of subsequent episodes) of an event. It may provide information on the heterogeneity of RISK in the population, and thus be useful for etiological studies. Observable in many areas of health (e.g., reproductive

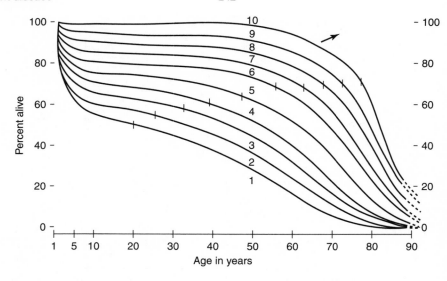

1. India, Male, 1901–1911. (Expectation of life at birth, 22.59 years)
2. Guatemala, Male, 1921. (25.59 years)
3. Mexico, Male, 1930. (33.02 years)
4. England and Wales, Male, 1861. (40.47 years)
5. Guatemala, Male, 1964. (48.51 years)
6. England and Wales, Male, 1921. (55.94 years)
7. Venezuela, Male, 1964. (63.74 years)
8. Netherlands, Male, 1947–49. (69.40 years)
9. Sweden, Male, 1964. (75.93 years)
10. Sweden, Female, 1974. (78.10 years)

Rectangularization of mortality. Survivorship curves by age and sex, selected countries, 1861–1974. Vertical bars show life expectancy at birth. Source: Basch PF.[673] With permission.

and perinatal events). High recurrence rates of certain health problems may result from interactions among genetic, epigenetic, and persistent environmental factors.[6,699,799]

RECURRENT DISEASE A bacteriologically confirmed disease episode needing retreatment after a patient was successfully treated or defaulted during a previous disease episode.[6,59,116,190,679,700] See also REINFECTION.

REDUCTION (of data)

1. (Syn: "collapsing") Reducing the number of categories of a set of data to simplify analysis. An important application is aggregation of small numbers and/or small areas in published tables from a national census in order to preserve the CONFIDENTIALITY of these localities and their residents.
2. Formation of composite (derived) variables based on several originally collected variables, using methods ranging from simple indexes to factor analysis.
3. Summarizing data by means of classification schemes and arithmetical manipulations.

REDUCTIONISM A philosophical concept of scientific investigation based on studying component parts of a system; e.g., proceeding from organs to tissues, to cells, to molecules. The reductionist view is that the whole can be explained in terms of the functioning of its parts. The discovery of the DNA structure can be viewed as a triumph for reductionist approaches. While some reductionist approaches have been fruitful, they may favor rigid compartmentalizing and fragmentation of sciences and hence delay progress. They may also favor MEDICALIZATION and GENETIZATION. Epidemiological studies that focus exclusively on individual RISK FACTORS are also a form of reductionism (not always wrong or irrelevant), which tends to disregard contextual influences on health. Clinical and molecular epidemiology are practiced with both reductionist and INTEGRATIVE approaches.[39,42,201,203,323,548] See also TRANSDISCIPLINARITY.

REED-FROST MODEL A mathematical model of infectious disease transmission and HERD IMMUNITY developed by Lowell Reed (1886–1966) and Wade Hampton Frost (1880–1938). The model gives the number of new cases, C, of an infectious disease that can be expected in a closed, freely mixing population of immunes and susceptibles in time period t to $t + 1$, with varying assumptions about the distribution of each in the population:

$$C_{t+1} = S_t \left[1 - (1 - p)_t^c \right]$$

where C_{t+1} is the number of cases between time t and $t + 1$, S_t is the number of susceptibles at time t, and p is the probability that any specified individual will have contact with any other specified individual in the population. Elaborations of the model provide the theoretical basis for IMMUNIZATION programs that control infectious diseases without necessarily achieving 100% immunization coverage.[67,110,527]

REFERENCE POPULATION The standard against which a population that is being studied can be compared.

REFINEMENT The process of identifying new subcategories of study variables for the purpose of more accurate or more detailed description of relationships. An example is refinement of the concept of serum cholesterol level into high-, low-, and very low density lipoproteins.

REGISTER, REGISTRY In epidemiology the term *register* is applied to the file of data concerning all cases of a particular disease or other health-relevant condition in a defined population such that the cases can be related to a population base. With this information, incidence rates can be calculated. If the cases are regularly followed up, information on remission, exacerbation, prevalence, and survival can also be obtained. The *register* is the actual document, and the *registry* is the system of ongoing registration.

In most developed countries all births and deaths are recorded through birth and death registration systems. Results and summaries are then tabulated and published. Examples of registries that have epidemiological value include the following:

Cancer registries, which secure reports of cancer patients as soon as possible after first diagnosis. The principal sources for these reports are the hospitals serving the community, but a few cases are not reported until death.

Twin registries, which have provided the basis for studies attempting to differentiate genetic from environmental factors in the etiology of cancer and other conditions where both genetic and environmental factors may be contributing causes.

Birth defect registries, which seek to document anomalies that are apparent at or soon after birth. They suffer from incompleteness owing to the omission of STILLBIRTHS and of anomalies that do not declare their presence until later in life, such as certain forms of congenital heart lesion, mental deficiency, and neurological disorders.

Many types of register—e.g., disease-specific, treatment-specific, "at risk," local (hospital- or clinic-based)—are not population based. Population-based registers are usually considered to be the most useful type for epidemiological purposes; clinic-based, disease-specific registers can be used as a source of cases for case-control studies.[8,24-26,701]

REGISTRATION The term *registration* implies something more than notification for the purpose of immediate action or to permit the counting of cases. A register requires that a permanent record be established, including identifying data. Cases may be followed up, and statistical tabulations may be prepared on both frequency and survival. In addition, the persons listed on a register may be subjects of special studies.

REGRESSAND In REGRESSION ANALYSIS, the variable whose mean values are studied in relation to regressors; the dependent variable.

REGRESSION

1. As used by Francis Galton (1822–1911) in his book *Hereditary Genius* (1869), the tendency of offspring of exceptional parents (unusually tall, unusually intelligent, etc.) to possess characteristics closer to the average for the general population. Hence "regression to the mean"; i.e., the tendency of individuals at the extremes to have values nearer to the mean on repeated measurement.
2. In statistics, the relation of mean values of a dependent or regressand variable to independent or regressor variables (covariates).[1,3,7,11,110,244,270,797]
3. A synonym for REGRESSION ANALYSIS.

REGRESSION ANALYSIS Given data on a regressand (dependent variable) Y and one or more regressors (covariates or independent variables) x_1, x_2, etc., regression analysis involves finding a mathematical model (within some restricted class of models) that adequately describes the average value of Y as a function of the x's, or that predicts y from the x's. The most common form of model for an unbounded continuous Y is a linear model; the logistic and proportional hazards models are the most common forms used when Y is binary or a survival time, respectively.[1,3,7,11,34,36,37,244,270,796]

REGRESSION CURVE, LINE, SURFACE, PLANE Diagrammatic presentation of a regression model as a curve on a graph, usually drawn with the regressor, x, as the abscissa and the predicted average of the dependent variable (regressand), Y, as ordinate. In the case of LINEAR REGRESSION, the curve reduces to a line. A model with three variables (two regessors and one regressand) can be shown diagrammatically on a three-dimensional plot or stereogram; the result is a regression surface, which in the case of MULTIPLE LINEAR REGRESSION reduces to a plane.

REGRESSION, LOGISTIC See LOGISTIC MODEL.

REGRESSION MODEL A MATHEMATICAL MODEL for the relation of the average value of a variable (the REGRESSAND) to other variables (the REGRESSORS). See also REGRESSION ANALYSIS.

REGRESSION TO THE MEAN See REGRESSION.

REGRESSOR In REGRESSION ANALYSIS, a variable used to predict the regressand (dependent) variable. An independent variable or regression covariate.

REINFECTION A second infection by the same agent or a second infection of an organ with a different agent or strain. In tuberculosis, DNA fingerprinting of *Mycobacterium tuberculosis* showed that some recurrences are not treatment failures (i.e., they are not a relapse).[56,59,67,110,116,188,190,196,217-219,702,703]

REINFORCING FACTORS See CAUSATION OF DISEASE, FACTORS IN.

RELAPSE

1. Return of a disease state after remission or apparent cure.
2. Insufficient bacteriological cure of a first episode. In tuberculosis the episode is caused by the same strain. In malaria, true relapses are caused by reactivation

of dormant liver stage parasites (hypnozoites) found in *Plasmodium vivax* and *P. ovale*.[56,59,116,190,347] See also RECURRENCE.

RELATIONSHIP See ASSOCIATION.

RELATIVE EFFECT A ratio of rates, proportions, or other measures of an effect. For example, the INCIDENCE RATE RATIO, calculated as the incidence rate in the exposed divided by the incidence rate in the unexposed, is a measure of relative effect.[1]

RELATIVE EXCESS RISK (RER) A measure that can be used in comparisons of adverse reactions to drugs (or other exposures), based solely on the component of risk due to the exposure or drug under investigation, removing the risk due to background exposure experienced by all in the population:

$$RER = (R_1 - R_0)/(R_2 - R_0)$$

where R_1 is the rate in the study population. R_2 is the rate in the comparison group, and R_0 is the rate in the general population.[704]

RELATIVE INDEX OF INEQUALITY A means of quantifying the degree of relative INEQUALITY in health in relation to another variable that can be ordered hierachically, typically socioeconomic status. It is the ratio of the extreme adjusted values of a health indicator by means of a regression model where the outcome is a health status indicator and the exposure or predictor is the relative rank of socioeconomic status. It can be interpreted as the relative difference in health between the top (relative rank 1) and the bottom (relative rank 0) of the socioeconomic scale. It only applies where there is linear variation in the health outcome.[705,706] See also CONCENTRATION INDEX; GINI COEFFICIENT; LORENZ CURVE; SLOPE INDEX OF INEQUALITY.

RELATIVE ODDS See ODDS RATIO.

RELATIVE POVERTY LEVEL The amount of income a person, family, or group needs to purchase a relative amount of basic necessities of life; these basic necessities are identified relative to each society and economy. See also ABSOLUTE POVERTY LEVEL.

RELATIVE RISK (RR) Usually, a synonym for RISK RATIO. However, the term is also commonly used to refer to the RATE RATIO and even to the ODDS RATIO (OR). To minimize confusion, it may be better to avoid this term in favor of more specific terms.

RELATIVE RISK REDUCTION (RRR)
1. The difference in event rates between two groups expressed as a proportion of the event rate in the untreated group. The RRR may be similar in populations with different risks. An estimate of the number of people spared the consequences of an exposure that has been eliminated or controlled. The amount by which a person's risk of disease is reduced by elimination or control of an exposure to risk.
2. Let ARC be the absolute risk of events in the control group and ART the absolute risk of events in the treatment group; then RRR = (ARC − ART) / ARC = 1 − Risk Ratio.[9,10,58] See also ABSOLUTE RISK; ABSOLUTE RISK REDUCTION; NUMBER NEEDED TO TREAT.
3. The RRR, ARC, and NNT are related as follows: NNT × RRR × ARC = 1. This equation is used to assess plausible benefits of an intervention in populations and individuals with different levels of baseline risk.[638]

RELEVANCE
1. The importance for existing ideas or practices. The degree to which a study, program, policy, or organization should theoretically change or can actually influence knowledge, beliefs, ideas, attitudes, decisions, actions, policies, structures, procedures,

techniques, or processes of all sorts (social, cultural, political, organizational, individual, medical, biological, etc.).

2. In epidemiology, a relevant study or program may be one that makes a practical or a theoretical contribution to the identification, characterization, understanding, or solution of a public health, environmental, social, clinical, biological, or technological problem. EPIDEMIOLOGICAL RESEARCH usually aims at having social, environmental, or public health relevance; epidemiological studies often also have clinical, biological, methodological, or technological relevance.

3. In clinical and epidemiological research, *relevance* is commonly used as a synonym of importance and of SIGNIFICANCE. Statistical significance must be distinguished from clinical and public health significance. A statistically significant effect may be found in a study with a large number of participants and yet lack clinical or public health significance (because the magnitude of the effect is small, for instance). Hence, statistical significance should never be assumed to equal *significance*, and *significance* encompasses more than statistical significance. Clinical studies usually aim at being clinically significant, important, or relevant for the care of patients. Sometimes, epidemiological and clinical studies are also mechanistically relevant; e.g., they produce knowledge on mechanisms of disease.[1-3,5-9,25,26,28,91,101,202,222] See also MECHANISTIC EPIDEMIOLOGY; MINIMALLY IMPORTANT DIFFERENCE; SIGNIFICANCE, CLINICAL.

RELIABILITY The degree of stability exhibited when a measurement is repeated under identical conditions. The extent to which scores for individuals (e.g., patients) who have not changed are the same for repeated measurement under several conditions; e.g., using different sets of items from the same health related-patient reported outcomes (HR-PRO) (INTERNAL CONSISTENCY); over time (test-retest); by different persons on the same occasion (inter-rater); or by the same persons (i.e., raters or responders) on different occasions (intra-rater). Lack of reliability may arise from divergences between observers or instruments of measurement or instability of the attribute being measured.[3,5,8,26,91,274] See also MEASUREMENT, TERMINOLOGY OF; OBSERVER VARIATION.

REMOTE SENSING The collection and interpretation of information at a distance from the phenomenon or object being observed, e.g., by aerial photography, satellite imaging. Remote sensing has provided valuable information about ecological zones hospitable to mosquitoes and other vectors, plankton blooms that can potentiate cholera outbreaks, etc.

REPEATABILITY (Syn: reproducibility) The value below which the absolute difference between two single test results may be expected to lie with a probability of 95%, when the results are obtained by the same method and equipment from identical test material in the same setting by the same operator within short intervals of time. A test or measurement is repeatable if the results are identical or closely similar each time it is conducted.[1-3,5-9,91] See also MEASUREMENT, TERMINOLOGY OF; RELIABILITY.

REPLACEMENT-LEVEL FERTILITY The level of fertility at which a cohort of women are having only enough daughters to replace themselves in the population. By definition, it is equal to a net reproduction rate of 1.00. The total fertility rate is also used as a measure of replacement level fertility. In the United States today, a total fertility rate of 2.12 is considered to be replacement level; it is higher than 2 because of mortality and because of a sex ratio greater than 1 at birth. The higher the female mortality rate, the higher is the replacement-level fertility. See also GROSS REPRODUCTION RATE.

REPLICATION The execution of an observational or experimental study more than once so as to confirm the findings, increase PRECISION, and obtain a closer estimation of sampling error. *Exact replication* should be distinguished from *consistency of results on replication*. Exact replication is often possible in the physical sciences, but in the health, life, and social sciences consistency of results on replication is often the best that can be attained.[1,2,6,25,39,42,91,206-208,270,273,533] Consistency of results on replication is perhaps the most important consideration in judgments of CAUSALITY.

REPORTING BIAS Selective revelation or suppression of information (e.g., about past medical history, smoking, sexual experiences) or of study results.[1,3,6,9,26,58,64,87,91,135-137,226,467,626] See also DATA DREDGING; PUBLICATION BIAS.

REPRESENTATIVENESS The degree to which the characteristics of a study (notably, of study subjects and setting, but sometimes also of exposures and outcomes) are similar to those of an external population that did not participate in the study. Representativeness is time-, place-, and context-specific. Although it is not necessary for studies with etiologic aims, it has an important place in health surveys and descriptive studies. Evidence-based health policies require population-representative information. It should neither be avoided nor uncritically sought.[1,3,474] See also GENERALIZABILITY; VALIDITY.

REPRESENTATIVE SAMPLE A sample that to a large extent resembles a population of interest. The term *representative* as it is commonly used is largely undefined in the statistical or mathematical sense. The use of probability sampling will not ensure that a sample will be representative of the population in all relevant aspects. It is unwarranted to assume that if the sample resembles the reference population on factors that have been checked, no differences exist in other relevant factors.[7,283] See also BIAS; GENERAL POPULATION.

REPRESSION BIAS Bias that results from failing to pursue a line of inquiry because the inquiry does not conform to certain social norms, vested interests, or scientific paradigms. It may lead to PUBLICATION BIAS. It may distort or delay the discovery of scientific knowledge on health risks, and compromise trust in science and administrative processes that aim at assessing and preventing exposure to hazards. See also PUBLICATION BIAS; SCIENTIFIC MISCONDUCT; SUPPRESSION BIAS.

REPRODUCIBILITY See REPEATABILITY.

REPRODUCTIVE ISOLATION Absence of interbreeding between populations.

REPRODUCTIVE SUCCESS In population genetics, quantitatively, the proportion of offspring surviving long enough to reproduce.

REPROGRAMMING In GENETICS and EPIGENETICS, the erasure and reestablishment of DNA methylation during mammalian development.

RESCUE BIAS A form of INTERPRETIVE BIAS that occurs in discounting data by finding selective faults in a study when the data are viewed unfavorably or by discounting faults when the data are viewed favorably. A deliberate attempt to evade evidence that contradicts expectation or interests.[99,561] See also AUXILIARY HYPOTHESIS BIAS; CONFIRMATION BIAS.

RESEARCH A class of activities designed to develop or contribute to knowledge. In applied science, the goal is generalizable knowledge, where the latter consists of theories, principles, relationships, products, or the accumulation of information on which these are based that can be corroborated by acceptable scientific methods of observation, inference, or experiment. When humans are the subjects of EPIDEMIOLOGICAL RESEARCH, ethical review is mandatory; however, there is a blurry boundary between research, which must undergo review, and common clinical or public health practice (e.g.,

SURVEILLANCE and epidemic control), to which the same rules may not apply, but that still must comply with ethical requirements.[1,3,5-9,26,202,270] See also INTEGRATIVE RESEARCH.

RESEARCH DESIGN The "architecture," "anatomy," or "physiology" of a study: its structure and procedures, the specific methods, details on the selection and management of the study population (e.g., follow-up), time frame, and ethical decisions. All of them should be explicitly stated in the research PROTOCOL.[1-3,5-9,25,26,197,202,270,795] Details of all aspects of the research design are essential to anyone seeking to replicate a study; thus, there may be an obligation to ensure that these details are in the public domain. They must be adhered to by all centers in a multicenter study.

RESEARCH ETHICS BOARD, COMMITTEE See INSTITUTIONAL REVIEW BOARD.

RESEARCH SUBJECT A person who is studied. Under some circumstances the word *subject* is perceived as demeaning, and other terms may be more socially acceptable, e.g., *study participant, volunteer*, or *patient*.

RESERVOIR OF INFECTION

1. Any person, animal, arthropod, plant, soil, or substance, or combination of these in which an infectious agent normally lives and multiplies, on which it depends primarily for survival, and where it reproduces itself in such a manner that it can be transmitted to a susceptible host.[56]

2. The natural habitat of the infectious agent.[20-22,56,217-219] See also ACCESSORY RESERVOIR.

RESILIENCE A process of positive ADAPTATION in the face of adversity; e.g., intrinsic and extrinsic factors confer educational, emotional, and behavioral resilience to children.[13,23,33,38]

RESIDUAL CONFOUNDING (Syn: uncontrolled confounding) Confounding that persists after ADJUSTMENT for the putatively measured confounders. It may have two components: UNMEASURED CONFOUNDING, and incorrect analysis (e.g., improper categorization, misspecified functional form, or other forms of model misspecification).[1-3,101,242,270,557,797] See also INVERSE PROBABILITY WEIGHTING; STANDARDIZATION.

RESOLUTION, RESOLVING POWER

1. The capacity of a system to distinguish between truly distinct things that are close together.

2. A component of a measuring instrument that helps determine PRECISION. The degree of refinement of the measuring process is commonly referred to as the "resolution" or the "resolving power of the system." The capability of distinguishing between things that are indeed separate or distinct from one another. See also POWER.

RESOURCE ALLOCATION The process of deciding how to distribute financial, material, and human resources among competing claimants for these resources. Resource allocation is an essential feature of all health planning everywhere.[302,707] Epidemiological evidence on need, demand, supply, and use of existing services is integral to the process, although factors such as political, commercial, and emotional considerations sometimes carry more weight than objective epidemiological evidence; ethical considerations should affect decisions about resource allocation.

RESPONSE BIAS Systematic error due to differences in characteristics between those who volunteer, choose, or accept to take part in a study and those who do not. See also REPRESENTATIVE SAMPLE; SELECTION BIAS.

RESPONSE RATE The number of completed or returned survey instruments (questionnaires, interviews, etc.) divided by the total number of persons who would have been surveyed if all had participated. Usually expressed as a percentage. Nonresponse can have several causes, e.g., death, removal from the survey community, and refusal.[1,24-26,30,160,551] See also BIAS; COMPLETION RATE; NONPARTICIPANTS.

RESPONSIVENESS The ability of an instrument to detect change accurately. The ability of a health related-patient reported outcomes (HR-PRO) instrument to detect change over time in the construct to be measured. It is usually quantified by a statistical or numerical score, such as an effect size statistic or a standardized response mean. *Internal responsiveness* is the ability of a measure to change over a prespecified time frame, and *external responsiveness* reflects the extent to which change in a measure relates to corresponding change in a reference measure of clinical or health status.[6,9,274,708,709] See also elasticity; immunity, specific.

RETROLECTIVE Pertaining to data gathered without planning for the needs of an investigation.[224,687] See also DIRECTIONALITY; PROLECTIVE.

RETROSPECTIVE STUDY A research design used to test etiological hypotheses in which inferences about exposure to the putative causal factor(s) are derived from data relating to characteristics of the persons under study or to events or experiences in their past. The essential feature is that some of the persons under study have the disease or other outcome condition of interest, and their characteristics and past experiences are compared with those of other, unaffected persons. Persons who differ in the severity of the disease may also be compared.[1-3,5,197,795] It is not a synonym for CASE-CONTROL STUDY.

RETROVIRUS This name is given to a family of RNA viruses characterized by the presence of an enzyme, reverse transcriptase, that enables transcription of RNA to DNA inside an affected cell. Thus retroviruses can make copies of themselves in host cells. The most important retrovirus is the human immunodeficiency virus (HIV); this makes copies of itself in host cells, such as T4 "helper" lymphocytes, and normal immune responses are disrupted.

REVERSE CAUSATION (Syn: reverse causality, retrocausality, backward causation) The biological, clinical, or social processes through which a causal relationship operates in a way opposite to that which is apparent; e.g., while the observed, apparent causal relationship is that F causes or alters Y (F→Y), the true, actual relationship is Y→F. Bidirectional effects (e.g., feedback between exposures) may also occur. For instance, it is possible both that religious service attendance may protect against depression and that depression may lead to lower levels of religious participation in some populations; seemingly protective associations between attendance at religious services and depression must consider that depressive disorders may influence subsequent discontinuation of such attendance.[710] Interpretation of the effects of prevalent (already present) exposures can be complicated, even when the study is longitudinal. Studies of incident exposure and changes in exposure can circumvent some of these problems, but may also be subject to CONFOUNDING, may require repeated measurements of the variables at etiologically relevant periods, and may need to allow for feedback between exposures and between exposures and intermediate or precursor outcomes. Analyses of change may actually be cross-sectional with respect to their outcomes if the exposure variable used in defining change is measured contemporaneously with the outcomes of interest.[1-3,5,101,710,791,792] When hypothesizing that a given association may be due to reverse causation, plausible and specific reasons or mechanisms for the hypothesis (e.g., DISEASE PROGRESSION BIAS) should be given. See also BIAS; TIME ORDER; VALIDITY.

REVERSE CAUSATION BIAS bias due to improper accounting for reverse causation.

REVERSE TRANSCRIPTION The process by which an RNA molecule is used as a template to make a single-stranded DNA copy.[549] This is the mode of action of the HUMAN IMMUNODEFICIENCY VIRUS when it attacks T4 helper lymphocytes, which maintain immune competence.

REVIEW BIAS In diagnostic accuracy studies, bias that occurs when the investigator knows the results of the new diagnostic test when the "gold standard" test is interpreted or when the investigator knows the results of the gold standard test when the new diagnostic test in interpreted.[9,58] See also QUADAS-2.

REVIEW, SYSTEMATIC See SYSTEMATIC REVIEW.

RIDIT (from Relative to an Identified Distribution) A method of presenting observed values, e.g., health measurement scale scores of a group, relative to a reference population. The average ridit for the group shows the probability that a member of the group differs from a member of the reference population. For example, if the average ridit for a group is 0.62, 62% of persons in the reference population have higher scores than a randomly chosen member of the group.[707]

RIDIT ANALYSIS A method proposed by Bross[711] for analyzing subjectively categorized or poorly recorded data. It consists of allocating scores relative to the identified distribution of the data based upon a transformation to the uniform distribution rather than the normal distribution.

RISK The probability of an adverse or beneficial event in a defined POPULATION over a specified time interval. In epidemiology and in clinical research it is commonly measured through the CUMULATIVE INCIDENCE and the INCIDENCE PROPORTION.[1-3,5,6,8,270] Other concepts and measures of risk are also relevant to study and control threats to human health.[14,38,106-108,212,248,279,303,304,332-336,361,539,603,712-718]

RISK ASSESSMENT

1. The qualitative or quantitative estimation of the likelihood of adverse effects that may result from exposure to specified health hazards or from the absence of beneficial influences. Risk assessment uses clinical, epidemiological, toxicological, environmental, and any other pertinent evidence.

2. The process of determining risks to health attributable to environmental or other hazards. The process consists of four steps:

Hazard identification: Identifying the agent responsible for the health problem, its adverse effects, the target population, and the conditions of exposure.

Risk characterization: Describing the potential health effects of the hazard, quantifying dose-effect and dose-response relationships.

Exposure assessment: Quantifying exposure (dose) in a specified population based on measurement of emissions, environmental levels of toxic substances, BIOLOGICAL MONITORING, etc.

Risk estimation: Combining risk characterization, dose-response relationships, and exposure estimates to quantify the risk level in a specific population. The end result is a qualitative and quantitative statement about the health effects expected and the proportion and number of affected people in a target population, including estimates of the uncertainties involved. The size of the exposed population must be known.[1-3,5,7,12-14,25,38,106-108,212,361] See also ATTRIBUTABLE FRACTION.

RISK ASSESSMENT PLOT See DISCRIMINATORY ACCURACY.

RISK-BENEFIT ANALYSIS The process of analyzing and comparing on a single scale the expected positive (benefits) and negative (risks, costs) results of an action or lack of an action.

RISK-BENEFIT RATIO The results of a risk-benefit analysis expressed as the ratio of risks to benefits.

RISK CHARACTERIZATION See RISK ASSESSMENT.

RISK DIFFERENCE (RD) The difference of two risks, usually risk in the exposed minus risk in the unexposed. For harmful exposures, the negative of the RISK DIFFERENCE is sometimes referred to as ABSOLUTE RISK REDUCTION (ARR). The reciprocal of the ARR is the NUMBER NEEDED TO TREAT (NNT).

RISK ESTIMATION See RISK ASSESSMENT.

RISK EVALUATION See RISK MANAGEMENT.

RISK FACTOR (Syn: determinant) A factor that is causally related to a change in the RISK of a relevant health process, outcome, or condition. The causal nature of the relationship is established on the basis of scientific evidence (including, naturally, evidence from EPIDEMIOLOGICAL RESEARCH) and CAUSAL INFERENCE. The causal relationship is inherently probabilistic, as it happens in many other spheres of nature and human life.[101] If the relationship is noncausal the factor is just a RISK MARKER. Examples of types of risk factors are offered throughout this book; they may be a socioeconomic characteristic, personal behavior or lifestyle, environmental exposure, inherited characteristic, or another TRAIT. Risk factors for human health often have individual and social components; even when individual and social risk factors can be separated, they often interact. A DETERMINANT that can be modified by intervention is a modifiable risk factor.

The term *risk factor* became popular after its frequent use in papers from the Framingham study.[719] To prevent MEDICALIZATION of life and IATROGENESIS, the RELEVANCE and SIGNIFICANCE of the factor-outcome risk relationship must be cautiously assessed; so must uncertainties and ambiguities in risk-related concepts, as well as different legitimate meanings of risk across and within cultures.[1-3,5,6,9,13,29,33,38,42,56,58,91,106-108,113,158,215,248,270,279,292,303,304, 332-336,350,361,426,539,600,603,712-718,795]

RISK INDICATOR A RISK FACTOR (if causally related with the risk of interest) or a RISK MARKER (if noncausally associated with RISK).

RISK MANAGEMENT The steps taken to alter (i.e., reduce) the levels of risk to which an individual or a population is subject. The managerial, decision-making, and active hazard control process to deal with environmental agents of disease, such as toxic substances, for which risk evaluation has indicated an unacceptably high level of risk.[12-14,25,28,38,56,139,267,359,361,449] The process consists of three steps:

1. RISK EVALUATION: Comparison of calculated risks or public health impact of exposure to an environmental agent with the risks caused by other agents or societal factors and with the benefits associated with the agent as a basis for deciding what is an ACCEPTABLE RISK.

2. EXPOSURE CONTROL: Actions taken to keep exposure below an acceptable maximum limit.

3. RISK MONITORING: The process of measuring reduction in risk after exposure control actions have been taken in order to reassess risks and initiate further control measures if necessary.

RISK MARKER A factor that is noncausally associated with the RISK of a disease or other specified outcome. It may be used as an indicator of such risk, but it is not a causal factor. Contrast with RISK FACTOR and RISK INDICATOR.

RISK MONITORING See RISK MANAGEMENT

RISK RATIO The ratio of two risks, usually of exposed and not exposed. See also CUMULATIVE INCIDENCE RATIO; INCIDENCE RATE RATIO; RELATIVE RISK.

RISK SET The set of people in the source population who are at risk of becoming a case at the time that each case is diagnosed. The population at risk at the time point when a new case occurs, from which the time-matched controls are sampled in a DENSITY CASE-CONTROL STUDY.[1]

ROBUSTNESS

1. A property of a statistical test or procedure that confers to it a certain degree of insensitivity to departures from the assumptions from which it is derived (e.g., that the data are normally distributed).[7,37,101,796] See also INFLUENCE ANALYSIS; MULTIPLE BIAS MODELING.

2. The resistance of genes to manipulations supposed to lead to a predicted phenotype. Essentially due to the fundamental regulatory role of interactions among genes, and to a common redundancy of functions and regulatory mechanisms converging toward a specific goal.[470,720] See also PLEIOTROPY.

ROUNDING The process of eliminating surplus digits, taking the nearest whole number, multiple of 10, etc., as an approximation of the value of a measurement. See also DIGIT PREFERENCE.

"ROUTINE" DATA, ROUTINELY COLLECTED DATA An ambiguous and potentially misleading term referring to data collected regularly (and sometimes indeed, routinely, yet often with considerable effort and expense to maximize VALIDITY), mostly by governmental organizations, such as data on births and deaths, disease registries, or VITAL STATISTICS.

RUBRIC Section or chapter heading. Used in epidemiology with reference to groups of diseases, e.g., in the INTERNATIONAL CLASSIFICATION OF DISEASES (ICD).

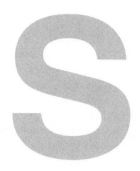

SAFETY FACTOR A multiplicative factor incorporated in risk assessments or safety standards to allow for unpredictable types of variation, such as variability from test animals to humans, random variation within an experiment, and person-to-person variability. Safety factors are often in the range of 10 to 1000 or even higher magnitudes.

SAFETY STANDARDS In occupational health, standards that require conditions, practices, methods, operations, or processes reasonably necessary to provide safe and healthful employment and places of employment.[14,571,572,643,644] Examples of safety standards include: Permissable Exposure Limits (PELs), Recommended Exposure Limits (RELs) or Threshhold Limit Values (TLVs). There are safety standards and infection control programs for dental hygienists, for food safety, for construction safety, for electrical safety in the workplace, for early education, for patient safety, and for many other sectors and activities.

SAMPLE A selected subset of a population. A sample may be random or nonrandom and may be representative or nonrepresentative.[1,7,25,34,37,270] Several types of sample can be distinguished, including the following:

1. *Area sample* See AREA SAMPLING.
2. *Cluster sample* Each unit selected is a group of persons (all persons in a city block, a family, etc.) rather than an individual. See also CLUSTER SAMPLING.
3. *Grab sample* (Syn: sample of convenience) These ill-defined terms describe samples selected by easily employed but basically nonprobabilistic (and probably biased) methods. "Man-in-the-street" surveys and a survey of blood pressure among volunteers who drop in at an examination booth in a public place are in this category. It is improper to generalize from the results of a survey based upon such a sample, for there is no way of knowing what sorts of BIAS may have been operating.
4. *Probability (random) sample* All individuals have a known chance of selection. They may all have an equal chance of being selected, or, if a stratified sampling method is used, the rate at which individuals from several subsets are sampled can be varied so as to produce greater representation of some classes than of others. A probability sample is created by assigning an identity (label, number) to all individuals in the "universe" population, e.g., by arranging them in alphabetical order and numbering in sequence, or simply assigning a number to each, or by grouping according to area of residence and numbering the groups. The next step is to select individuals (or groups) for study by a procedure such as use of a table of random numbers (or comparable procedure) to ensure that the chance of selection is known.

5. *Simple random sample* In this elementary kind of sample each person has an equal chance of being selected out of the entire population. One way of carrying out this procedure is to assign each person a number, starting with 1, 2, 3, and so on. Then numbers are selected at random, preferably from a table of random numbers, until the desired sample size is attained.

6. *Stratified random sample* This involves dividing the population into distinct subgroups according to some important characteristic, such as age or socioeconomic status, and selecting a random sample out of each subgroup. If the proportion of the sample drawn from each of the subgroups, or strata, is the same as the proportion of the total population contained in each stratum (e.g., age group 40–59 constitutes 20% of the population, and 20% of the sample comes from this age stratum), then all strata will be fairly represented with regard to numbers of persons in the sample.

7. *Systematic sample* The procedure of selecting according to some simple, systematic rule, such as all persons whose names begin with specified alphabetical letters, born on certain dates, or located at specified points on a master list. A systematic sample may lead to errors that invalidate generalizations. For example, persons' names more often begin with certain letters of the alphabet than with other letters, e.g., in English, A and S are common starting letters while Q and X are not, and are related to ethnic origin. A systematic alphabetical sample is therefore likely to be biased.

SAMPLE DESIGN The set of rules and specifications for the drawing of a sample. The characteristics of a study sample, including a sample survey. The term *sampling plan* may be restricted to mean steps taken in selecting the sample; the term *sample design* may cover, in addition, the method of estimation; and *survey design* may cover also other aspects of the survey (e.g., choice and training of interviewers, plans for analyses). See also RESEARCH DESIGN.

SAMPLE, **EPSEM** ("equal probability of selection method") A sample selected in such a manner that all the population units have the same probability of selection. A simple random sample is an EPSEM sample; a stratified sample is not unless the probability of selection is the same for all strata.

SAMPLE SIZE DETERMINATION The mathematical process of deciding, before a study begins, how many subjects should be studied. The factors to be taken into account include the incidence or prevalence of the condition being studied, the estimated or putative relationship among the variables in the study, the POWER that is desired, and the maximum allowable magnitude of TYPE I ERROR.[1,6-8,26,58]

SAMPLE SPACE In applied statistics, the collection of all possible data sets that could be (or could have been) generated by a particular study design. For example, in a study that performs random sampling of exactly n persons of a population of size N and in which participation is assured, the sample space consists of all possible data sets from samples of size n from that population. In practice, however, many of those samples may be unattainable due to the fact that some persons would refuse to participate or could not be located if selected. Because not all such persons could be identified without sampling the entire population, the true sample space would remain unknown. See also REPRESENTATIVENESS; SAMPLING; SAMPLING FRACTION; SAMPLING UNIT; SELECTION BIAS.

SAMPLING The process of selecting a number of subjects from all the subjects in a particular group, or "universe." Statistical inference based on sample results may be attributed only to the population sampled. Any extrapolation or GENERALIZATION to a larger or different population involves judgments about population differences, along with any available data pertaining to the difference, and is not part of conventional statistical inference; BAYESIAN STATISTICAL METHODS can incorporate some of these issues.[1,7,25,26,34,37]s See also REPRESENTATIVENESS; SAMPLING FRACTION; SAMPLING UNIT; SELECTION BIAS.

SAMPLING BIAS See GENERALIZABILITY.

SAMPLING ERROR That part of the total estimation error caused by random influences on who or what is selected for study.

SAMPLING FRACTION The fraction of SAMPLING UNITS selected for study from a candidate population of such units. In a study that selects n units of a population of size N, this fraction is n/N. See also SAMPLE SPACE; SAMPLING.

SAMPLING UNIT The units into which a sampled population is divided for purposes of selection for study. These units are often persons (individual sampling), but may be regions (e.g., census tracts, counties), families, households, or other aggregates or entities. See also AREA SAMPLING; CLUSTER SAMPLING; SAMPLE SPACE.

SAMPLING VARIATION If, as is usually the case, the inclusion of individuals in a sample is partly determined by chance, the results of analysis in two or more samples will differ in part by chance. This is known as "sampling variation" or more precisely as "random sampling variation."[1,34,37]

SANITARY CORDON See CORDON SANITAIRE.

SANTAYANA SYNDROME The neglect of what might be learned from the many blunders and errors contained in medical and scientific history.[721,722] A term coined and used by A. R. Feinstein in remembrance of a sentence from George Santayana (1863–1952), a philosopher and poet: "Those who cannot remember the past are condemned to repeat it."[723] See also INTERPRETIVE BIAS.

SARTWELL'S INCUBATION MODEL Philip Sartwell (1908–1999) found that the incubation periods for many COMMUNICABLE DISEASES tend to have a log-normal distribution, and that the "incubation" periods for certain cancers following certain well-defined external causes also tend to have a log-normal distribution.[724] This model is useful but should not be assumed to hold universally. See also INCUBATION PERIOD; LATENCY PERIOD.

"SATELLITE EPIDEMIOLOGY" The use of data and images derived from geospatial technologies (e.g., satellites) for the study of the occurrence and distribution of health-related events in specified populations, and the application of this knowledge to control the health problems.[725] See also DISEASE MAPPING; GEOGRAPHICAL INFORMATION SYSTEM; GEOMATICS; MEDICAL GEOGRAPHY; SPATIAL EPIDEMIOLOGY.

SCALE A device or system for measuring a characteristic or property.[1,26] See also MEASUREMENT SCALE.

SCAN STATISTIC A test for detection of CLUSTERING over time. A technique used in SURVEILLANCE epidemiology to detect an unusual rate of occurrence of a disease by comparing observed number of cases with the expected number on the basis of experience in a recent defined period.

SCATTER DIAGRAM, PLOT (Syn: scattergram) A graphic method of displaying the DISTRIBUTION of two variables in relation to each other. The values for one variable are measured on the horizontal axis and the values for the other on the vertical axis.[1,3,37,102-108,505]

SCENARIO-BASED HEALTH RISK ASSESSMENT A variant of population health risk assessment in which the exposure input is not an actual measured or measurable exposure but a plausible, preferably model-generated scenario of future exposure. It is particularly relevant in using existing epidemiological knowledge to prepare plans for the future

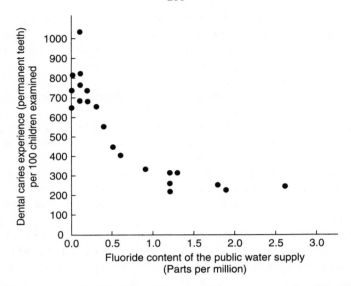

Scatter plot. Relationship between the number of dental caries in permanent teeth and fluoride content in the public water supply. Source: Lilienfeld DE.[726]

health impacts of anticipated environmental changes, such as climate change and stratospheric ozone depletion.[13,14,33,213,360,426]

SCENARIO BUILDING A method of predicting the future that relies on a series of assumptions about alternative possibilities rather than on simple extrapolation of existing trends.[727] TREND lines for demographic composition, morbidity and mortality rates, etc., can then be modified by allowing for each assumption in turn, or combinations of assumptions. The method is claimed to lead to greater flexibility in long-range health planning than simple forecasting that relies only upon extrapolation of trends.[426]

SCIENCE Systematic observation and experiment to explain and predict natural phenomena with the goal of establishing, enlarging, or confirming knowledge. Science uses observations and/or experiments to make logical inferences, formulate and test hypotheses, and arrive at generalizable conclusions, expressed as testable laws and principles. Science advances through conjecture or intuition, hypothesis, refutation of deductions from hypotheses, and verification of hypotheses and theories by induction.[38,39,42,50,135,206,267,537,579,728] Occasionally science undergoes a paradigm shift as long-established principles and laws are overturned by new discoveries.[648] A characteristic of vigorous science is ongoing tests of hypotheses and theories that are taken as "established" in order to detect failings. This activity stems from a point distinguishing science from other systems of knowledge: the idea that all knowledge of the real world is fallible at some level and must not be allowed to become completely unassailable dogma. See also EPISTEMIC COMMUNITIES; FALSE DISCOVERY RATE (FDR); HYPOTHETICO-DEDUCTIVE METHOD; KNOWLEDGE CONSTRUCTION; RESEARCH; SOCIOLOGY OF SCIENTIFIC KNOWLEDGE.

SCIENTIFIC MISCONDUCT A class of ethical violations in the conduct of research, generally taken to include falsification, fabrication, fraud, or plagiarism in the proposal, design, implementation, reporting, or review of research. May also include violation of the rights and dignity of participants in research, misuse of research funds, mistreatment of scientific colleagues (e.g., in PEER REVIEW), and failure to report undesired findings.[26,64,117,118,135,467,626] See also DATA DREDGING; ETHICS; PUBLICATION BIAS; REPRESSION BIAS; SUPPRESSION BIAS.

SCIENTOMETRICS The measurement of scientific output and the impact of scientific findings (e.g., on knowledge, public health policies, clinical practice).[132,133]

SCREENING The presumptive identification of unrecognized disease or defect by the application of tests, examinations, or other procedures which can be applied rapidly. Screening tests sort out apparently well persons who probably have a disease from those who probably do not. A screening test is not intended to be diagnostic. Persons with positive or suspicious findings must be referred to their physicians for diagnosis and necessary treatment.[5,6,8,9,24,26,28,302,462,729]

The initiative for screening usually comes from an agency or organization rather than from a patient with a complaint. Screening is usually concerned with chronic illness and aims to detect disease not yet under medical care. Screening may identify risk factors, genetic predisposition, and precursors, or early evidence of disease.

There are different types of medical screening, each with its own aim:

1. *Mass screening* usually means the screening of a whole population.
2. *Multiple* or *multiphasic screening* involves the use of a variety of screening tests on the same occasion or sequentially.
3. *Prescriptive screening* has as its aim the EARLY DETECTION in presumptively healthy individuals of specific diseases that can be controlled better if detected early in their natural history.[532] An example is the use of mammography to detect breast cancer.

The characteristics of a screening test must include ACCURACY, estimates of yield, PRECISION, reproducibility, sensitivity and specificity, and validity.[6,9,58,349] See also CASE FINDING; DETECTABLE PRECLINICAL PERIOD; PREVENTION.

SCREENING LEVEL The normal limit or cutoff point at which a screening test is regarded as positive.

SEASONAL VARIATION Change in physiological status or in disease occurrence that conforms to a regular seasonal pattern.

SECONDARY ATTACK RATE The number of cases of an infection that occur among contacts within the incubation period following exposure to a primary case in relation to the total number of exposed contacts; the denominator is restricted to susceptible contacts when these can be determined. It is a measure of contagiousness and is useful in evaluating control measures. While the traditional terminology includes "rate," it is often a proportion. See also ATTACK RATE; BASIC REPRODUCTIVE RATE.

SECONDHAND TOBACCO SMOKE See INVOLUNTARY SMOKING; ENVIRONMENTAL TOBACCO SMOKE.

SECOND-LINE DRUGS (SLDs) See DRUG RESISTANCE, MULTIPLE.

SECTOR In the language used by UN agencies (WHO, UNICEF, etc.), a sector is a defined component of the body politic, such as the health sector, the education sector, the housing sector.

SECULAR TREND (Syn: temporal trend) Changes over a long period of time, generally years or decades. Examples include the decline of tuberculosis mortality and the rise, followed by a decline, in coronary heart disease mortality in many industrial countries in the past 50 years.[24]

SEDENTARY LIFESTYLE A LIFESTYLE that lacks vigorous physical exercise, characterized by sitting, reading, watching television, or using a computer for much of the day.

SELECTION

1. In epidemiology, the process and procedures for choosing individuals for study. See also SAMPLE; SAMPLING.
2. In genetics, the force that brings about changes in the frequency of alleles and genotypes in populations through differential reproduction.

SELECTION BIAS Bias in the estimated association or effect of an exposure on an outcome that arises from the procedures used to select individuals into the study or the analysis. When the selection involves conditioning on a factor that is affected by the exposure or a cause of the exposure, and also affected by the outcome or a cause of the outcome, selection bias can arise even in the absence of a causal effect of exposure on outcome, i.e., under the CAUSAL NULL HYPOTHESIS.[1-3,5-9,25,101,269,270,678] One example of selection bias is BERKSON'S BIAS. Other examples: the estimated effect of cigarette smoking on heart disease will be biased if study participants are volunteers and the decision to volunteer is affected by smoking status and by having a family history of heart disease; the estimated effect of the exposure on the outcome will be biased if losses to follow-up occur differentially across exposure groups and depend on prognostic factors (also known as ATTRITION BIAS).[730,731] Often "selection bias" is used to refer to systematic differences between the characteristics of the study population and those of other populations (i.e., SAMPLING BIAS). These differences may make it problematic to transport the inferences from the study population to the other populations. Because such uses of "selection bias" do not imply lack of INTERNAL VALIDITY, it is more appropriate to use the expressions "lack of GENERALIZABILITY" or "low EXTERNAL VALIDITY." Examples: surveys limited to volunteers or to persons present in a particular place at a particular time; studies based on disease survivors; hospital-based studies that cannot include patients who die before hospital admission due to acute illness or that do not include persons with mild conditions; systematic differences among participants and nonparticipants in CLINICAL TRIALS. Selection biases may not be independent of CONFOUNDING and INFORMATION BIASES; i.e., these types of biases are often interrelated, overlap, and interact with each other.[1-3,6,9,42] Selection bias is a common and commonly overlooked problem in clinical and microbiological or preclinical research. Selection bias is difficult to address analytically; however, it can sometimes be adjusted for if the selection probabilities can be obtained or estimated under plausible assumptions (e.g., in follow-up bias, where INVERSE PROBABILITY WEIGHTING can be used under certain assumptions). Selection bias is not exclusively a causal issue, it also occurs in descriptive disease surveys, as when a simple rate is distorted because cases participate more than noncases. See also BERKSON'S BIAS; COLLIDER; CONTROLS, HOSPITAL; IGNORABILITY; INCEPTION COHORT; M-BIAS; SAMPLE SPACE; SIMPSON'S PARADOX.

SEMI-INDIVIDUAL DESIGN Individual-level studies (e.g., COHORT STUDIES, CROSS-SECTIONAL STUDIES, CASE-CONTROL STUDIES) in which outcome and covariates are measured at the individual level while exposure is characterized on the aggregate (or ecological) level. Used either because groups share the same exposure or because individual-level exposure measures are not available. Frequently used in environmental epidemiology to describe exposure to air, water, or soil pollutants. Not to be confused with ECOLOGICAL STUDIES, for which exposure and outcome variables are both aggregates.[295,732,795]

SEMIOLOGY See SYMPTOMATOLOGY.

SENSITIVE PERIOD (Syn: critical period) A time during the development of a tissue, organ, or system when it can be permanently changed by harmful influences (e.g., undernutrition, chemicals, hypoxia, stress). It often coincides with a period of rapid cell division and, for many tissues and systems, occurs before birth. The brain and liver are the main organs that remain plastic after birth.[161] The adverse or protective effects on health of exposures during a sensitive period may be apparent many years later.[32] See also DEVELOPMENTAL ORIGINS OF HEALTH AND DISEASE; PLASTICITY; PROGRAMMING; VULNERABILITY.

SENSITIVITY ANALYSIS A method to determine the ROBUSTNESS of an assessment by examining the extent to which results are affected by changes in methods, models, values of unmeasured variables, or assumptions.[1,3,7,733,734] The aim is to display the extent to which results are dependent on questionable or unsupported assumptions. See also BIAS ANALYSIS; INFLUENCE ANALYSIS; OUTLIERS; MULTIPLE BIAS MODELING; UNCERTAINTY ANALYSIS.

SENSITIVITY AND SPECIFICITY (of a SCREENING test, of a DIAGNOSTIC TEST):

1. *Sensitivity* is the probability that a diseased person (case) in the population tested will be identified as diseased by the test (syn: true positive probability). Sensitivity is thus the probability of correctly diagnosing a case or the probability that any given case will be identified by the test (syn: true-positive rate).

2. *Specificity* is the probability that a person without the disease (noncase) will be correctly identified as nondiseased by the test. It is thus the probability of correctly identifying a nondiseased person with a test (syn: true-negative probability).

The relationships are shown in the following fourfold table, in which the letters a, b, c, and d represent the numbers in the table below. The predictive value of a positive test result may be called the *yield*. Sensitivity and specificity may also be applied to screening for an exposure.[3,6,8,9,24,26,58,322,796] See also LIKELIHOOD RATIO; PREDICTIVE VALUE.

Screening test results	True status		Total
	Diseased	Not diseased	
Positive	a	b	a + b
Negative	c	d	c + d
Total	a + c	b + d	a + b + c + d

a. Diseased individuals detected by the test (true positives)
b. Nondiseased individuals positive by the test (false positives)
c. Diseased individuals not detectable by the test (false negatives)
d. Nondiseased individuals negative by the test (true negatives)

$$\text{Sensitivity} = \frac{a}{a+c} \quad \text{Specificity} = \frac{d}{b+d}$$

$$\text{Predictive value of a positive test result} = \frac{a}{a+b}$$

$$\text{Predictive value of a negative test result} = \frac{d}{c+d}$$

$$\text{Accuracy} = \frac{a+d}{a+b+c+d}$$

SENSITIVITY TESTING A study of how the final outcome of an analysis changes as a function of varying one or more of the input parameters in a prescribed manner.[3] See also SENSITIVITY ANALYSIS.

SENTINEL HEALTH EVENT A condition that can be used to assess the stability or change in health levels of a population, usually by monitoring mortality statistics. Thus, death due to acute head injury is a sentinel event for a class of severe traffic injury that may be reduced by such preventive measures as use of seat belts and crash helmets.

SENTINEL INITIATIVE An electronic system launched by the U.S. Food and Drug Administration (FDA) in 2008 to monitor the safety of its regulated products once they reach the market. The Initiative aims to develop and implement a proactive system that enables FDA to actively query diverse automated health care data holders (e.g., electronic health record systems, administrative and insurance claims databases, and registries).[735]

SENTINEL PHYSICIAN, SENTINEL PRACTICE In family medicine, a physician or practice that undertakes to maintain SURVEILLANCE for and to report certain specific predetermined events, such as cases of certain COMMUNICABLE DISEASES or adverse drug reactions.[24,48]

SENTINEL SURVEILLANCE Surveillance based on selected population samples chosen to represent the relevant experience of particular groups. This approach is useful in dealing with sensitive issues such as HIV/AIDS or when cooperation levels can be improved through participation of professional organizations, such as colleges or NETWORKS of family physicians, for the early detection of influenza epidemics. In sentinel surveillance, standard case definitions and protocols must be used to ensure VALIDITY of comparisons across time and sites despite lack of statistically valid sampling.[1,12,48,56,69,160,188,366,550,735] Sentinel SURVEILLANCE may include the use of animal sentinels to detect circulation of arboviruses.

SEQUENTIAL ANALYSIS A statistical method that allows an experiment to be ended as soon as an answer of the desired precision is obtained. Study and control subjects are randomly allocated in pairs or blocks. The result of the comparison of each pair of subjects, one treated and one control, is examined as soon as it becomes available and is added to all previous results.[7]

SERENDIPITY The accidental or fortuitous discovery of important evidence by a sagacious and reflective individual or team; the "happy accident" or "pleasant surprise" of a relevant finding while not specifically searching for it, often made by integrating disparate types of evidence. See also INTEGRATION.

SERIAL INTERVAL (Syn: generation time) The period of time between analogous phases of an infectious illness, in successive cases of a chain of infection, that is spread from person to person.

SEROEPIDEMIOLOGY Epidemiological study or activity based on serological testing of characteristic changes in the serum level of specific antibodies. Latent, subclinical infections and CARRIER states can thus be detected in addition to clinically overt cases.

SEROLOGY The branch of science dealing with the measurement and characterization of antibodies and other immunological substances in body fluids, particularly serum.

SET A defined group of events, objects, or data that is distinguishable from other groups.

SET THEORY Branch of mathematics and logic dealing with the characteristics and relationships of sets.

SEX RATIO The ratio of one sex to the other. Usually defined as the RATIO of males to females (or of the rates observed in males and females).

SF36 Acronym for the 36-item questionnaire derived from the longer set of questions used in household interview surveys conducted by the U.S. National Center for Health Statistics. The SF36 questions measure eight multi-item variables: physical function, social function, role limitation, mental health, energy, vitality, pain, and general perception of health. The instrument has been widely adopted, although some authors have raised doubts about its validity.

SHARPS A jargon term for any sharp object used in a health care setting that is capable of penetrating the skin (e.g., hypodermic needles, scalpel blades, broken glass vials).

"SHOE-LEATHER" EPIDEMIOLOGY Gathering information for epidemiological studies by direct inquiry among the people, e.g., walking from door to door and asking questions of every householder (wearing out shoe leather in the process).[72,678] John Snow (1813–1858) did this when he was investigating the sources of water supply to households in the cholera epidemic in London in 1854; the method has been successfully used in many subsequent epidemic investigations. It is especially useful in investigations of sexually transmitted diseases. Much of the work of the Epidemic Intelligence Service (EIS) is based on shoe-leather epidemiology. EIS officers have a club tie displaying the sole of a shoe with a hole in it. See also NATURAL EXPERIMENT.

SHRINKAGE ESTIMATION (Syn: Stein estimation, penalized estimation) In statistics, a family of procedures to improve the overall accuracy of multiple estimates. This improvement is made by moving the estimates toward values judged or estimated to be more probable than most of the possible values for the parameters being estimated. The value chosen is often zero, whence the procedures make the estimates smaller, or "shrunk" toward zero. Most shrinkage methods are equivalent to EMPIRICAL-BAYES METHODS.[7]

SIBLINGS Children borne by the same mother.

SIBSHIP All the brothers and sisters borne by the same mother.

SICKNESS See DISEASE.

SICKNESS ABSENCE Nonattendance to work attributed to incapacity due to illness or injury that is not necessarily work-related. It is often necessary for the recovery of ill workers, part of the medical treatment, and as such it may be certified or prescribed by a physician.[358,736,737] See also ABSENTEEISM; PRESENTEEISM.

SICKNESS "CAREER" The process of decisions and actions made by and/or for a person as she becomes symptomatic, defined as sick, seeks informal and professional care, and becomes a patient. It takes place in specific settings, in interaction with other people who, in accordance with their assessment of the problem and taking into account their own needs and the opportunities for alternative courses of action, apply the social norms of their group and set expectations for behavior.[332-336] See also ACCESS; DISEASE LABEL; SEMIOLOGY.

SIDE EFFECT An effect, other than the intended one, produced by a preventive, diagnostic, or therapeutic procedure or regimen. Not necessarily harmful.

SIDESTREAM SMOKE Smoke from combusted tobacco products, usually cigarettes, that is not filtered through the cigarette or the smoker's respiratory system but directly enters the air, where its toxic and irritant effects on nonsmokers can lead to adverse health effects.[13,179] See also ENVIRONMENTAL TOBACCO SMOKE; INVOLUNTARY SMOKING.

SIGNAL-TO-NOISE RATIO

1. In statistics and signal processing, the RATIO of explained variation to unexplained (error) variation.
2. A jargon term for the relationship of pertinent findings to that which is extraneous or irrelevant because measurement methods or other procedures are insufficiently sensitive.

SIGNIFICANCE, CLINICAL Importance, RELEVANCE, or meaning for the care of individuals, who often are—in clinical research—patients. A difference in effect size considered to be important (e.g., by a patient or a professional) in medical decisions regardless of the degree of statistical significance. statistical significance can never be taken to equal clinical significance. For example, when large numbers of subjects are studied, some differences will be statistically significant even if their magnitude or size is small; hence they will be of little importance for patient care. Conversely, when small numbers of subjects are studied, some differences will not be statistically significant even if their magnitude is large; hence they may be of importance for patient care.[1,3,6,9,25,26,38,58,91,202,203,225] See also MINIMALLY IMPORTANT DIFFERENCE.

SIGNIFICANCE, PUBLIC HEALTH Importance, RELEVANCE, or meaning from a public health perspective; e.g., if exposure to an environmental factor that causes a small increase in the individual risk of a disease is common in a population, the factor may have public health significance or importance because of its impact on the BURDEN OF DISEASE in the population.[12,28,83,101,366,426] See also STRATEGY.

SIGNIFICANCE, STATISTICAL

1. The probability of the observed or a larger value of a test statistic under the NULL HYPOTHESIS. Often equivalent to the probability of the observed or larger degree of association under the null hypothesis. This usage is synonymous with P VALUE.[1,7,101,270]

2. The event of the P value falling below a prespecified cutoff or ALPHA LEVEL for declaring a result "statistically significant", typically 0.05. This event should not be confused with clinical, public health, or scientific SIGNIFICANCE. See also CHI-SQUARE TEST; RELEVANCE.

SIGN TEST A DISTRIBUTION-FREE TEST that can be used in combining results of several studies. The test considers the direction of results of individual studies (i.e., whether the associations demonstrated are positive or negative).[7]

SILENCING, GENE See gene silencing.

SIMPSON'S PARADOX An example proposed by Edward H. Simpson (b. 1922) in 1951,[738] which illustrates the need to consider the causal structure linking exposure, outcome, and a third variable before deciding whether to adjust for the third variable.[739] Simpson's original example presents two 2 × 2 tables in which the stratifying variable is either a CONFOUNDER (which needs to be adjusted for to eliminate CONFOUNDING) or a COLLIDER (which should not be adjusted for in order to prevent SELECTION BIAS), depending on the labeling of the three variables involved. Simpson's paradox was redefined by Blyth in 1972[740] as a reversal of the association between exposure and outcome upon stratification by a third variable, a reversal that was not contemplated by Simpson himself. The confusion about the definition of Simpson's paradox has been further compounded by subsequent definitions that conflate the concepts of CONFOUNDING and COLLAPSIBILITY.[101] See also CONFOUNDING BIAS; SELECTION BIAS.

SIMULATION The use of a model system (e.g., a mathematical model or an animal model) to approximate the functioning or action of a real system; often used to study the properties of a real system. See also MONTE-CARLO STUDY.

SINGLE NUCLEOTIDE POLYMORPHISM (SNP) DNA sequence variations that occur when a single nucleotide (adenine, thymine, cytosine, or guanine) in the genome sequence is altered.[54]

SINGLE-PATIENT TRIAL See N-OF-ONE STUDY.

SITUATION ANALYSIS Study of a situation that may require improvement. This begins with a definition of the problem and an assessment or measurement of its extent, severity, causes, and impacts upon the community; it is followed by appraisal of interactions between the system and its environment and evaluations of performance.

SKEW DISTRIBUTION An older and less recommended term for an asymmetrical frequency distribution. If a unimodal DISTRIBUTION has a longer tail extending toward lower values of the variate, it is said to have negative skewness; if the longer tail extends toward higher values, it is said to have positive skewness.[7,34,37] An example is the LOG-NORMAL DISTRIBUTION.

SLOPE INDEX OF INEQUALITY A means of quantifying the degree of absolute INEQUALITY in health in relation to another variable that can be ordered hierarchically, typically socioeconomic status. It is the absolute difference in the extreme adjusted values of a health indicator by means of a regression model where the outcome is a health status indicator and the exposure or predictor is the fractional rank of socioeconomic status. It can be interpreted as the absolute difference in health between the top (relative rank 1) and bottom (relative rank 0) of the socioeconomic scale. It only applies where there is linear variation in the health outcome. See also CONCENTRATION INDEX; GINI COEFFICIENT; LORENZ CURVE; RELATIVE INDEX OF INEQUALITY.

SLOW VIRUS DNA- or RNA-based agents hypothesized to causing degenerative (often, neurological) diseases characterized by a long incubation period and a prolonged, slowly progressive course. Most slow-virus hypotheses have been superseded by PRION hypotheses.

SMALL AREA VARIATIONS See MEDICAL PRACTICE VARIATIONS.

SMALL FOR GESTATIONAL AGE (SGA) See BIRTH WEIGHT.

SMOOTHING General term for methods of minimizing irregularities in a set of data. Examples include ROUNDING, KRIGING, and MOVING AVERAGES.

SNOWBALL SAMPLING A method of selecting for study the members of "hidden" populations, e.g., illicit drug users. Those initially identified are asked to name acquaintances who are added to the SAMPLE; these, in turn, are asked to name further acquaintances, and so on until enough numbers are accumulated to give adequate power to the proposed study. The sample is, of course, not random. Compare CAPTURE-RECAPTURE METHOD.

SOCIAL CAPITAL

1. The resources—for example, trust, norms, and the exercise of sanctions—available to members of social groups. The social group can take different forms, such as a work place, a voluntary organization, or a tightly-knit residential community. The salient feature of this approach is that social capital is conceptualized as a group attribute.[741]

2. The resources—for example, social support, information channels, social credentials— that are embedded within an individual's social networks. In this approach, social

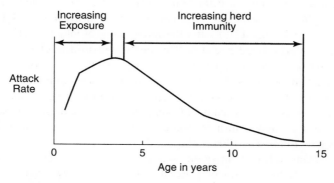

Skew diagram. Skew distribution of attack rate of measles in relation to age. Source: Lilienfeld DE.[726]

capital is conceptualized as an individual attribute as well as a property of the collective.[742]

Empirical research on social capital has stimulated a vigorous debate regarding its conceptualization and definition. Two points of contention are whether social capital ought to be considered as an individual or as a group attribute, and as social cohesion or as resources embedded in networks.[303,741-746]

SOCIAL CLASS A stratum in society composed of individuals, families, and groups of equal socioeconomic standing or position. A method of socially stratifying populations according to occupation, education, or income.[93,255,308,375,469,663,747,748] See also CLASS; LIFE COURSE; SOCIOECONOMIC CLASSIFICATION.

SOCIAL DRIFT Downward social class mobility as a result of impaired health, sometimes due to reduced earning potential, mental disorders, or substance abuse. The "social drift hypothesis" also suggests that persons with poor mental health are more likely to move to neighborhoods with poor-quality environments.

SOCIAL EPIDEMIOLOGY A branch or subspecialty of epidemiology that studies the role of social structures, processes, and factors in the production of health and disease in populations. It uses epidemiological knowledge, reasoning, and methods to study why and how the distribution of health states is influenced by factors as ethnicity, socioeconomic status and position, social class, or environmental and housing conditions. It may use a LIFE COURSE approach.[28,93,158,279,303-308,357,358,407,649,741,746,749,750] See also CAUSES IN PUBLIC HEALTH SCIENCES; ETHNOEPIDEMIOLOGY.

SOCIAL MARKETING The use of marketing theory, skills, and practice to achieve social change; to promote health or other public health objectives; to influence a target audience to voluntarily accept, reject, modify, or abandon a behavior for the benefit of individuals, groups or society as a whole.[751] In the social marketing model, "targeted behavior change" itself is the "product." Thus, the competition in social marketing comes from the current or preferred behavior of the target market and the perceived benefits of that behavior. Social marketing seeks to influence social behavior to benefit not the marketer but the target audience and the general society.

SOCIAL MEDICINE The practice of medicine concerned with health and disease as a function of group living. Social medicine is concerned with the health of people in relation to their behavior in social groups; as such, it involves care of the individual patient as a member of a family and of other significant groups in everyday life. It is also concerned with the health of these groups and with that of the whole community. The "father of social medicine" was Johann Peter Frank (1745–1821), who described many features of this discipline in *System einer vollständigen medicinischen Polizey* (A System of Complete Medical Police, 1779). After the appointment of John Ryle (1889–1950) as the first professor of social medicine at the University of Oxford, this became the preferred term to describe academic departments dealing with this range of disciplines in the United Kingdom; in the 1970s, the preferred term became community medicine. The Acheson Report (1988) advocated the term PUBLIC HEALTH MEDICINE, which was for some years adopted by the Faculty of Community Medicine of the UK Royal Colleges of Physicians and many British academic departments; it later became the Faculty of Public Health (FPH). The FPH is the standard setting body for specialists in public health in the United Kingdom; a joint Faculty of the three Royal Colleges of Physicians of the United Kingdom (London, Edinburgh, and Glasgow). See also COMMUNITY MEDICINE; PUBLIC HEALTH.

SOCIAL NETWORK The NETWORK of individuals, groups, organizations, institutions, and social resources to which individuals and groups are connected to or isolated from. Health status has been found to be positively associated with the extent of social networks.[27]

SOCIETAL RISK Probability of harm to the human population, including probability of adverse health effects to descendants and probability of disruption resulting from loss of services, such as industrial plant, loss of material goods, electricity.

SOCIOECONOMIC CLASSIFICATION Arrangement of persons into groups according to characteristics such as prior education, occupation, and income. Social class is a reliable and consistent predictor of health experience and status; analyses often reveals strong connections with average length of life or risk of dying from specific causes.[93,212,357,407,469,741,747] One such classification that is epidemiologically useful is the occupational classification developed in 1911 by the Registrar-General of England and Wales. This classified all occupations into five groups—the five "occupational social classes" (social class III is often further subdivided into nonmanual and manual groups) as follows: (I) Professional occupations; (II) Intermediate occupations; (IIIN) Nonmanual skilled occupations; (IIIM) Manual skilled occupations; (IV) Partly skilled occupations; and (V) Unskilled occupations.

There have been attempts to develop more refined classifications; however, most refinements require the collection of more detailed information. For example, Hollingshead's scale requires details about education and income as well as occupation. One's prestige in society and attitudes or values (e.g., setting a high value on getting a good education) are generally an integral part of social class, socioeconomic status, or socioeconomic position. Attitudes toward health are often part of the set of values and may explain part of the observed difference in health between social classes.

SOCIOECONOMIC STATUS Descriptive term for a person's position in society, which may be expressed on an ORDINAL SCALE using such criteria as income, level of education attained, occupation, value of dwelling place, etc.

SOCIOLOGY OF EPIDEMIOLOGY The application of the scientific principles and methods of sociology to the science, discipline, and profession of epidemiology in order to improve understanding of the wider social causes and consequences of epidemiologists' professional and scientific organization, patterns of practice, ideas, knowledge, and cultures (e.g., institutional arrangements, academic norms, scientific discourses, defense of identity, and epistemic authority). It also addresses the patterns of interaction of epidemiologists with other branches of science and professions (e.g., clinical medicine, public health, the other health, life, and social sciences), and with social agents, organizations, and systems (e.g., the economic, political, and legal systems). The tradition of sociology *in* epidemiology is rich; the sociology *of* epidemiology is virtually uncharted (in the sense of not mapped neither surveyed) and unchartered (i.e., not furnished with a charter or constitution). See also EPIDEMIOLOGY, DEMARCATION OF; EPISTEMIC COMMUNITIES; KNOWLEDGE CONSTRUCTION.

SOCIOLOGY OF SCIENTIFIC KNOWLEDGE An approach to the understanding of science that focuses on the social causes of the scientists' convictions, knowledge, and beliefs. It centers on *science as knowledge*, by contrast with the "constructivist approach," which is more interested in the constructive elements of scientific production (i.e., it considers *science as practice*). Both approaches tend to agree that the content of natural science is accessible by way of empirical sociological analysis and should be subjected to it; science is not to be investigated merely as a social institution; science's epistemic core is a matter of investigation in its own right and should not be studied only by philosophers of science.[579] See also EPISTEMIC COMMUNITIES; EPISTEMOLOGY; INTERPRETIVE BIAS; KNOWLEDGE CONSTRUCTION; PUBLICATION BIAS.

SOJOURN TIME (Syn: detectable preclinical period) The interval between detectability at screening and clinical presentation of a condition—i.e., the interval during which the condition is potentially detectable but not yet diagnosed.[752]

SOUNDEX CODE A sequence of letters used for recording names phonetically, especially in RECORD LINKAGE.

SOURCE OF INFECTION The person, animal, object, or substance from which an infectious agent passes to a host. Source of infection should be clearly distinguished from source of CONTAMINATION, such as overflow of a septic tank contaminating a water supply or an infected cook contaminating a salad.[20-22,56,188,196,217-219] See also RESERVOIR OF INFECTION.

SPATIAL AUTOCORRELATION A clustering pattern in the spatial DISTRIBUTION of a variable. The magnitude to which a variable is spatially correlated with itself. Positive autocorrelation (or clustering) occurs when neighboring observations tend to be more similar, while negative autocorrelation (or dispersion) occurs when neighboring observations tend to differ.[1,7,8]

SPATIAL EPIDEMIOLOGY A branch or subspecialty of epidemiology that studies the spatial variation in disease risk or incidence. See also DISEASE MAPPING; GEOGRAPHICAL INFORMATION SYSTEM; LANDSCAPE EPIDEMIOLOGY; MEDICAL GEOGRAPHY; SATELLITE EPIDEMIOLOGY.

SPATIAL WEIGHT MATRIX (Syn: contiguity matrix, connectivity matrix, or adjacency matrix) A representation of the spatial relationship among different features in a dataset which can be used to generate a matrix of spatial weights used in an analysis.[753] There are different types, including Queen's case contiguity, Rook's case contiguity, first-order neighbors, and second-order (or higher-order) neighbors.

SPEARMAN'S RANK CORRELATION See CORRELATION COEFFICIENT.

SPECIFICATION

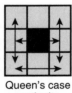

Queen's case
contiguity

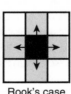

Rook's case
contiguity

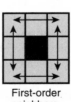

First-order
neighbors

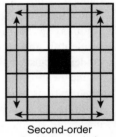

Second-order
(or higher-order)
neighbors

■	Central spatial unit of interest
▢	Adjacent spatial units of interest

Spatial weight matrix. Different types of spatial weight matrixes. Central cell is black and neighboring cells used in calculations are in light gray. Source: adapted from Lloyd CD.[753]

1. The process of selecting a particular functional form or model for the relationships to be analyzed in a study.
2. The process of selecting variables for inclusion in the analysis of an effect or association. This process may lead to the identification of variables that are EFFECT MODIFIERS and CONFOUNDING VARIABLES. See also STRATIFICATION.

SPECIFICITY (OF A TEST) See SENSITIVITY AND SPECIFICITY.

SPECTRUM BIAS A problem that may affect a study of diagnostic accuracy when it fails to account for the variation or heterogeneity of the test performance across population subgroups. Failure to recognize and address such heterogeneity will lead to estimates of test performance that are not generalizable to the relevant clinical populations. Bias may occur when diagnostic test performance varies across patient subgroups and the study does not adequately include all subgroups.[6,9,26,203,224] For instance, overestimation of the sensitivity and specificity of the test will occur when the study includes a healthy group and a group with overt disease. Originally described as a BIAS,[754] the variation is no longer considered to necessarily create a bias; rather, the spectrum of patients is considered a clinically relevant piece of information to be reported accurately and analyzed appropriately (e.g., by stratification). The term *spectrum bias* would hence be less appropriate than *spectrum effect*, which reflects the inherent variation in test performance among population subgroups.[755] In interpreting results of a diagnostic study, assessing the spectrum of patients included will help determine whether results are generalizable to other populations. See also WORKUP BIAS; QUADAS-2.

SPECTRUM OF DISEASE The full range of manifestations of a disease; e.g., from precursor states, to subclinical and mild cases, to florid and fulminating disease. The natural history of a disease from onset to resolution.[6,203,250] See also INCEPTION COHORT; INDUCTION PERIOD.

SPELL OF SICKNESS An episode of sickness with a well-defined onset and termination. As used in the monitoring or SURVEILLANCE of disease, the spell is often defined by the duration of absence from work or school. See also DISEASE; SICKNESS "CAREER."

SPILLOVER EFFECTS See EXTERNAL EFFECTS.

SPLEEN RATE A term used in malaria epidemiology to define the frequency of enlarged spleens detected on survey of a population in which malaria is prevalent. In association with the Hackett spleen classification, it summarizes the severity of malaria endemicity.

SPLINE A mathematical function used for interpolation or smoothing.

SPLINE MODELS Methods for flexible regression modeling of high dimensional data. Their use allows to combine the advantages of categorical and power models. The boundaries between categories of the regressor are called the *knots* or *joint points* of the spline.[1]

SPORADIC Occurring irregularly, haphazardly, from time to time, and generally infrequently (e.g., cases of certain infectious diseases).

SPOT MAP Map showing the geographic location of people with a specific attribute (e.g., cases of a disease or elderly persons living alone). The making of a spot map is a common procedure in the investigation of a localized outbreak of disease. Inferences from such a map depend on the assumption that the population at risk of developing the disease is fairly evenly distributed over the area or that at least the heterogeneities are known and can be considered in interpreting the map. A refinement is to indicate multiple cases at a single location by a series of short horizontal bars, as John Snow did to mark the location of cases of cholera in the epidemic in London in 1849; the method has been used by innumerable field epidemiologists ever since.[24]

STABLE POPULATION A population that has constant fertility and mortality rates, no migration, and consequently a fixed age distribution and constant growth rate; a population with stable structure. See also STATIONARY POPULATION.

STANDARD Something that serves as a basis for comparison; a technical specification or written report drawn up by experts based on the consolidated results of scientific study, technology, and experience, aimed at optimum benefits and approved by a recognized and representative body.

STANDARD DEVIATION A measure of dispersion or variation. It is the most widely used measure of dispersion of a frequency DISTRIBUTION. It is equal to the positive square root of the VARIANCE. The mean tells where the values for a group or for an estimator are centered in terms of the overall mass of their distribution. The standard deviation is a summary of how widely dispersed the values are around this center.[7,34,37]

STANDARD ERROR The standard deviation of an estimator, or the estimate of this standard deviation.[3,7,37] Used to calculate CONFIDENCE INTERVALS.

STANDARD GAMBLE See VON NEUMANN-MORGENSTERN STANDARD GAMBLE.

STANDARDIZATION A set of techniques, based on weighted averaging, used to remove as much as possible the effects of differences in age or other confounding variables in comparing two or more populations.[1] It is practically used (e.g., in the analysis of routinely collected data as vital statistics and governmental surveys) to adjust rates and any other measures of occurrence (e.g., prevalence) or effect (e.g., prevalence ratios or differences) for

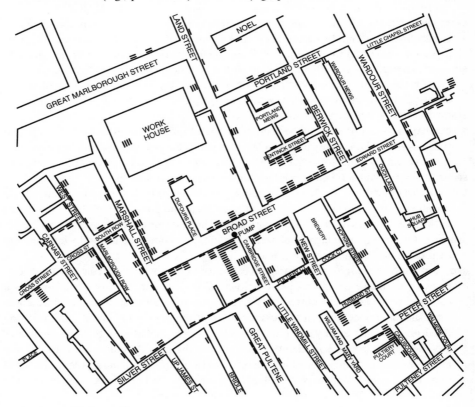

Spot map. Source: Snow J.[621]

factors such as age, ethnicity, area of residence, or socioeconomic position. The common method uses weighted averaging of rates specific for age, sex, or some other potential CONFOUNDING variable(s) according to some specified DISTRIBUTION of these variables. There are two main methods, as follows:

Direct method: The specific rates in a study population are averaged, using as weights the distribution of a specified standard population. The directly standardized rate represents what the crude rate would have been in the study population if that population had the same distribution as the STANDARD POPULATION with respect to the variable(s) for which the adjustment or standardization was carried out. INVERSE PROBABILITY WEIGHTING can be seen as a generalization.

Indirect method: This is used to compare study populations for which the specific rates are either statistically unstable or unknown. The specific rates in the standard population are averaged, using as weights the distribution of the study population. The RATIO of the crude rate for the study population to the weighted average so obtained is the standardized mortality (or morbidity) ratio, or SMR. The indirectly standardized rate itself is the product of the SMR and the crude rate for the STANDARD POPULATION, but this product is rarely used in etiological studies. A problem that arises with indirect standardization is that different SMRs are based on different weighting schemes (one for each study population) and so are not fully standardized for comparison to one another. As a result, comparisons of SMRs (or indirectly standardized rates) may remain partially confounded by the adjustment variables.[1,2,7,8]

STANDARDIZED INCIDENCE RATIO (Syn: Standardized Morbidity Ratio) The ratio of the incident number of cases of a specified condition in the study population to the incident number that would be expected if the study population had the same incidence rate as a standard or other population for which the incidence rate is known; this RATIO is sometimes expressed as a PERCENTAGE.[1] See also STANDARDIZATION (indirect).

STANDARDIZED MORTALITY RATIO (SMR) The ratio of the number of deaths observed in the study group or population to the number that would be expected if the study population had the same specific rates as the standard population.[1,5,793] Often multiplied by 100. See also STANDARDIZATION (indirect).

STANDARDIZED RATE RATIO (SRR) A rate ratio in which the numerator and denominator rates have been standardized (weighted) to the same (standard) population distribution. See also STANDARDIZATION (direct).

STANDARD METROPOLITAN STATISTICAL AREA Because of the extensive interactions between a city and its surrounding areas, a unit encompassing both is needed as a base for statistical description. The concept of a standard metropolitan statistical area (SMSA) was introduced in the United States to furnish such a unit. To qualify as an SMSA, an area has to meet criteria related to size, social and economic integration of the city and surrounding county or counties, minimum population density, and minimum proportion of the labor force engaged in nonagricultural work.

STANDARD POPULATION
1. A population in which the age and sex composition is known precisely as a result of a census or by an arbitrary means (e.g., an imaginary population, the "standard million," in which age/sex composition is arbitrary). A standard population is used as a comparison group in the actuarial procedure of standardization of mortality rates.
2. A population used as the reference in STANDARDIZATION.

STANDARD INSTRUMENTAL VARIABLE ESTIMATOR See G-ESTIMATOR.

STARD Standards for Reporting of Diagnostic Accuracy. A consensus checklist and flow diagram aimed at improving the accuracy and completeness of reporting of studies of diagnostic accuracy.[276,423,756,757] See also CONSORT; EQUATOR; PRISMA; QUADAS-2; STROBE; TREND.

STATIONARY POPULATION A stable population that has a zero growth rate with constant numbers of births and deaths each year.

STATISTIC A summary value of some attribute of a sample, usually but not necessarily as an estimator of some population parameter. It is calculated by applying a function to the values of the items of the sample.

STATISTICAL ERROR See ERROR.

STATISTICAL INFERENCE See INFERENCE.

STATISTICAL MODEL

1. A MATHEMATICAL MODEL for distribution of samples or data.[1,7,34,37,270]
2. The set of all statistical and other mathematical assumptions embodied in the DISTRIBUTION used to derive a statistical procedure or result.

STATISTICAL SIGNIFICANCE See SIGNIFICANCE, STATISTICAL.

STATISTICAL TEST A procedure intended to decide whether a statistical hypothesis (which may be about the distribution of one or more populations or variables or the size of an association or effect) should be rejected or not. Statistical tests may be parametric or nonparametric.[1,7,34,37] There are important objections to such procedures. See also HYPOTHESIS TESTING, STATISTICAL; *P* VALUE; SIGNIFICANCE, STATISTICAL.

STATISTICS

1. The science of collecting, summarizing, and analyzing data. Data may or may be not subject to random variation.[7,34,37,38]
2. The data themselves and summarizations of the data.

STEIN ESTIMATION See SHRINKAGE ESTIMATION

STEM-AND-LEAF DISPLAY A method of presenting numbers in a form resembling a HISTOGRAM, with multiples of 10 along the "stem" and the integers forming the "leaves." [37] See also BOX-AND-WHISKERS PLOT.

0	6 9
1	7
2	0 0 1 1 2 3 3 4 5 8 8
3	1 3 7 4
4	0 1 4 4 9
5	0 0 1 2 4 7 8
6	1 7 8 9
7	9
8	1
9	

Stem-and-leaf display. Stem-and-leaf plot showing the percentage of literate females in 37 African countries. The column to the left of the line is known as the "stem," while the numbers on the right of the line are the "leaves." The stem represents the "tens" and the leaves the "digits." For example, the row beginning with "6" has the digits "1," "7," "8," and "9." Therefore we know there are observations of 61, 67, 68, and 69 among the data. Source: Diamond I, et al.[758] With permission.

STEPPED WEDGE DESIGN A form of CLUSTER RANDOMIZED CONTROLLED TRIAL in which the intervention is administered in a random sequence to all clusters over time, so that all clusters will have received the intervention at the end of the trial. Each time point at which a new cluster receives the intervention is called a "step". Before and after each step, the dependent variable of interest is measured in all clusters. The analysis of data from such a design involves the comparison of the intervention "wedge" (i.e., data from the clusters that have received the intervention during a step) with the control wedge.[759]

STEWARDSHIP The ethical use of common resources in pursuit of socially efficient outcomes. The concept can be applied to health, the environment, economics, information, etc. Responsibility for the sustainable management and use of a particular resource or place.[139] The health system stewardship function can encourage decision making in the public sector that is ethical, fair and economically efficient.[760]

STILLBIRTH See FETAL DEATH.

STOCHASTIC PROCESS A process (usually a temporal sequence) that incorporates some element of randomness.

STOPPING RULES In randomized controlled trials and other forms of systematic experiments, stopping rules are laid down in advance, specifying conditions or criteria under which the trial or experiment shall cease or be terminated. For example, in a RANDOMIZED CONTROLLED TRIAL, the unequivocal demonstration of superiority of one regimen over another is the most obvious reason for terminating the trial; a less frequent situation is the demonstration that a regimen causes harm to participants in the trial. The rule must be based on appropriate statistical tests to ensure that the empirically observed results are not due to chance.

STRATEGY

1. In public health, a set of essential measures (e.g., social, sanitary, environmental) proven to be effective or efficient to control a health problem.[252,302,405,681] A mid- and long-term plan to improve chances of success for adoption and implementation of HEALTHY PUBLIC POLICIES.

2. In PREVENTIVE MEDICINE, seminal work by Geoffrey Rose helped establish the important distinction between the "HIGH-RISK" STRATEGY and the "POPULATION" STRATEGY.[211,426]

3. In politics, the means that policymakers choose to attain desired ends. A course of action, an overall plan for achieving specified goals.[38,665] See also POLICY; TACTICS.

STRATEGY, "HIGH-RISK" A clinically oriented approach to PREVENTIVE MEDICINE that focuses on individuals with the highest levels of the RISK FACTOR and utilizes the established framework of medical services. "A targeted rescue operation for vulnerable individuals".[211] The aim is to help each person reduce the high level of exposure to a cause or to some intermediate variable. Main strengths of this strategy include that the intervention may be matched to the needs of the individual; it may avoid interference with those who are not at a special risk; it may be accommodated within the ethical and cultural values, organization, and economics, of the health care system; selectivity may increase the likelihood of a cost-effective use of resources. Main weaknesses are that prevention may become medicalized; success may be palliative and temporary; the contribution to overall (population) control of a disease may be small; the preventive intervention may be behaviorally or culturally inadequate or unsustainable; it has a relatively low ability to predict which individuals will benefit from the intervention.[211]

STRATEGY, "POPULATION" A public health-oriented approach to PREVENTIVE MEDICINE and PUBLIC HEALTH predicting that a shift in the population distribution of a risk factor will prevent more BURDEN OF DISEASE than targeting people at high risk. It starts with the recognition that the occurrence of common exposures and diseases reflects the functioning of society as a whole.[211] The approach is more relevant to decrease exposure to (1) certain environmental agents that individuals have little capacity to detect than to (2) risk factors that individuals may generally decide to avoid. Main strengths of this strategy include that it may be radical ("only the social and political approach confronts the root causes"); the societal effects of a distributional shift may be large; it may be more culturally appropriate and sustainable to seek a general change in behavioral norms and in the social values that facilitate their adoption than to attempt to individually change behaviors that are socially conditioned.[211] Main limitations of the population strategy are that it offers only a small benefit to each participating individual, which may be wiped out by a small risk; it requires major changes in the economics and mode of functioning of society, which often makes changes unlikely. Individuals generally prefer to pay as late as possible and to enjoy the benefits as soon as possible. Social benefits— which are often achieved through processes with the opposite timing of costs and benefits—may thus be scarcely attractive to the individual. Nevertheless, shared values and targets do exist at the community level.[35,213,334,426,661] See also COMMON GOOD.

STRATIFICATION The process of or result of separating a sample into several subsamples according to specified criteria, such as age groups, socioeconomic status, etc. The effect of confounding variables may be controlled by stratifying the analysis of results. For example, lung cancer is known to be associated with smoking. To examine the possible association between urban atmospheric pollution and lung cancer, controlling for smoking, the population may be divided into strata according to smoking status. The association between air pollution and cancer can then be appraised separately within each stratum. Stratification is used not only to control for confounding effects but also as a way of detecting modifying effects. In this example, stratification makes it possible to examine the effect of smoking on the association between atmospheric pollution and lung cancer.[1-3,7,37,270] See also ADJUSTMENT; EFFECT MODIFICATION; STANDARDIZATION.

STRATIFIED RANDOMIZATION A randomization procedure in which strata are identified and subjects randomly allocated within each. This produces a situation intermediate between paired allocation and simple random allocation.[26,37,58,73-77] See also BLOCKED RANDOMIZATION; POSITIVITY; RANDOM ALLOCATION.

STREGA Strengthening the Reporting of Genetic Association Studies. A supplement and extension to the Strengthening the Reporting of Observational Studies in Epidemiology (STROBE). Additions concern POPULATION STRATIFICATION, genotyping errors, modeling haplotype variation, HARDY-WEINBERG EQUILIBRIUM, REPLICATION, SELECTION of participants, statistical methods, and other issues important in genetic association studies.[423] See also CONSORT; EQUATOR; PRISMA; QUOROM; STARD; STROBE; STREGA.

STRENGTH OF AN ASSOCIATION See HILL'S CONSIDERATIONS FOR CAUSATION; MEASURE OF ASSOCIATION.

STRESS The result of a process through which environmental demands challenge, strain, and exceed the adaptive capacity of a person or community, resulting in psychological, physiological, or clinical changes that place persons at risk for adverse health events. Distributions of stress depend on structural, interpersonal, cognitive, biological, and physical processes. Responses to stressors may favor survival and adaptation.[572]

STROBE Strengthening the Reporting of Observational Studies in Epidemiology. An evidence-based and structured approach to reporting of analytical OBSERVATIONAL STUDIES. Recommendations on what should be included in an accurate and complete report of cohort studies, case-control studies, and cross-sectional studies.[276,423,761] See also CONSORT; EQUATOR; PRISMA; STARD; STREGA; TREND.

STRUCTURAL NESTED MODELS A model for the effect of treatment defined, for example, as the difference in mean counterfactual outcomes (structural mean model), or the ratio of counterfactual survival times (structural nested accelerated failure time model) under different levels of treatment. For time-varying treatments, it models the effect of a small increment ("blip") of treatment on the outcome. The parameters of structural nested models are estimated by G-ESTIMATION.[2]

STRUCTURED ABSTRACT An abstract or summary of a scientific article or report that is organized or structured in well-defined sections. A typical sequence of sections includes some or all of the following: "Objectives" or "Aims," "Design," "Setting," "Subjects," "Main outcome measures," "Results," and "Conclusions." The structured abstract is intended to be comprehensive and to provide a logical order for the presentation of a scientific communication. Structured abstracts are required by many journals.

STUDY BASE The persons or PERSON-TIME in which the outcomes of interest are observed. The population experience actually captured ("harvested") by a study. In case-control studies, cases and controls should be representative of the same base experience.[1,25] Some authors, like Oli Miettinen (b.1936)[270] distinguish between primary and secondary bases; in the former, the POPULATION experience is defined in time and place; in the latter, the cases are defined before the study base is or can be defined. In a clinical trial, the base is the follow-up experience of the patients actually enrolled in the study.

STUDY DESIGN See RESEARCH DESIGN.

STUDY MONITOR An organization or individual responsible for the independent oversight and monitoring of the conduct of a research study to ensure the safety of participants and the validity and integrity of the data.[37,58,59,73-77,117]

SUBCLINICAL DISEASE See DISEASE, SUBCLINICAL.

SUFFICIENT CAUSE A set of conditions, factors, or events sufficient to produce a given outcome. A complete causal mechanism that does not require the presence of any other determinant in order for an outcome to occur.[1-3,5,8,39,42,84,101,206-210,253,406,407,433,798] See also ASSOCIATION; CAUSALITY; CAUSATION OF DISEASE, FACTORS IN; COMPONENT CAUSES; DISEASES OF COMPLEX ETIOLOGY; EVANS'S POSTULATES; HILL'S CONSIDERATIONS FOR CAUSATION; NECESSARY CAUSE.

SUMMATIVE RATING A rating scale based on measurements of individually scaled items that are monotonically related to an underlying attribute or attributes; the sum of the item scores is approximately linearly related to the attribute.

SUPERINFECTION Fresh infection in a host already infected with a PARASITE of the same species; a term mainly used in malaria epidemiology.[56]

SUPERIORITY TRIAL A trial designed to show that a treatment is superior to a comparison treatment.[73,76,77] See also NON-INFERIORITY TRIAL.

SUPPRESSION BIAS Bias that results when actions aimed at obstructing the conduct or publication of research produce a bias in the available evidence.[1,64,467,626] It may lead to PUBLICATION BIAS. See also REPRESSION BIAS; SCIENTIFIC MISCONDUCT.

SUPPRESSOR VARIABLE A variable that is causally related to the outcome of interest and, because of its association with the exposure variable of interest, suppresses the study association between the exposure and the outcome.[1,2] One variety of CONFOUNDING VARIABLE. For example, smoking can be a suppressor variable of the association between pesticide exposure and Parkinson's disease.[762]

SURROGATE MARKER A pathological sign or symptom, biomarker, or other parameter associated with a health state, which is more feasible or efficient to measure or monitor than a more valid and fundamental but less easily quantified measure (clinical or of some other nature). The validity or relevance of the surrogate needs to be well justified.[59,146,551,612-615]

SURVEILLANCE

1. Systematic and continuous collection, analysis, and interpretation of data, closely integrated with the timely and coherent dissemination of the results and assessment to those who have the right to know so that action can be taken. It is an essential feature of epidemiological and public health practice. The final phase in the surveillance chain is the application of information to health promotion and to disease prevention and control. A surveillance system includes a functional capacity for data collection, analysis, and dissemination linked to public health programs.[1,12,28,48,49,56,160,188,217-219,550,735,763] It is often distinguished from MONITORING by the notion that surveillance is continuous and ongoing, whereas monitoring tends to be more intermittent or episodic.

2. Continuous analysis, interpretation, and feedback of systematically collected data, generally using methods distinguished by their practicality, uniformity, and rapidity rather than by ACCURACY or completeness. By observing TRENDS in time, place, and persons, changes can be observed or anticipated and appropriate action, including investigative or control measures, can be taken. Sources of data may relate directly to disease or to factors influencing disease. Thus they may include mortality and morbidity reports based on death certificates, hospital records, general practice sentinels, or notifications; laboratory diagnoses; outbreak reports; vaccine uptake and side effects; sickness absence records; changes in disease agents, vectors, or reservoirs; serological surveillance through serum banks. The latter can also be seen as an example of BIOLOGICAL MONITORING.

SURVEY An observational investigation, usually descriptive, in which information is systematically collected. A population survey may be conducted by face-to-face inquiry, self-completed questionnaires, telephone, postal service, via the Internet or other ways. Each method has advantages and disadvantages; e.g., a face-to-face (interview) survey may be a better way than a self-completed questionnaire to collect information on attitudes or feelings, but it is more costly. Existing medical, occupational or other records may contain accurate information, but not about a REPRESENTATIVE SAMPLE.[1,8,110,160,167,518,519] See also FIELD SURVEY; GENERALIZABILITY.

SURVEY INSTRUMENT The interview schedule, questionnaire, medical examination record form, etc., used in a survey.

SURVIVAL ANALYSIS A class of statistical procedures for estimating the SURVIVAL FUNCTION and related quantities, such as the HAZARD RATE, and for making inferences about the relation to these quantities of treatments, other exposures, prognostic factors, and other covariates. The PROPORTIONAL HAZARDS MODEL and the KAPLAN-MEIER ESTIMATE are examples of tools for survival analysis.[1,3,5,8,11,37,764]

SURVIVAL CURVE A curve that starts at 100% of the study population and shows the percentage of the population still surviving at successive times for as long as information is available. May be applied not only to survival as such but also to the persistence of freedom from a disease or complication or some other endpoint.[11]

SURVIVAL FUNCTION (Syn: survival distribution) A function of time, usually denoted by $S(t)$, that starts with a population 100% well at a particular time and provides the percentage of the population still well at later times. Survival functions may be applied to any discrete event; for example, disease incidence or relapse, death, or recovery after onset of disease (in which case the population is initially 100% diseased, and the "survival" function gives the percentage still diseased).[7,11,37] See also KAPLAN-MEIER ESTIMATE.

SURVIVAL PROPORTION (Syn: cumulative survival rate, survival rate) The proportion of a CLOSED POPULATION at risk for a disease that does not become diseased during a specified interval; i.e., 1 minus the INCIDENCE PROPORTION.[1] The proportion of survivors in a group (e.g., of patients studied and followed over a specified period). May be studied by current or cohort LIFE TABLE methods.[11]

SURVIVAL RATIO The probability of surviving between one age and another; when computed for age groups, the ratios correspond to those of the person-years-lived function of a life table.

SURVIVAL, RELATIVE Adjustment of survival rate for independent cause(s) of death. Multiple regression models of relative survival take into account the mortality from all other causes in each area, permitting better comparisons of survival within and between populations with different life expectancies.[5,11,764,765]

SURVIVORSHIP STUDY Use of a cohort LIFE TABLE to provide the probability that an event, such as death, will occur in successive intervals of time after diagnosis and, conversely, the probability of surviving each interval. The multiplication of these probabilities of survival for each time interval for those alive at the beginning of that interval yields a cumulative probability of surviving for the total period of study.

SUSCEPTIBILITY

1. Vulnerability; lack of resistance to disease; the dynamic state of being more likely or liable to be harmed by a health determinant.
2. The condition or status of having one of two interacting causes already and therefore being susceptible to the effect of the other.[1]
3. A process occurring over time during which host factors (both inherited and learned or otherwise acquired and embodied) increase the likelihood that an exposure will produce disease. Susceptibility to positive influences and beneficial outcomes also exists.[23,67,110,248,332,336,365] Sometimes used as a synonym for VULNERABILITY.

In many living organisms, including humans, a clinically and epidemiologically meaningful increase in susceptibility to disease cannot be assumed only on the basis of mechanistic studies (since, for instance, studies often lack design characteristics required to estimate baseline risk and risk differences, and because significant changes in phenotype are prevented by ROBUSTNESS, redundancy, and compensatory mechanisms).[5,24,54,470,720,766,767] Assessment of the biological, clinical, and epidemiological COHERENCE of research findings helps to prevent overestimates of susceptibility to disease. See also LIFE COURSE; NONMALEFICENCE; SENSITIVE PERIOD.

SUSCEPTIBLE VARIABLE A variable that is potentially confounding in that it is subsequent, not antecedent, to the variable whose effect is being studied. It may or may not be an intermediate variable as well; if it is, special tools such as MARGINAL STRUCTURAL MODELS must be used to adjust for its confounding effects.

SUSTAINABILITY The ability to continue economic, social, cultural, and environmental aspects of human society and the nonhuman environment. Sustainable development is development that "meets the needs of the present without compromising the ability of future generations to meet their own needs."[768] Common principles in action programs to achieve sustainable development include dealing transparently and SYSTEMICALLY with risk, uncertainty, and irreversibility; ensuring appropriate valuation, appreciation, and restoration of nature; integration of environmental, social, human, and economic goals in policies and activities; equal opportunity; community participation; conservation of biodiversity and ecological integrity; intergenerational equity; commitment to best practices; no net loss of human capital and natural capital; and good governance. The COSTS OF INACTION is an example of approaches to the political economy of sustainable development.[13,17,33,139,213,267,286,287,310,350-352,359,360]

SYMBIOSIS The biological association of two or more species to their mutual benefit.

SYMPTOMATOLOGY (Syn: semiology) The study of signs and symptoms of disease. While their relevance to the practice of clinical medicine has long been recognized, signs and symptoms are important also to epidemiology-related activities like HEALTH SERVICES RESEARCH (e.g., when quality assurance programs monitor intervals from first symptom of disease to first medical consultation, diagnosis, and treatment), research on the QUALITY OF LIFE and PATIENT-REPORTED OUTCOMES. Symptoms and signs are also relevant to etiological research because they often reflect underlying pathophysiological processes that may alter levels of the exposures under study (e.g., when disease progression entails metabolic changes that alter exposure BIOMARKERS). The analysis of the attribution of meaning to signs and symptoms is essential to understand the SICKNESS "CAREER" [248,332,336] and hence to PREVENTIVE MEDICINE and EARLY CLINICAL DETECTION. See also DISEASE PROGRESSION BIAS; SYNDROME.

SYNDROME A complex of signs and symptoms that tend to occur together, often characterizing a DISEASE.

SYNERGISM, SYNERGY (Opposite: ANTAGONISM)

1. One of two main types of *effect modification* or INTERACTION: the EFFECT MODIFIER enhances the effect of the putatively causal variable. Under an additive model, a situation in which the combined effect of two or more factors is greater than the sum of their solitary effects.[1-3,620,798]

2. In a BIOASSAY, two factors act synergistically if there are persons who will get the disease when exposed to both factors but not when exposed to either alone. Under this definition and definition 2 of ANTAGONISM, two factors may act synergistically in some persons and antagonistically in others.

SYSTEM A set of interacting and interdependent elements connected in an organized (sometimes, stable and coherent) way to produce as a whole functions and outputs that none of such components alone could archive; the properties of the different levels of the system are qualitatively different from the properties of the components; the components are affected by the system and the behavior of the system is altered by changes in the components.[13,33,48,38,213,359,360,432,769]

SYSTEMATIC ERROR See BIAS.

SYSTEMATIC REVIEW A review of the scientific evidence which applies strategies that limit bias in the assembly, critical appraisal, and synthesis of all relevant studies on the specific topic. Systematic reviews differ from traditional narrative reviews, which tend to be mainly descriptive, do not involve a systematic search of the literature, and thus can suffer from selection bias.[6,9,25,26,52,58,230,231,294,300,340,485,504,689,691,770] See also GRADE.

SYSTEMIC

1. Relating to a whole system, rather than to just a particular component, that (dys)regulates or otherwise affects (often, positively) key structural or functional networks of and, hence, a whole body, organism, organization, set of functions, region, sector or society.[13,33,213,673] See also CAUSES IN PUBLIC HEALTH SCIENCES; DETERMINANT(S); DYSREGULATION; GLOBAL HEALTH GLOBAL HEALTH; SUSTAINABILITY; PUBLIC HEALTH.

2. In medicine, a process affecting the body as a whole, rather than individual organs (e.g., when an infection or an autoimmune disease is systemic rather than localized). The systemic circulation is the system of blood vessels that supplies all parts of the body except the lungs.[190]

SYSTEMS ANALYSIS

1. The systemic examination of the key networks of a body, organization, set of functions, region, or population to ascertain whether the possible causes of—and solutions to—a process or problem will effect an overall improvement in the system.

2. A formal comprehensive analysis to suggest a course of action by systematically examining the objectives, costs, effectiveness, and risks of alternative policies or strategies and designing additional ones if those examined are found wanting.[13,17,213]

T

TABLE See TWO-WAY TABLE.

TACTICS The detailed directions and instructions designed to achieve an aim or target. See STRATEGY.

TAGSNP (Syn: tagging SNP) A SINGLE NUCLEOTIDE POLYMORPHISM (SNP) that is used to "tag" (label, identify, mark) a particular haplotype in a region of the genome. As a subset of all of the SNPs in the genome, tagSNPs can be useful for testing the association of a marker locus with a qualitative or quantitative TRAIT locus in that it may not be necessary to genotype all the SNPs.[54]

TARGET An aspired outcome that is explicitly stated. What a health policy or program will achieve by a specified date; for example, reduced unwanted pregnancy rates, lower teenage smoking rates, enhanced QALYs. Usually but not necessarily expressed in quantitative terms.

TARGET POPULATION
1. The collection of individuals, items, measurements, etc., about which inferences are desired. The term is sometimes used to indicate the population or group from which a sample or study population is drawn and sometimes to denote a reference population about which inferences are desired. See also GENERALIZABILITY; REPRESENTATIVENESS.
2. The group to which inference from the study is directed.
3. The group of persons for whom an intervention is planned.[1,7]

TAU² A measure of the among-study variance for random-effects META-ANALYSES.[229,230,258]

TAXON (plural, taxa) The general term for a group or entity; e.g., a species or family in a taxonomy.

TAXONOMY A systematic CLASSIFICATION into related groups.

TAXONOMY OF DISEASE The orderly CLASSIFICATION of diseases into appropriate categories on the basis of relationships among them, with the application of names. See also NOSOGRAPHY, NOSOLOGY.

_t_-DISTRIBUTION, _t_-TEST The t-distribution is the DISTRIBUTION of a quotient of independent random variables, the numerator of which is a standardized normal variate and the denominator of which is the positive square root of the quotient of a chi-square distributed variate and its number of degrees of freedom. The t-test uses a statistic that, under the null hypothesis, has the t-distribution to test whether two means differ, or to test linear regression or correlation coefficients. It is an EXACT TEST under the assumption that the distributions being compared are normal with the same variance.[1,7,34,37] The t-distribution and the t-test were developed by William S. Gosset (1876 – 1937), who published under the pseudonym "Student," as required by his employers at the Guinness brewery.

TEMPORALITY See TIME ORDER.

TERATOGEN A substance that produces abnormalities in the embryo or fetus by disturbing maternal homeostasis or acting directly on the fetus in utero.

TEST OF SIGNIFICANCE See P VALUE; SIGNIFICANCE, STATISTICAL.

TEST HYPOTHESIS In statistics, the hypothesis subject to a statistical test, such as a SIGNIFICANCE test. A test hypothesis may concern any possible value for the measure under study; e.g., it may test whether a RISK RATIO is 0.5, 1, 2, 4, or any other value of interest. The NULL HYPOTHESIS is a special case of a test hypothesis in which the hypothesis tested is one of no association or no effect.[1,7,270]

TEST STATISTIC In HYPOTHESIS TESTING, a number computed from the data, which is used to compute a p VALUE for the TEST HYPOTHESIS, or which is compared to a value that the statistic has a probability of exceeding equal to the ALPHA LEVEL chosen for the test if the test hypothesis is true.[1]

THEORETICAL EPIDEMIOLOGY The study of theories on the population occurrence of phenomena of interest in the health sciences[215,270] The development of mathematical models and theories to explain and predict the occurrence of diseases and other health-related events in defined populations. With some infectious diseases, for instance, MODELS have been proposed to elucidate the reasons for epidemics and to predict their course once control measures are implemented. See also MECHANISTIC EPIDEMIOLOGY.

THERAPEUTIC TRIAL See CLINICAL TRIAL; RANDOMIZED CONTROLLED TRIAL.

THRESHOLD DOSE The dose above which effects occur.[14]

THRESHOLD LIMIT VALUE See SAFETY STANDARDS.

THRESHOLD PHENOMENA Events or changes that occur only after a certain level of a characteristic is reached.[14,33]

THRIFTY PHENOTYPE HYPOTHESIS The hypothesis proposed by Nick Hales and David Barker in 1992, that an undernourished fetus becomes thrifty.[771] Fetal undernutrition leads to impaired development of the pancreas, liver, and other tissues (e.g., muscle), leading to low insulin secretion and insulin resistance, which maintains high levels of sugar in the fetal bloodstream to preserve brain development, but may trade off muscle development. Once adopted, this thrifty behavior becomes permanent and, combined with adiposity in later life, leads to type 2 diabetes. It has been superceded by evidence on the DEVELOPMENTAL ORIGINS OF HEALTH AND DISEASE. See also "BRAIN SPARING."

THURSTONE SCALING An indirect measurement method that establishes preferences by making direct pairwise comparisons or rankings. This and comparable methods based on ordinal responses are embedded in a theory of human information processing and have been applied in areas such as consumer marketing research, political science, transportation research, and environmental economics. The major advantage of the response task in the Thurstone scaling model is that it is based on a basic human cognitive process, the ability to discriminate. Thurstone scaling may demand less cognitive resources than other measurement methods and, thus, may prove useful in patients suffering processes as dementia.[772,773]

TIME CLUSTER See CLUSTERING.

TIME ORDER Of all possible PROPERTIES OF A CAUSE, the only one that is necessary: a cause must precede an effect. Conceptually obvious as it may seem, assessment of the temporal relationship must be strictly based on an objective analysis of study characteristics (e.g., when using cross-sectional data, to assess DISEASE PROGRESSION BIAS and other causes of REVERSE CAUSATION), as well as on an in-depth understanding of substantive matter (e.g., pathophysiology of the disease, clinical pharmacology of the drug, self-care and health care referral processes, clinical reasoning, social and individual reasons of exposure to preventive and toxic agents, cultural processes).[1,3,5,12,25,39,101,208,270,272,710] See also CAUSALITY.

TIME-PLACE CLUSTER See CLUSTERING.

TIME SEQUENCE See TIME ORDER.

TIME SERIES A single-group research design in which measurements are made at several different times, thereby allowing TRENDS to be detected. An interrupted time series features several measurements both before and after an intervention and is usually more valid than a simple pretest-posttest design. A multiple time series involves several groups, including a control group.[1,7]

TIME-TO-PREGNANCY (TTP) The number of menstrual cycles required to achieve a pregnancy in healthy non-contracepting sexually active couples. The accuracy of TTP data can be assured only in a prospective study, but adequate data have been collected retrospectively by interview. In reproductive epidemiology, TTP is particularly useful in studies of environmental and occupational exposures.[1,7] See also FECUNDABILITY.

TIME TRADE-OFF A method of determining health-related changes in QUALITY OF LIFE in which members of a panel express preferences either for normal life expectancy in a defined suboptimal health state or reduced life expectancy in good health.[356] The magnitude of reduced life expectancy is varied until there is EQUIPOISE between the choices.

TOLERANCE In toxicology and pharmacology, the adaptive state characterized by diminished effects of a particular dose of a substance.

TORT A legal term for the harmful consequence of an act. Such acts are tried in courts of law, and damages are awarded if wrong or harm is demonstrated. A "toxic tort" is a lawsuit centered around a claim for harm due to a toxic chemical. Epidemiologists sometimes have to testify in legal cases involving tort.

TOTAL FERTILITY RATE (TFR) The average number of children that would be born per woman if all women lived to the end of their childbearing years and bore children according to a given set of age-specific fertility rates. It is computed by summing the age-specific fertility rates for all ages and multiplying by the interval into which the ages are grouped. The TFR is an important fertility measure, providing the most accurate answer to the question "How many children does a woman have on average?"

TOWNSEND SCORE An index of social deprivation developed by the British social scientist Peter Townsend (b.1928), used mainly in the United Kingdom; based on numbers economically active but unemployed, households with no car, households not owner-occupied, households overcrowded. The Townsend score uses readily available census data and can be used to rank administratively defined jurisdictions. See also JARMAN SCORE; OVERCROWDING.[774]

TOXICOLOGY The scientific discipline involving the study of actual or potential hazards of chemicals on living organisms and ecosystems; of the relationship of their harmful effects to exposure; and of the mechanisms of action, diagnosis, prevention, and treatment of acute and chronic intoxications.[13,14,450] Toxicology and epidemiology intensely interact.

TRACER DISEASE METHOD Tracer or indicator conditions are easily diagnosed, reasonably frequent illnesses or health states whose outcomes are believed to be affected by health care and that, taken in aggregate, should reflect the gamut of patients and health problems encountered in a medical practice.[775] The extent to which the recorded care of these conditions concurs with preset standards of care is used as an index of the quality of care delivered. However, it should first be shown that the preset standards contribute to a favorable outcome. See also SENTINEL HEALTH EVENT.

TRAIT An observable or measurable characteristic of an organism (e.g., height, skin colour). Traits can be influenced by genes, the environment, and GENE-ENVIRONMENT INTERACTIONS. The genetic contribution to a trait is the GENOTYPE. The outward expression of the genotype is the PHENOTYPE. [52,57,86,183-185,245,316,349,409-414,454,473,477,481,549,601,657]

TRANSCRIPTION Copying of a strand of DNA to generate a complementary strand of RNA.

TRANSDISCIPLINARITY The philosophical concept of scholarly inquiry that overlooks conventional boundaries among ways of thinking about and solving problems.[776] It is based on recognition of the complexity of many problems confronting humans and seeks to mobilize all pertinent scholarly disciplines: physical, biological, social, and behavioral sciences; ethics; moral philosophy; communication sciences; economics; politics; and the humanities. Many problems in public health have required transdisciplinary analyses and solutions. Epidemiology thus has a long tradition of transdisciplinary analysis of complex problems, of INTEGRATIVE RESEARCH (i.e., research that integrates multiple disciplines and levels of analysis), and of multidimensional intervention on the population and individual DETERMINANTS on health. The ecological impact of global climate change—which includes the epidemiological impact—is a current, relevant example of the important contributions of epidemiology to transdisciplinary research.[13,28,33,213,309,359,548] Sometimes it may be practically opposed to—but it is not an antonym of—REDUCTIONISM.

TRANSMISSION OF INFECTION The process, mechanisms, and DETERMINANTS by which an infectious agent or an infectious disease are spread from a source or reservoir to another person or across communities and countries. Such mechanisms are defined as follows:[56,67,110,188,240]

1. Direct transmission. Direct and essentially immediate transfer of infectious agents to a receptive portal of entry through which human or animal infection may take place. This may be by direct contact such as touching, kissing, biting, or sexual intercourse or by the direct projection (droplet spread) of droplet spray onto the conjunctiva or the mucous membranes of the eyes, nose, or mouth. It may also be by direct exposure of susceptible tissue to an agent in soil, compost, or decaying vegetable matter or by the bite of a rabid animal. Transplacental transmission is another form of direct transmission.

2. Indirect transmission. *Vehicle-borne:* Contaminated inanimate material or objects (fomites) such as toys, handkerchiefs, soiled clothes, bedding, cooking or eating utensils, and surgical instruments or dressings (indirect contact); water, food, milk; biological products including blood, serum, plasma, tissues, or organs; or any substance serving as an intermediate means by which an infectious agent is transported and introduced into a susceptible host through a suitable portal of entry. The agent may or may not have multiplied or developed in or on the vehicle before being transmitted. *Vector-borne:* (a) *Mechanical:* Includes simple mechanical carriage by a crawling or flying insect through soiling of its feet or proboscis or by passage of organisms through its gastrointestinal tract. This does not require multiplication or development of the organism. (b) *Biological:* Propagation (multiplication), cyclic development, or a combination of these (cyclopropagative) is required before the arthropod can transmit the infective form of the agent to humans. An incubation period (extrinsic) is required following infection before the arthropod becomes

infective. The infectious agent may be passed vertically to succeeding generations (transovarian transmission); transstadial transmission is its passage from one stage of the life cycle to another, as nymph to adult. Transmission may be by saliva during biting or by regurgitation or deposition on the skin of feces or other material capable of penetrating subsequently through the bite wound or through an area of trauma from scratching or rubbing. Transmission by an infected nonvertebrate host must be differentiated for epidemiological purposes from simple mechanical carriage by a vector in the role of a vehicle. An arthropod in either role is termed a *vector*.

Airborne: The dissemination of microbial aerosols to a portal of entry, usually the respiratory tract. Microbial aerosols are suspensions in the air of particles consisting partially or wholly of microorganisms. Particles in the range of 1 to 5 µm are easily drawn into the alveoli of the lungs and may be retained there. They may remain suspended in the air for long periods.

Airborne transmission includes:

Droplet nuclei: residues that result from evaporation of fluid from droplets emitted by an infected host. Droplet nuclei also may be created purposely by a variety of atomizing devices, or accidentally, as in microbiology laboratories or in abattoirs, rendering plants, or autopsy rooms. They usually remain suspended in the air for long periods.

Dust: The small particles of widely varying size that may arise from soil (fungus spores) or from clothes, bedding, or contaminated floors.

See also ACQUAINTANCE NETWORK; AIRBORNE INFECTION; CARRIER; COMMON VEHICLE SPREAD; CONTACT; CONTAMINATION; DROPLET NUCLEI; NETWORK.

TRANSMISSION PARAMETER (r) In infectious disease epidemiology, the proportion of total possible contacts between infectious cases and susceptibles that lead to new infections.[56,188,196]

TRANSOVARIAL TRANSMISSION See VECTOR-BORNE INFECTION.

TRANSPORTABILITY See GENERALIZABILITY.

TRANSPORT HOST See PARATENIC HOST.

TRAP, DEMOGRAPHIC See DEMOGRAPHIC ENTRAPMENT.

TRAVEL MEDICINE The field of medicine that seeks to prevent and manage illnesses and injuries occurring to travelers. It is also aims to control negative impacts of tourism on health.[777] See also EMPORIATRICS.

TREND A basic and explicit mathematical form that summarizes the pattern of association of an outcome measure (such as a frequency or a mean) across levels of a characteristic or an exposure. It often refers to a MONOTONIC trend, a special case of which is a linear trend, in which a plot of the outcome measure against the exposure follows a straight line. NONMONOTONIC trends include quadratic trends, in which there is one reversal in direction of the plot (from upward to downward, or from downward to upward), and more complex shapes such as cyclical trends (in which direction may reverse with season, time of day, or other cyclical quantities).[1,37]

TREND (STATEMENT) A proposal for a structured approach to reporting and evaluating studies of behavioral and public health interventions that use nonrandomized designs.[276,423,778] SEE ALSO CONSORT; EQUATOR; QUADAS-2, PRISMA; QUOROM; STARD; STROBE.

TREND LINE The line that best fits the distribution of a set of values plotted on two axes.

TRIAGE The process of selecting for care or treatment those of highest priority or, when resources are limited, those thought most likely to benefit. From the French *trier*, to separate, choose. See also RAPID EPIDEMIOLOGICAL ASSESSMENT.

TRIAL See CLINICAL TRIAL.

TRIAL PROFILE See CONSORT.

"TRIMMING" (data trimming)

1. The statistical practice of eliminating outlier effects by dropping equal number of outliers from both extremes of a distribution before computing means. Trimming all but the central one or two observations results in the median.[7]

2. The practice—which can be viewed as a form of scientific fraud or misrepresentation—of excluding from analysis observations or measurements that lie outside the range the investigator expects; the grounds for exclusion are that these outlying observations would distort the results. Data trimming is permissible only when rules written in advance in the research protocol specify circumstances in which it may be done. Even then it should be done with caution, and openly. See also OUTLIERS.

TRIPLE BLIND STUDY A study in which subjects, observers, and analysts are blinded as to which subjects received what interventions.[58,73-77] See also BLINDED STUDY.

TRUE-POSITIVE RATE See SENSITIVITY AND SPECIFICITY.

TRUE-NEGATIVE RATE See SENSITIVITY AND SPECIFICITY.

TUBERCULIN SKIN TEST (Syn: Mantoux tuberculin skin test) The standard method of determining whether a person has a tuberculosis infection. It is an intradermal injection of 0.1 ml of tuberculin purified protein derivative (PPD) in the inner surface of the forearm. The interpretation of the result depends on the measurement in millimeters of the induration and the person's risk of being infected with tuberculosis and of progression to disease if infected.[779]

TUBERCULOSIS A chronic disease since Neolithic times, afflicting an estimated 0.17% of the world's population (12 million prevalent cases). Caused by *Mycobacterium tuberculosis*.[780] It continues to present an epidemiological challenge.[20,22,56,69,188,217-219,781,782] See also HENLE-KOCH POSTULATES.

TUKEY'S METHOD See MULTIPLE COMPARISON TECHNIQUES.

TWIN STUDY A method of detecting genetic etiology in human disease. The basic premise of twin studies is that monozygotic twins, being formed by the division of a single fertilized ovum, carry identical genes, while dizygotic twins, being formed by the fertilization of two ova by two different spermatozoa, are genetically no more similar than two siblings born after separate pregnancies.[5] See also CONCORDANT; HERITABILITY; GENETIC EPIDEMIOLOGY.

TWO-BY-TWO TABLE See TWO-WAY TABLE.

TWO-SIDED TEST A statistical significance test based on the assumption that deviation from the TEST HYPOTHESIS in either direction is of interest. Sometimes called a "two-tailed test," although that term has other meanings. See also ONE-SIDED TEST.

TWO-WAY TABLE A contingency table for categorical variables. A table with r rows and c columns in which the entry in each cell represents the frequency for each outcome. Such a table is called an r-by-c table (e.g., a 3-by-4 table). If r = 2 and c = 2 then it is called a two-by-two table.[1,37]

TYPE I ERROR See ERROR, TYPE I.

TYPE II ERROR See ERROR, TYPE II.

TYPE III ERROR See ERROR, TYPE III.

"TYPHOID MARY" A slang expression for an individual who unwittingly transmits infection to others. The original Typhoid Mary, Mary Mallon, was an itinerant cook and an infamous CARRIER of typhoid in New York City and environs early in the twentieth century.[5]

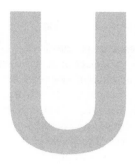

UNBIASED ESTIMATOR An estimator that, for all sample sizes, has an expected value equal to the parameter being estimated. If an estimator tends to be unbiased as sample size increases it is called asymptotically unbiased.

UNCERTAINTY ANALYSIS A form of analysis that recognizes and attempts to quantify the effects of several kinds of error and uncertainty that might affect the applicability of study findings to a public health problem in a specified population and setting. Such factors may include random and systematic errors, and uncertainty about levels of exposure in the population of interest.[116,734] See also BIAS ANALYSIS; INFLUENCE ANALYSIS; MULTIPLE BIAS MODELING; OUTLIERS; SENSITIVITY ANALYSIS.

UNCONTROLLED CONFOUNDING See RESIDUAL CONFOUNDING.

UNDERFIVE MORTALITY RATE OR RATIO A health indicator computed by dividing the death count of children under age 5 by the count of live births in the same year and expressing the result per thousand. Therefore, it is not an age-specific mortality rate but in fact a ratio, because the denominator is not the size of the child population under age 5. For global estimates, this indicator is preferable to the INFANT MORTALITY RATE, which is more difficult to determine in communities where the age of young children may not be known precisely.

UNDERLYING CAUSE OF DEATH The disease or injury that initiated the train of events leading directly to death, or the circumstances of the accident or violence that produced the fatal injury. See DEATH CERTIFICATE.

UNDERREPORTING Failure to identify and/or count all cases, leading to reduction of the numerator in a rate. See also ERROR.

UNICEF United Nations Children's Fund. The acronym originally stood for United Nations International Children's Emergency Fund. The acronym is unchanged.

UNIVERSAL PRECAUTIONS Procedures to be followed when health workers anticipate the possibility of infection by a patient who may harbor a highly contagious, dangerous pathogen. Universal precautions may include segregation of the patient in a private room; use of gloves, gown, mask, Perspex shield (eye protection); and rigorous attention to ensuring that no blood or other body fluid from such a patient can come into contact with the skin or mucous membranes of the health care worker.[56,188,217,218] See also BARRIER NURSING; NEEDLE STICK.

UNIVERSE, UNIVERSE POPULATION The entire population from which a sample is selected for study. The term is seldom used and is preferably avoided outside of theoretical discussions. See also GENERALIZABILITY; REPRESENTATIVENESS.

UNMEASURED CONFOUNDING CONFOUNDING that persists (i.e., RESIDUAL CONFOUNDING) because of lack of data on or imperfect measurement of confounders.[1-3,101,242,270,557]

UNOBTRUSIVE MEASURES A set of methods for assessing behavior without actually asking people how they behave or examining them physically to determine the effects of their behavior.[783] For example, the cigarette smoking behavior of groups can be assessed by studying cigarette sales.

UTILITY The value of a particular health state, usually expressed on a scale from 0 to 1; it is used in defining QUALITY-ADJUSTED LIFE YEARS (QALYS) and HEALTH-ADJUSTED LIFE EXPECTANCY. Utility is determined from preferences expressed by an individuals in a VON NEUMANN–MORGENSTERN STANDARD GAMBLE, TIME TRADE-OFF, or other related technique.[7] See also COST-UTILITY ANALYSIS.

UTILITY-BASED UNITS In the context of QUALITY-ADJUSTED LIFE YEARS (QALYs), utility-based units relate to a person's level of well-being estimated on the basis of the total life years gained from a procedure or intervention.

UTILITY, CLINICAL Risks and benefits associated with the introduction of a screening or diagnostic test into clinical practice.[6,9,58,91,202,435,454,475-478] See also SIGNIFICANCE, CLINICAL.

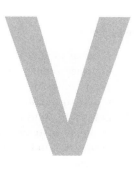

VACCINATION Strictly speaking, vaccination refers to inoculation (from Latin *in oculus*, into a bud) with vaccinia virus against smallpox. Nowadays the word is broadly used synonymously with procedures for IMMUNIZATION against all infectious disease. The original use of the word was confined to vaccination against smallpox. This was the first method of preventing a lethal disease by immunizing humans. It was introduced by Edward Jenner (1749–1823). Jenner's discovery led to the worldwide eradication of smallpox. Immunization is a more semantically and etymologically correct word than vaccination.[48,56,67,69,110,188,240]

VACCINE Immunobiological substance used for active immunization by introducing into the body a live modified, attenuated, or killed inactivated infectious organism or its toxin. The vaccine is capable of stimulating an immune response by the host, who is thus rendered resistant to infection. The word *vaccine* was originally applied to the serum from a cow infected with vaccinia virus (cowpox; from Latin *vacca*, "cow"); it is now used of all immunizing agents.[48,56,67,110,188,240]

VACCINE EFFICACY (Syn: protective efficacy) The proportion of persons in the placebo group of a vaccine trial who under ideal conditions would not have become ill if they had received the vaccine. Alternatively, the percentage reduction of cases among vaccinated individuals. The term has been used to refer to outcomes other than clinical outcomes (e.g., carriage). Different types of vaccine effectiveness and efficacy can be calculated (e.g., for disease, infectiousness, susceptibility, colonization, progression, conditional on exposure).[56,67,69,110,188,240]

VALIDATION The process of establishing that a method is sound or that data are correctly measured.[7,8,91]

VALIDITY The degree to which inferences drawn from a study are valid.[1,3,5-7,24,25,58,91,269,270] Two fundamental types of study validity must be distinguished:

1. INTERNAL VALIDITY The degree to which a study is free from BIAS or systematic error. Contrast with PRECISION, the relative lack of random error. As a principle, in etiological research internal validity must take precedence over PRECISION. However, small amounts of bias are often inevitable, and in some cases gains in efficiency and precision may be worth risking some limited bias. Internal validity depends on methods used to select the study subjects, collect the relevant information, and conduct analyses. For instance, the index and comparison groups must be selected and compared in such a manner that the observed outcome differences between groups, apart from sampling error, be attributed only to the exposure of interest.

Internal validity also depends on subject-matter knowledge; e.g., the identification and measurement of confounders, the choice of valid and relevant windows of exposure or of valid intervals and procedures for outcome detection. Internal validity is usually a prerequisite for external validity.

2. EXTERNAL VALIDITY (Syn: generalizability, transportability) The degree to which results of a study may apply, be generalized, or be transported to populations or groups that did not participate in the study. A study is externally valid if it allows unbiased inferences regarding some other specific target population beyond the subjects in the study.

Valid conclusions about the internal and external validity of a study require wisdom and rigor to apply expert judgment based on knowledge of the subject matter and of methodology; methodological knowledge may be slightly more important to judge internal validity, whilst substantive knowledge may be somewhat more relevant to judge external validity, but these nuances must not obscure the need to integrate both types of knowledge.[1-3,6,9,36,58,83,101,268,270,422] The epidemiological definitions of internal and external validity do not correspond exactly to some definitions in the social sciences. See also ACCURACY; BIAS; CRITICAL APPRAISAL; EVIDENCE-BASED MEDICINE; FEASIBILITY; GENERALIZABILITY; MEASUREMENT, TERMINOLOGY OF; REPRESENTATIVENESS; REVERSE CAUSATION.

VALIDITY, ANALYTICAL The ability of a test to correctly identify a property or characteristic in a specimen. This term encompasses both "analytical sensitivity" and "analytical specificity."

VALIDITY, CLINICAL The ability of a test to correctly identify a person who does or does not have the disease of interest.[6,58,203,224,270,349] This term encompasses both "clinical sensitivity" and "clinical specificity."

VALIDITY, INTERNAL See VALIDITY.

VALIDITY, EXTERNAL See VALIDITY.

VALIDITY, MEASUREMENT An expression of the degree to which a measurement measures what it purports to measure.[3,5,7] Several varieties are distinguished:

1. *Construct validity* The extent to which the measurement corresponds to theoretical concepts (constructs) concerning the phenomenon under study. For example, if on theoretical grounds the phenomenon should change with age, a measurement with construct validity would reflect such a change.

2. *Content validity* The extent to which the measurement incorporates the domain of the phenomenon under study. For example, a measurement of functional health status should embrace activities of daily living (occupational, family, and social functioning, etc.).

3. *Criterion validity* The extent to which the measurement correlates with an external criterion of the phenomenon under study; ideally, a GOLD STANDARD. Two aspects of criterion validity can be distinguished:

    a. *Concurrent validity* The measurement and the criterion refer to the same point in time. An example is a visual inspection of a wound for evidence of infection validated against bacteriological examination of a specimen taken at the same time.

    b. *Predictive validity* The measurement's validity is expressed in terms of its ability to predict the criterion. An example is an academic aptitude test that is validated against subsequent academic performance.

4. *Face validity* The extent to which a measurement or a measurement instrument appears reasonable on superficial inspection.

See also MEASUREMENT, TERMINOLOGY OF.

VALUES

1. In the health, life, and social sciences, what we believe in, what we hold dear about the way we live. Values influence the behavior of persons, groups, communities, cultures. They are strong influences on the health of individuals and populations (scientists are here included as well).[6,28,58,248,260-265,290,336,365]

2. Concepts used to explain how and why things matter. Values are involved wherever we distinguish between things good and bad, better or worse. Values are pervasive in human activities, including EPIDEMIOLOGICAL RESEARCH and PUBLIC HEALTH.[117,118]

3. In statistics, the magnitudes of measurements, statistics, or parameters.

VARIABLE Any quantity that can have different values across individuals or other study units.

VARIABLE, CONFOUNDING See CONFOUNDER.

VARIABLE, CONTROL Independent variable other than the "hypothetical causal variable" that has a potential effect on the outcome variable and is subject to control by analysis.

VARIABLE, DEPENDENT See DEPENDENT VARIABLE.

VARIABLE, DICHOTOMOUS See DICHOTOMOUS VARIABLE.

VARIABLE, INDEPENDENT See INDEPENDENT VARIABLE.

VARIABLE, INTERVENING See INTERMEDIATE VARIABLE.

VARIABLE, PASSENGER See PASSENGER VARIABLE.

VARIABLE, POLYTOMOUS See POLYTOMOUS VARIABLE.

VARIABLE, UNCONTROLLED A (potentially) CONFOUNDING VARIABLE that has not been brought under control by design or analysis. See also RESIDUAL CONFOUNDING.

VARIANCE

1. A measure of the variation shown by a set of observations, defined by the sum of the squared deviations from the mean, divided by the number of DEGREES OF FREEDOM in the set of observations.[1,7,34,37] This is an empirical measure and is usually called the *sample variance* or *empirical variance*.

2. The mean of the squared difference between an ESTIMATOR of a quantity or parameter and the estimator's mean. This is a theoretical measure of variation. See also MEAN SQUARED ERROR.

VARIATE See RANDOM VARIABLE.

VECTOR

1. In infectious disease epidemiology, an insect or any living CARRIER that transports an INFECTIOUS AGENT from an infected individual or its wastes to a susceptible individual, its food, or its immediate surroundings. The organism may or may not pass through a developmental cycle within the vector.[20-22,56,188,217-219] See also COMMUNICABLE DISEASE; CONTAGION.

2. In statistics, an ordered set (list) of numbers representing the values of an ordered set of variables (which is a vector of variables).[1,7]

VECTOR-BORNE INFECTION Several classes of vector-borne infections are recognized, each with epidemiological features determined by the interaction between the INFECTIOUS AGENT and the human host on the one hand and the vector on the other. Therefore environmental factors, such as climatic and seasonal variations, influence the epidemiological pattern by virtue of their effects on the vector and its habits.[20,22,56,67,110,188,217-219]

The terms used to describe specific features of vector-borne infections are as follows:

1. BIOLOGICAL TRANSMISSION Transmission of the infectious agent to susceptible host by the bite of a blood-feeding (arthropod) vector, as in malaria, or by other inoculation, as in *Schistosoma* infection.
2. EXTRINSIC INCUBATION PERIOD Time necessary after acquisition of infection by the (arthropod) vector for the infectious agent to multiply or develop sufficiently that it can be transmitted by the vector to a vertebrate host.
3. HIBERNATION A possible mechanism by which the infected vector survives adverse cold weather by becoming dormant.
4. INAPPARENT INFECTION Response to infection without developing overt signs of illness. If this is accompanied by viremia or bacteremia in a high proportion of infected animals or persons, the receptor species is well suited as an epidemiologically important host in the transmission cycle.
5. MECHANICAL TRANSMISSION Transport of the infectious agent between hosts by arthropod vectors with contaminated mouthparts, antennae, or limbs. There is no multiplication of the infectious agent in the vector.
6. OVERWINTERING Persistence of the infectious microorganism in the vector for extended periods, such as the cooler winter months, during which the vector has no opportunity to be reinfected or to infect a vertebrate host. Overwintering is an important concept in the epidemiology of vector-borne diseases, since the annual recrudescence of viral activity after periods (winter, dry season) adverse to continual transmission depends on a mechanism for local survival of an infectious microorganism or its reintroduction from outside the endemic area. To some extent, the risk of a summertime epidemic may be determined by the relative success of microorganism survival in the local winter reservoir. Since overwinter survival may in turn depend upon the level of activity of the microorganism during the preceding summer and autumn, outbreaks sometimes occur for 2 or more successive years.
7. TRANSOVARIAL INFECTION (Syn: transovarial transmission) Transmission of the infectious microorganism from the affected female arthropod to her progeny.

VECTOR SPACE The entire collection of possible values for a VECTOR (ordered list) of variables.

VEHICLE OF INFECTION TRANSMISSION The mode of transmission of an INFECTIOUS AGENT from its reservoir to a susceptible host. This can be person-to-person, via food, vector-borne, etc.[56,110,188]

VENN DIAGRAM A pictorial presentation of the extent to which two or more quantities or concepts overlap.[102-106]

VERBAL "AUTOPSY" A procedure for gathering information that may make it possible to determine the cause of death in situations where the deceased has not been medically attended. It is based on the assumption that most common and important causes of death have distinct symptom complexes that can be recognized, remembered, and reported by lay respondents. It is promoted as a useful way of enhancing the quality of mortality statistics in developing countries.[784]

VERIFICATION The process aimed at converting speculative ideas and hypotheses into facts. It usually results either in the rejection of false hypotheses by deduction (see DEDUCTIVE LOGIC) or the acceptance and consensus by induction (see INDUCTIVE REASONING). A most illustrative case history is William Harvey's confirmation of his hypothesis of the circulation of the blood, now universally recognized. In its broadest sense, verification is a summary of a process of CAUSAL INFERENCE.

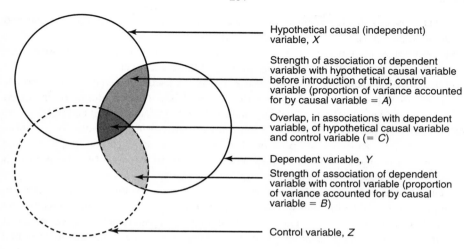

Hypothetical causal (independent) variable, X

Strength of association of dependent variable with hypothetical causal variable before introduction of third, control variable (proportion of variance accounted for by causal variable = A)

Overlap, in associations with dependent variable, of hypothetical causal variable and control variable (= C)

Dependent variable, Y

Strength of association of dependent variable with control variable (proportion of variance accounted for by causal variable = B)

Control variable, Z

Venn diagram. Source: Susser MW.[50]

VERIFICATION BIAS In studies evaluating screening and diagnostic tests, this bias occurs when some patients with negative test results are not evaluated with the "gold standard" test. While sensitivity can be overestimated and specificity underestimated, the final bias depends on the variables associated with receiving or not receiving the gold standard. When the gold standard is invasive, clinicians will tend to perform it on patients whose experimental test results increase the probability of disease and to refrain from performing it in those whose experimental test results decrease the probability of disease.[3,9,115,340,349,689] See also WORKUP BIAS.

VERTICAL TRANSMISSION (Syn: intergenerational transmission) The TRANSMISSION OF INFECTION from one generation to the next, especially of HIV infection from mother to infant prenatally, during delivery, or in the postnatal period via breast milk.[20,22,56,188,217-219]

VETERINARY EPIDEMIOLOGY (Syn: epizoology, epizootiology) The study and control of disease occurrence in animal populations.[20-22]

VIOLENCE Harm caused by the use of force. Harm may take the form of traumatic injury or death. Violence can be unintentional (e.g., in traffic, sport) and intentional (e.g., in warfare, domestic settings). The intentional use of physical force or power, threatened or actual, against oneself, another person, a group or community, that results in or has a high likelihood of resulting in injury, death, psychological harm, deprivation, or other health effects.[785]

VIRGIN POPULATION A population that has never been exposed to a particular infectious agent.

VIRULENCE The degree of pathogenicity; the disease-evoking power of a microorganism in a given host. Numerically expressed as the RATIO of the number of cases of overt infection to the total number infected as determined by immunoassay. When death is the only criterion of severity, this is the case-fatality rate.

VIRUS A microscopic INFECTIOUS AGENT composed of a piece of genetic material (RNA or DNA) surrounded by a protein coat. To replicate, a virus must infect a living cell: viruses can reproduce only by entering a host cell and using the translational system of the cell to initiate the synthesis of viral proteins and to undergo replication.

VITAL RECORDS Certificates of birth, death, marriage, and divorce required for legal and demographic purposes.[24] Literally, "to do with living."

VITAL STATISTICS Systematically tabulated information concerning births, marriages, divorces, separations, and deaths based on registrations of these vital events.[8]

VON NEUMANN–MORGENSTERN STANDARD GAMBLE Procedure used to assess the risk a seriously ill person is prepared to take when the trade-off is between potentially enhanced QUALITY OF LIFE and a finite possibility that the treatment regimen will be fatal.[786]

VULNERABILITY A position of relative disadvantage; e.g., owing to impaired nutrition, cognition, or socioeconomic position. The extent to which a person, population, or ecosystem is unable or unlikely to respond or adapt to threats.[13] May be used as a synonym for SUSCEPTIBILITY. See also ROBUSTNESS; RESILIENCE.

VULNERABLE POPULATION A population at risk of coercion, abuse, exploitation, discrimination, imposition of unjust burdens of risk, infection, disease, or poorer health outcomes by reason of diminished competence or decision-making capacity, lack of power or social standing, fragile health, deprivation, or limited access to basic needs, including public health and medical care. Similar acts may be construed to be coercive in a vulnerable population which would not be so in other, well-situated populations.[117,118]

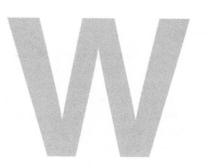

WASHOUT PHASE That stage in a study, especially a therapeutic trial, when symptomatic treatment is withdrawn so that its effects disappear and the subject's characteristics return to their baseline state.[9,26,691] An effective washout phase is essential in a CROSSOVER EXPERIMENT.

WEBER EFFECT A phenomenon of increased volume of reported adverse events for new drugs within their first years of approval. Older drugs are thought to be better understood as they have been around for longer time and, therefore, clinicians feel there is less need to report adverse events. This may lead to biases when comparing medications with different periods since marketing.[654,787,788] See also PHARMACOEPIDEMIOLOGY; POSTMARKETING SURVEILLANCE.

WEB OF CAUSATION (Syn: causal web) In epidemiology and public health, a popular METAPHOR for the theory of sequential and linked multiple causes of diseases and other health states (MULTIPLE CAUSE THEORY). The term appears in several monographs on epidemiology published in the early 1960s,[406] and was probably first published in 1959 by Dawber et al.[719] and in 1960 by Brian MacMahon (1923–2007) et al.[789] Originally deployed mainly for an epidemiology practiced at the individual level of organization (although not necessarily confined to it), the metaphor can be extended to incorporate a sequence of multiple dimensions.[254] See also ASSOCIATION; CAUSAL DIAGRAMS; DISEASES OF COMPLEX ETIOLOGY; ECOEPIDEMIOLOGY; MULTILEVEL ANALYSIS; MULTIPLE CAUSATION; PROBABILITY OF CAUSATION.

WEIBULL MODEL Dose-response model of the form

$$P(d) = 1 - \exp(-bd^m)$$

where $P(d)$ is the probability of response due to a continuous dose rate d; b and m are constants. The model is useful for extrapolating from high- to low-dose exposures—e.g., animal to human or occupational to environmental.[7,11] Also used to model SURVIVAL PROPORTIONS.

WEIGHTED AVERAGE An average calculated after assigning nonnegative weights to individual measurements or estimates. The sum of the products of each value by its weight divided by the sum of the weights is the weighted average.[24] See also META-ANALYSIS.

WEIGHTED SAMPLE A sample in which each SAMPLING UNIT has been assigned a weight for use in subsequent analysis. Common uses include survey weights to adjust for intentional oversampling of some units relative to others. For example, a sample that has intentionally selected two persons under age 60 for every person age 60 or more may assign a weight of ½ to those under 60 and a weight of 1 to those 60 or more when estimating population means. This is a special case of INVERSE PROBABILITY WEIGHTING.[1,7]

WESTERN BLOT See BLOT.

WHO World Health Organization.

WHOLE GENOME ASSOCIATION STUDY **(WGA STUDY)** See GENOME-WIDE ASSOCIATION STUDY (GWAS).

"WHISTLE-BLOWING" Informing authorities or the media when fraud or misrepresentation of research results or any other form of wrongdoing is suspected.[9,26]

WILD TYPE The normal, nonaltered sequence of a gene; the opposite is a mutated sequence.

WONCA World Organization of National Colleges, Academies, and Academic Associations of General Practitioners/Family Physicians, the World Organization of Family Doctors.[559] See also INTERNATIONAL CLASSIFICATION OF PRIMARY CARE, SECOND EDITION REVISED (ICPC-2-R).

WOOLF-HALDANE CORRECTION A modification of the observed data that avoids division by zero in statistical analysis when one or more cells in a data table have a value of zero. An increment close to zero (e.g., 0.5) is added to all the cells to enable computation of the stratum-specific odds ratio and other quantities.[269] Now largely obsolete owing to the availability of packaged software for methods that require no such correction (e.g., FISHER'S EXACT TEST, MANTEL-HAENSZEL ODDS RATIO, SHRINKAGE ESTIMATION).

WORKING CONDITION An agent, situation, or context to which workers are exposed during the performance of their working tasks, including physical conditions (e.g., structural insecurity, deficient lighting), physical stress (e.g., lifting heavy weights, repetitive movements), physical agents (e.g., noise, vibration, radiation), chemicals (e.g., pesticides, solvents), biological agents (e.g., bacteria, viruses), or psychosocial stressors (e.g., low control over job tasks, poor communication with workmates).[13,267,358,571,572] See also JOB STRAIN MODELS; EMPLOYMENT CONDITIONS.

WORK-RELATED DISEASE Disease or health disorder related to exposure to WORKING CONDITIONS with a weaker association with such conditions than an OCCUPATIONAL DISEASE. See also OCCUPATIONAL INJURY.

WORKUP BIAS Bias due to incorrectly or incompletely diagnosed cases being more numerous in one of the study groups than in the other. Usually because patients with a positive screening-level test receive a more thorough workup with diagnostic ("GOLD STANDARD") tests than those whose screening-level test was negative.[6,9,754] It is a form of VERIFICATION BIAS. See also DETECTION BIAS; PERFORMANCE BIAS; QUADAS-2; SPECTRUM BIAS.

WORLD HEALTH ASSEMBLY (WHA) The supreme decision-making body for the WHO. It meets once a year and is attended by delegations from all of WHO's over 190 Member States.

WORM COUNT A method of SURVEILLANCE of helminth infection of the gut that depends upon counts of worms, or cysts or ova, in quantitatively titrated samples of feces. Other terms to describe this form of surveillance are *egg count, cyst count*, and *parasite count*.

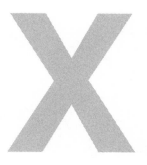

XDR (EXTENSIVELY DRUG-RESISTANT TUBERCULOSIS) See DRUG-RESISTANT TUBERCULOSIS, EXTENSIVELY.

XENOBIOTIC

1. A chemical compound that is foreign to a biological or an ecological system. A substance, typically a synthetic chemical, that is foreign to the body. Examples include many synthetic pesticides and their derivatives, food additives, or persistent toxic substances such as dioxins and polychlorinated biphenyls (PCBs).[13,80,183-186,415,416,482] See also CARCINOGEN.

2. (Syn: commensal, symbiosis) Pertaining to an association of two animal species, usually insects, in the absence of a dependency relationship, as opposed to parasitism. Contrast ENDOBIOTIC. See also COMMENSAL.

XENODIAGNOSIS Detection of a (human) pathogenic organism by allowing a noninfected vector (e.g., mosquito) to consume infected material and then examining this vector for evidence of the pathogen.

X-LINKED (Syn: sex-linked) Heritable characteristic transmitted by a gene located on the X CHROMOSOME. In an X-linked or sex-linked disease, it is usually males who are affected because they have a single copy of the X chromosome that carries the mutation. In females, the effect of the mutation may be masked by the second healthy copy of the X chromosome.

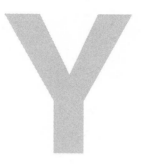

YATES'S CORRECTION An adjustment proposed by Frank Yates (1902–1994) in the chi-square calculation for a 2 × 2 table that brings the DISTRIBUTION based on discontinuous frequencies closer to the continuous CHI-SQUARE DISTRIBUTION from which the published tables for testing chi-squares are derived.[7,37]

YEARS OF POTENTIAL LIFE LOST (YPLL) See POTENTIAL YEARS OF LIFE LOST.

YIELD The number or proportion of cases of a condition accurately identified by a screening test.

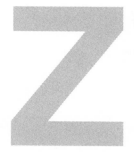

Zelen design (Syn: prerandomization design, post-randomized consent) A modified double-blind RANDOMIZED CONTROLLED TRIAL design proposed by Marvin Zelen (b. 1927).[790] The essential feature of the Zelen design is randomization before informed consent procedures, which are claimed to be needed only for the group allocated to receive the experimental regimen. Many ethicists disagree, holding that it is necessary to obtain the INFORMED CONSENT of all participants regardless of the group to which they are allocated.[7]

Zero population growth The status of a population in which there is no net increase of numbers; the number of births (plus immigrants) equals the number of deaths (plus emigrants).

Zero reporting Reporting of the absence of cases of a disease under SURVEILLANCE; this ensures that participants have not merely forgotten to report.

Zero-sum game A situation in which one participant can "gain" only at the expense of or to the detriment of another.

Zero-time shift The selection of a starting point for the measurement of survival following the detection of disease. It denotes the movement "backward" (toward the starting point of a disease) of time between onset and detection that may accompany use of a screening procedure.

Zoonosis A DISEASE, INFECTION, or INFESTATION transmitted under natural conditions from vertebrate animals to humans. Examples include rabies and plague. May be enzootic or epizootic.[20-22]

Z score Score expressed as a deviation from the mean value in standard deviation units; the term is used in analyzing continuous variables, such as heights and weights, of a sample, to express results of behavioral tests, etc. The use of Z scores has been criticized for reducing interpretability and comparability of results from different studies or populations.[1]

Bibliography

....

This bibliography complements the numbered references mentioned in the text, which can be found in the next section. The 125 books in epidemiology and biostatistics that were most cited in the biomedical literature in the past 50 years can be found in Porta M, Vandenbroucke JP, Ioannidis JPA, et al. Trends in citations to books on epidemiological and statistical methods in the biomedical literature. PLoS One 2013; 8(5): e61837. doi:10.1371/journal.pone.0061837.

Dictionaries, glossaries, general reference works

For many types of language and subject dictionaries: Oxford Reference: www.oxfordreference.com

Abercrombie N, Hill S, Turner BS, eds. *The Penguin Dictionary of Sociology*. 5th. ed. London: Penguin; 2006.

Bailey J. *The Concise Dictionary of Medical-Legal Terms: A General Guide to Interpretation and Usage*. New York: Parthenon; 1998.

Bannock MRG, Baxter RE, Davis E. *The Penguin Dictionary of Economics*. 8th. ed. London: Penguin; 2011.

Biron PJ. *A World Bank - UNICEF Glossary: Terminology of Water Supply and Environmental Sanitation* [English-French, French-English]. 2nd. ed. Washington, DC: World Bank; 1990.

Breslow L, ed. *Encyclopedia of Public Health*. New York: Macmillan; 2002.

Campbell RJ, ed. *Campbell's Psychiatric Dictionary*. 9th. ed. New York: Oxford University Press; 2009.

Everitt BS, Skrondal A. *The Cambridge Dictionary of Statistics*. 4th. ed. Cambridge: Cambridge University Press; 2010.

Florey C du V, editor. EPILEX. A Multilingual Lexicon of Epidemiological Terms. v. 4.0; 2013. http://www.personal.dundee.ac.uk/~cdvflore/Welcome

Forbis P, Bartolucci S. *Stedman's Medical Eponyms*. 2nd. ed. Baltimore: Williams & Wilkins; 2005.

Froom J. An International glossary for primary care. J Fam Pract 1981; *13*: 673–681.

Goldstein AS. *Dictionary of Health Care Administration*. Rockville, MD: Aspen; 1989.

Gunton T, ed. *The Penguin Dictionary of Information Technology*. London: Penguin Books; 1994.

International Programme on Chemical Safety (IPCS). *Glossary of Terms on Chemical Safety for Use in IPCS Publications.* Geneva: WHO; 1989.

Jammal A, Allard R, Loslier G, eds. *Dictionnaire d'Épidémiologie.* Ste-Hyacinthe, Maloine, Paris: Edisem; 1988.

King RC, Mulligan PK, Stansfield WD. *A Dictionary of Genetics.* 8th. ed. New York: Oxford University Press; 2013.

Kohn GC, ed. *Encyclopedia of Plague and Pestilence.* New York: Facts on File; 2008.

Kotz S, Johnson NL, Read CB, eds. *Encyclopedia of Statistical Sciences.* New York: Wiley; 2012. http://onlinelibrary.wiley.com/book/10.1002/0471667196

Leclerc A, Papoz L, Bréart G, Lellouch J. *Dictionnaire d'épidémiologie.* Paris: Frison-Roche; 1990.

Meadows AJ, Gordon M, Singleton A. *A Dictionary of New Information Technology.* London: Century; 1982.

Millar D. *The Cambridge Dictionary of Scientists.* 2nd. ed. Cambridge: Cambridge University Press; 2002.

Oxford Dictionary of English. 3rd. ed. Oxford: Oxford University Press; 2010.

Pressat R. *Dictionnaire de Démographie (The Dictionary of Demography).* English translation edited by Christopher Wilson. Oxford: Blackwell; 1985.

Segen JC, ed. *Dictionary of Modern Medicine.* Camforth, UK, and Park Ridge, NJ: Parthenon; 1992.

Stedman TL. *Stedman's Medical Dictionary.* 28th. ed. Baltimore: Lippincott Williams & Wilkins; 2006.

Thériault Y, Beauregard E, Charuest M. *Statistics and Surveys Vocabulary*; Terminology Bulletin No. 208. Ottawa: Secretary of State; 1992.

Vogt WP. *Dictionary of Statistics and Methodology: A Nontechnical Guide for the Social Sciences.* 4th. ed. London: Sage; 2011.

Wolman BB, ed. *Dictionary of Behavioral Science.* 2nd. ed. San Diego: Academic Press; 1989.

World Bank. *A World Bank Glossary: Population Terminology* [English, French, Spanish]. Washington, DC: World Bank; 1986.

World Health Organization. Glossary of Globalization, Trade and Health Terms. http://www.who.int/trade/glossary/en/

World Health Organization. Health Impact Assessment (HIA). Glossary of Terms. http://www.who.int/hia/about/glos/en/

World Health Organization. Health Systems Strengthening Glossary. http://www.who.int/healthsystems/hss_glossary/en/

World Health Organization. Human Genetics Programme. Glossaries of Genetic Terminology. http://www.who.int/genomics/glossary/en/

Epidemiology, biostatistics, public health, preventive medicine*

Abramson JH. *Research Methods in Community Medicine.* 6th. ed. Chichester: Wiley; 2008.

Abramson JH, Abramson ZH. *Making Sense of Data. A Self-Instruction Manual of the Interpretation of Epidemiological Data.* 3rd. ed. New York: Oxford University Press; 2001.

---

* This bibliography complements the references mentioned in the text, which can be found after this section.

Armenian HK. *The Case-Control Method: Design and Applications*. Oxford: Oxford University Press; 2009.

Armenian HK, Shapiro S. *Epidemiology and Health Services*. New York: Oxford University Press; 1998.

Aschengrau A, Seage GR. *Essentials of Epidemiology in Public Health*. Burlington, MA: Jones and Bartlett; 2014.

Atkinson W, Wolfe C, Hamborsky J, eds. *Epidemiology and Prevention of Vaccine-preventable Diseases*. 12th. ed. Washington, D.C.: Public Health Foundation; 2011.

Babbie E. *The Practice of Social Research*. 13th. ed. Belmont, Calif.: Wadsworth Cengage Learning; 2013.

Bailar III JC, Hoaglin DC. *Medical Uses of Statistics*. 3rd. ed. Hoboken: Wiley; 2009.

Baker D, Nieuwenhuijsen M, eds. *Environmental Epidemiology: Study Methods and Applications*. Oxford: Oxford University Press; 2008.

Bambra C. *Work, Worklessness, and the Political Economy of Health*. New York: Oxford University Press; 2011.

Barker DJP, Cooper C, Rose G. *Epidemiology in Medical Practice*. 5th. ed. New York: Churchill Livingstone; 1998.

Bayer R, Gostin LO, Jennings B, Steinbock B. *Public Health Ethics*: *Theory, Policy, and Practice*. New York: Oxford University Press; 2006.

Beaglehole R, Bonita R. *Global Public Health*: *A New Era*. 2nd. ed. New York: Oxford University Press; 2009.

Beaglehole R, Bonita R. *Public Health at the Crossroads: Achievements and Prospects*. 2nd. ed. Cambridge: Cambridge University Press; 2004.

Begley AC, Lairson DR, Morgan RO, et al. *Evaluating the Healthcare System: Effectiveness, Efficiency and Equity*. 4th. ed. Chicago: Health Administration Press; 2013.

Berridge V. *Marketing Health: Smoking and the Discourse of Public Health in Britain, 1945-2000*. New York: Oxford University Press; 2007.

Bland JM. *An Introduction to Medical Statistics*. 3rd. ed. New York: Oxford University Press; 2000.

Bland JM, Peacock J. *Statistical Questions in Evidence-Based Medicine*. New York: Oxford University Press; 2000.

Breslow NE, Day NE. *Statistical Methods in Cancer Research:* Vol. 1. *The Analysis of Case-Control Data*. Lyon: IARC; 1980. Vol. 2. *The Design and Analysis of Cohort Studies*. Lyon: IARC; 1987.

Coggon D, Rose G, Barker DJP. *Epidemiology for the Uninitiated*. 5th. ed. London: BMJ; 2003.

Dawson-Saunders B, Trapp RG. *Basic & Clinical Biostatistics*. 4th. ed. New York: Lange Medical Books; 2004.

Elliott P, Cuzick J, English D, Stern R. *Geographical and Environmental Epidemiology. Methods for Small-Area Studies*. New York: Oxford University Press; 1996.

Elston RC, Olson JM, Palmer L, eds. *Biostatistical Genetics and Genetic Epidemiology*. New York: Wiley; 2002.

Elwood M. *Critical Appraisal of Epidemiological Studies and Clinical Trials*. 3rd. ed. New York: Oxford University Press; 2007.

Exworthy M, Stuart M, Blane D, Marmot M. *Tackling Health Inequalities Since the Acheson Inquiry*. Bristol: The Joseph Rowntree Foundation & The Policy Press; 2003.

Farmer R, Miller D, Lawrenson R. *Lecture Notes on Epidemiology and Public Health Medicine.* 5th. ed. Oxford: Blackwell; 2004.

Fayers PM, Hays RD, eds. *Quality of Life Assessment in Clinical Trials.* 2nd. ed. Oxford: Oxford University Press; 2005.

Fleiss JL, Levin B, Paik MC. *Statistical Methods for Rates and Proportions.* 3rd. ed. Hoboken: Wiley; 2003.

Friedman GD. *Primer of Epidemiology.* 5th. ed. New York: McGraw-Hill; 2004.

Friis RH. *Epidemiology 101.* Sudbury, MA: Jones & Bartlett; 2010.

Friis RH, Sellers TA. *Epidemiology for Public Health Practice.* 5th. ed. Sudbury, MA: Jones & Bartlett; 2014.

Goodman KW. *Ethics and Evidence-Based Medicine: Fallibility and Responsibility in Clinical Science.* Cambridge: Cambridge University Press; 2003.

Gore SM, Altman DG. *Statistics in Practice.* London: British Medical Journal Publications; 1982.

Green A. *An Introduction to Health Planning for Developing Health Systems.* New York: Oxford University Press; 2007.

Greenberg RS, Daniels SR, Flanders WD, et al. *Medical Epidemiology.* 4th. ed. New York: McGraw-Hill; 2005.

Guest C, Ricciardi W, Kawachi I, et al., eds. *Oxford Handbook of Public Health Practice.* 3rd. ed. Oxford: Oxford University Press; 2013.

Haddix AC, Teutsch SM, Corso PS. *Prevention Effectiveness: A Guide to Decision Analysis and Economic Evaluation.* 2nd. ed. New York: Oxford University Press; 2003.

Hartzema AG, Tilson HH, Chan KA, eds. *Pharmacoepidemiology and Therapeutic Risk Management.* 4th. ed. Cincinnati: Harvey Whitney Books; 2008.

Hasselhorn HM, Toomingas A, Lagerström M, eds. *Occupational Health for Health Care Workers: A Practical Guide.* New York: Elsevier; 1999.

Hill A, Griffiths S. *Public Health and Primary Care.* New York: Oxford University Press; 2007.

Holford TR. *Multivariate Methods in Epidemiology.* New York: Oxford University Press; 2002.

Hosmer DW, Lemeshow S, Sturdivant RX. *Applied Logistic Regression.* 3rd. ed. Hoboken: Wiley; 2013.

Kalbfleisch JD, Prentice RL. *The Statistical Analysis of Failure Time Data.* 2nd. ed. New York: Wiley; 2002.

Katz DL, Wild D, Elmore JG, et al. *Jekel's Epidemiology, Biostatistics, Preventive Medicine, and Public Health.* 4th. ed. Philadelphia: Elsevier / Saunders; 2014.

Kawachi I, Kennedy BP. *The Health of Nations: Why Inequality Is Harmful to Your Health.* New York: The New York Press; 2002.

Kawachi I, Wamala S. *Globalization and Health.* New York: Oxford University Press; 2006.

Keating C. *Smoking Kills: The Revolutionary Life of Richard Doll.* Oxford: Signal Books; 2009.

Kleinbaum DG, Klein M. *Logistic Regression: A Self-Learning Text.* 3rd. ed. New York: Springer; 2010.

Kleinbaum DG, Klein M. *Survival Analysis: A Self-Learning Text.* 2nd. ed. New York: Springer; 2005.

Kleinbaum DG, Kupper LL, Nizam A, Rosenberg ES. *Applied Regression Analysis and Multivariable Methods.* 5th. ed. Stamford, CT: Cengage Learning; 2013.

Kleinbaum DG, Sullivan KM, Barker ND. *ActivEpi Companion Textbook. ActivEpi CD-ROM.* 2nd. ed. New York: Springer; 2013.

Kleinbaum DG, Sullivan KM, Barker ND. *A Pocket Guide to Epidemiology.* New York: Springer; 2007.

Kogevinas M, Pearce N, Susser M, Boffetta P, eds. *Social Inequalities and Cancer.* IARC Scientific Publications no. 138. Lyon: International Agency for Research on Cancer; 1997.

Kreis IA, Busby A, Leonardi G, et al. *Essentials of Environmental Epidemiology for Health Protection. A handbook for Field Professionals.* New York: Oxford University Press; 2013.

Lang T, Barling D, Caraher M. *Food Policy: Integrating Health, Environment and Society.* New York: Oxford University Press; 2009.

Lasky T, ed. *Epidemiologic Principles and Food Safety.* New York: Oxford University Press; 2007.

Levy BS, Sidel VW. *Terrorism and Public Health.* 2nd. ed. New York: Oxford University Press; 2011.

Loue S. *Case Studies in Forensic Epidemiology.* Dordrecht: Kluwer; 2002.

MacMahon B, Trichopoulos D. *Epidemiology: Principles and Methods.* 2nd. ed. Boston, MA: Little, Brown & Co; 1996.

Margetts B, Nelson M. *Design Concepts in Nutritional Epidemiology.* 2nd. ed. New York: Oxford University Press; 1997.

McDowell I. *Measuring Health: A Guide to Rating Scales and Questionnaires.* 3rd. ed. New York: Oxford University Press; 2006.

McMichael AJ. *Human Frontiers, Environments and Diseases. Past Patterns, Uncertain Futures.* Cambridge: Cambridge University Press; 2001.

Miettinen OS. *Up from Clinical Epidemiology and EBM.* New York: Springer; 2011.

Miettinen OS. *Epidemiological Research: Terms and Concepts.* New York: Springer; 2011.

Norell S. *Workbook of Epidemiology.* New York: Oxford University Press; 1995.

Oleske DM, ed. *Epidemiology and the Delivery of Health Care Services.* 3rd. ed. New York: Springer; 2009.

Olsen J, Saracci R, Trichopoulos D. *Teaching Epidemiology: A Guide for Teachers in Epidemiology, Public Health and Clinical Medicine.* 3rd. ed. New York: Oxford University Press; 2010.

Pfeiffer DU, Robinson TP, Stevenson M, et al., eds. *Spatial Analysis in Epidemiology.* New York: Oxford University Press; 2008.

Pickles A, Maughan B, Wadsworth M, eds. *Epidemiological Methods in Life Course Research.* New York: Oxford University Press; 2007.

Prince M, Stewart R, Ford T, Hotof M, eds. *Practical Psychiatric Epidemiology.* New York: Oxford University Press; 2003.

Rhodes R, Battin MP, Silvers A, eds. *Medicine and Social Justice: Essays on the Distribution of Health Care.* 2nd. ed. New York: Oxford University Press; 2012.

Robertson L. *Injury Epidemiology: Research and Control Strategies.* 3rd. ed. New York: Oxford University Press; 2007.

Rothman KJ. *Epidemiology: An Introduction.* 2nd. ed. Oxford: Oxford University Press; 2012.

Saracci R. *Epidemiology: A Very Short Introduction.* New York: Oxford University Press; 2010.

Siegrist J, Marmot M. *Social Inequalities in Health*. New York: Oxford University Press; 2006.

Smith TJ, Kriebel D. *A Biologic Approach to Environmental Assessment and Epidemiology*. New York: Oxford University Press; 2010.

Spasoff RA. *Epidemiologic Methods for Health Policy*. New York: Oxford University Press; 1999.

Steenland K, ed. *Case Studies in Occupational Epidemiology*. New York: Oxford University Press; 1993.

Thomas DC. *Statistical Methods in Genetic Epidemiology*. New York: Oxford University Press; 2004.

Valente TW. *Evaluating Health Promotion Programs*. New York: Oxford University Press; 2002.

VanderWeele TJ. *Explanation in Causal Inference: Methods for Mediation and Interaction*. New York: Oxford University Press; 2015.

Venables K. *Current Topics in Occupational Epidemiology*. New York: Oxford University Press; 2013.

Walker AM. *Observation and Inference: An Introduction to the Methods of Epidemiology*. Baltimore: Williams & Wilkins; 1991.

Wallace RB, ed. *Maxcy Rosenau-Last Public Health and Preventive Medicine*. 15th. ed. New York: McGraw-Hill; 2008.

Weiss NS. *Clinical Epidemiology: The Study of the Outcome of Illness*. 3rd. ed. New York: Oxford University Press; 2006.

Wilcox AJ. *Fertility and Pregnancy. An Epidemiologic Perspective*. New York: Oxford University Press; 2010.

Willett W. *Nutritional Epidemiology*. 3rd. ed. New York: Oxford University Press; 2012.

Yarnell J, O'Reilly D. *Epidemiology and Disease Prevention. A Global Approach*. 2nd. ed. New York: Oxford University Press; 2013.

History of epidemiology, logic and philosophy of science

Buck C, Llopis A, Nájera E, Terris M, eds. *The Challenge of Epidemiology: Issues and Selected Readings* [Spanish edition: *El desafío de la epidemiología. Problemas y lecturas seleccionadas*]. Washington, DC: Pan American Health Organization; 1988.

Bulger RE, Heitman E, Reiser SJ, eds. *The Ethical Dimensions of the Biological Sciences*. 2nd. ed. Cambridge: Cambridge University Press; 2002.

Daniels N, Kennedy B, Kawachi I. *Is inequality bad for our health?*. Boston: Beacon Press; 2000.

Jenicek M. *A Physician's Self-Paced Guide to Critical Thinking*. Chicago: American Medical Association (AMA Press); 2006.

Jenicek M, Hitchcock DL. *Evicence-Based Practice: Logic and Critical Thinking in Medicine*. Chicago: American Medical Association (AMA Press); 2005.

Knorr-Cetina K. *The Manufacture of Knowledge: An Essay on the Constructivist and Contextual Nature of Science*. Oxford: Pergamon Press; 1981.

Knorr-Cetina K. *Epistemic Cultures: How the Sciences Make Knowledge*. Cambridge, MA: Harvard University Press; 1999.

Pickering A, ed. *Science as Practice and Culture*. Chicago: University of Chicago Press; 1992.

Silverman WA. *Human Experimentation: A Guided Step into the Unknown*. Oxford: Oxford University Press; 1985.

White KL, Frenk J, Ordóñez C, et al., eds. *Health Services Research: An Anthology*. Washington, DC: Pan American Health Organization; 1992.

References

....

1. Rothman KJ, Greenland S, Lash TL, eds. Modern Epidemiology. 3rd. ed. Philadelphia: Lippincott-Raven; 2008.
2. Hernán MA, Robins JM. Causal Inference. New York: Chapman & Hall / CRC; 2014.
3. Szklo M, Nieto FJ. Epidemiology: Beyond the Basics. 3rd. ed. Sudbury, MA: Jones & Bartlett, 2014.
4. UNICEF. http://www.unicef.org/sowc96/define.htm.
5. Gordis L. Epidemiology. 4th. ed. Amsterdam: Elsevier; 2009.
6. Fletcher RH, Fletcher SW, Fletcher GS. Clinical Epidemiology. The Essentials. 5th. ed. Baltimore: Lippincott, Williams & Wilkins; 2014.
7. Armitage P, Colton T, eds. Encyclopedia of Biostatistics. 2nd. ed. Chichester: Wiley; 2005.
8. Gail MH, Benichou J, eds. Encyclopedia of Epidemiologic Methods. Chichester: Wiley; 2000.
9. Haynes RB, Sackett DL, Guyatt GH, et al. Clinical Epidemiology: How to Do Clinical Practice Research. 3rd. ed. Philadelphia: Lippincott, Williams & Wilkins, 2006.
10. Barratt A, Wyer PC, Hatala R, et al. Tips for Learners of Evidence-Based Medicine: 1. Relative Risk Reduction, Absolute Risk Reduction and Number Needed to Treat. Can Med Assoc J 2004; 171: 353–358.
11. Hosmer DW, Lemeshow S, May S. Applied Survival Analysis: Regression Modeling of Time to Event Data. 2nd. ed. New York: Wiley; 2008.
12. Aldrich T, Griffith J, Cooke C. Environmental Epidemiology and Risk Assessment. Hoboken: Wiley; 2002.
13. European Environment Agency. Late Lessons from Early Warnings: Science, Precaution, Innovation. EEA Report No 1/2013. Copenhagen: European Environment Agency; 2013. http://www.eea.europa.eu/publications/late-lessons-2
14. Asante-Duah K. Public Health Risk Assessment for Human Exposure to Chemicals. Dordrecht: Kluwer; 2002.
15. Ricketts TC, Goldsmith LJ. Access in health services research: the battle of the frameworks. Nurs Outlook 2005; 53: 274–280.
16. Mayberry RM, Mili F, Ofili E. Racial and ethnic differences in access to medical care. Med Care Res Rev 2000; 57 (Suppl 1):108–145.
17. World Health Organization. Health Systems Strengthening Glossary. http://www.who.int/healthsystems/hss_glossary/en/

18. Andersen RM. Revisiting the behavioral model and access to medical care: does it matter? J Health Soc Behav 1995; 36: 1–10.

19. Gwatkin DR, Bhuiya A, Victora CG. Making health systems more equitable. Lancet 2004; 364: 1273–1280.

20. Toma B, Vaillancourt JP, Dufour B, et al. Dictionary of Veterinary Epidemiology. Ames, Iowa: Iowa State University Press; 1999.

21. Toma B, Bénet JJ, Dufour B, Eloit M, et al. Glossaire d'Épidémiologie Animale. Maisons-Alfort, France: Editions du Point Vétérinaire; 1991.

22. Association pour l'Étude de l'Épidémiologie des Maladies Animales (AEEMA). Terminologie en épidémiologie animale. Maisons-Alfort (France): AEEMA, École Nationale Vétérinaire d'Alfort; 2014. http://aeema.vet-alfort.fr/

23. Kuh D, Ben-Shlomo Y, Lynch J, Hallqvist J, Power C. Life course epidemiology. J Epidemiol Community Health 2003; 57: 778–783.

24. Koepsell TD, Weiss NS. Epidemiologic Methods: Studying the Occurrence of Illness. New York: Oxford University Press; 2003.

25. Savitz DA. Interpreting Epidemiologic Evidence: Strategies for Study Design and Analysis. New York: Oxford University Press; 2003.

26. Hulley SB, Cummings SR, Browner WS, et al. Designing Clinical Research. 4th. ed. Philadelphia: Lippincott, Williams & Wilkins; 2013.

27. Christakis NA, Fowler JH. The collective dynamics of smoking in a large social network. N Engl J Med 2008; 358: 2249–2258.

28. Detels R, Beaglehole T, Lansang MA, Gulliford M, eds. Oxford Textbook of Public Health. 5th. ed. Oxford: Oxford University Press; 2009.

29. Katz S, Ford AB, Moskowitz RW, et al. Studies of illness in the aged: The index of ADL, a standardized measure of biological function. JAMA 1963; 185: 914–919.

30. Streiner DL, Norman GR. Health Measurement Scales: A Practical Guide to Their Development and Use. 3rd. ed. New York: Oxford University Press; 2003.

31. McLaren L, Hawe P. Ecological perspectives in health research. J Epidemiol Community Health 2005; 59: 6–14.

32. Gluckman PD, Hanson MA, Bateson P, et al. Towards a new developmental synthesis: adaptive developmental plasticity and human disease. Lancet 2009; 373: 1654–1657.

33. Rockström J, Steffen W, Noone K, et al. A safe operating space for humanity. Nature 2009; 461: 472–475.

34. Wasserman L. All of Statistics: A Concise Course in Statistical Inference. New York: Springer; 2004.

35. Marinker M, ed. From Compliance to Concordance: Toward Shared Goals in Medicine Taking. London: The Royal Pharmaceutical Society of Great Britain; 1997.

36. Greenland S. Modeling and variable selection in epidemiologic analysis. Am J Public Health 1989; 79: 340–349.

37. Armitage P, Berry G, Matthews JNS. Statistical Methods in Medical Research. 4th. ed. Oxford: Blackwell; 2002.

38. Kahneman D. Thinking, Fast and Slow. New York: Farrar, Straus and Giroux, 2011.

39. Greenland S, ed. Evolution of Epidemiologic Ideas: Annotated Readings on Concepts and Methods. Chestnut Hill, MA: Epidemiology Resources; 1987.

40. Susser M, Stein Z. Eras in Epidemiology: The Evolution of Ideas. New York: Oxford University Press; 2009.

41. Almeida-Filho N. La Ciencia Tímida. Ensayos de Deconstrucción de la Epidemiología. Buenos Aires: Lugar; 2000.

42. Morabia A. A History of Epidemiologic Methods and Concepts. Basel: Birkhäuser / Springer; 2004. http://www.epidemiology.ch/history.

43. Sentell TL, Halpin HA. Importance of adult literacy in understanding health disparities. J Gen Intern Med 2006; 21: 862–866.

44. National Cancer Institute. NCI Thesaurus (version 13.10b, 2013). http:// ncit.nci.nih.gov/ncitbrowser/ConceptReport.jsp?dictionary=NCI%20 Thesaurus&code=C41331 and http://ncit.nci.nih.gov

45. Vandenbroucke JP, Psaty BM. Benefits and risks of drug treatments: how to combine the best evidence on benefits with the best data about adverse effects. JAMA 2008; 300: 2417–2419.

46. Cutler DM, Zeckhauser RJ. Adverse selection in health insurance. In: Garber AM, ed. Frontiers in Health Policy Research, Vol. 1. Cambridge, MA: The MIT Press, 1998.

47. Mooney G, Ryan M. Agency in health care: getting beyond first principles. J Health Economics 1993; 12: 125–135.

48. World Health Organization. Epidemiological Surveillance. Alert, Response, and Capacity Building Under the International Health Regulations (IHR). http://www. who.int/ihr/lyon/surveillance/en/

49. Report of CIOMS/WHO Working Group on Vaccine Pharmacovigilance. Definition and Application of Terms for Vaccine Pharmacovigilance. Geneva: Council for International Organizations of Medical Sciences, World Health Organization; 2012. http://www.cioms.ch/index.php/publications/available-publications

50. Susser MW. Causal Thinking in the Health Sciences. New York: Oxford University Press; 1973.

51. Ioannidis JP. Calibration of credibility of agnostic genome-wide associations. Am J Med Genet B Neuropsychiatr Genet 2008; 147B: 964–972.

52. Ioannidis JP, Ntzani EE, Trikalinos TA, et al. Replication validity of genetic association studies. Nat Genet 2001; 29: 306–309.

53. Hunter DJ. Lessons from genome-wide association studies for epidemiology. Epidemiology 2012; 23: 363–367.

54 Pearson A, Manolio TA. How to interpret a genome-wide association study. JAMA 2008; 299: 1335–1344.

55. Hirschhorn JN, Lohmueller K, Byrne E, et al. A comprehensive review of genetic association studies. Genet Med 2002; 4: 45–61.

56. Mandell GL, Bennett JE, Dolin R, eds. Principles and Practice of Infectious Diseases. 7th. ed. Philadelphia: Churchill Livingstone; 2010.

57. Calafell F, Malats N. Glossary: basic molecular genetics for epidemiologists. J Epidemiol Community Health 2003; 57: 398-400. Malats N, Calafell F. Basic glossary on genetic epidemiology. J Epidemiol Community Health 2003; 57: 480–482. Malats N, Calafell F. Advanced glossary on genetic epidemiology. J Epidemiol Community Health 2003; 57: 562–564.

58. Straus S, Richardson WS, Glasziou P, et al. Evidence-Based Medicine: How to Practice and Teach It. 4th. ed. Edinburgh: Elsevier / Churchill Livingstone; 2011.

59. Lackie J. A Dictionary of Biomedicine. New York: Oxford University Press; 2010.

60. McEwen BS. Brain on stress: How the social environment gets under the skin. Proc Natl Acad Sci USA 2012; 109 (Suppl 2): 17180–17185.

61. www.worldmapper.org.

62. GRID-Arendal. Environment and Poverty Times 2000; 1: 1. http://www.grida.no/graphicslib/detail/world-economy-cartogram_1551.

63. Vandenbroucke JP. In defense of case reports and case series. Ann Internal Med 2001; 134: 330–334.

64. Landis SC, Amara SG, Asadullah K, et al. A call for transparent reporting to optimize the predictive value of preclinical research. Nature 2012; 490: 187–191.

65. Kim JY, Kim HH, Na BK, et al. Estimating the malaria transmission of Plasmodium vivax based on serodiagnosis. Malar J 2012; 11: 257.

66. Van der Weele TJ, Robins JM. Four types of effect modification. A classification based on directed acyclic graphs. Epidemiology 2007; 18: 561–568.

67. Plotkin SA, Orenstein WA, Offit PA, eds. Vaccines. 6th. ed. Philadelphia: Elsevier / Saunders; 2013.

68. Palese P, Young JF. Variation of influenza A, B, and C viruses. Science 1982; 215: 1468–1473.

69. Pollock G. An Epidemiological Odyssey: The Evolution of Communicable Disease Control. Dordrecht: Springer; 2012.

70. Hargrove J, Nguyen HB. Bench-to-bedside review: outcome predictions for critically ill patients in the emergency department. Crit Care 2005; 9: 376–383.

71. Casey BM, McIntire DD, Leveno KJ. The continuing value of the Apgar score for the assessment of newborn infants. N Engl J Med 2001; 344: 467–471.

72. Brownson RC, Petitti DB, eds. Applied Epidemiology: Theory to Practice. 2nd. ed. New York: Oxford University Press; 2006.

73. Meinert CL. Clinical Trials: Design, Conduct and Analysis. 2nd. ed. New York: Oxford University Press; 2012.

74. Pocock SJ. Clinical Trials: A Practical Approach. Chichester: John Wiley & Sons; 2002.

75. Friedman LM, Furberg CD, DeMets DL. Fundamentals of Clinical Trials. 4th. ed. New York : Springer; 2010.

76. Meinert CL. Clinical Trials Dictionary. 2nd. ed. Hoboken: Wiley; 2012.

77. Day S. Dictionary for Clinical Trials. 2nd. ed. Chichester: Wiley; 2007.

78. Vineis P, Schatzkin A, Potter JD. Models of carcinogenesis: an overview. Carcinogenesis 2010; 31: 1703–1709.

79. Armitage P, Doll R. The age distribution of cancer and a multi-stage theory of carcinogenesis. Br J Cancer 1954; 8: 1-12 (Reprinted: Int J Epidemiol 2004; 33: 1174–1179).

80. Hanahan D, Weinberg RA. Hallmarks of cancer: the next generation. Cell 2011; 144: 646–674.

81. Adami HO, Hunter D, Trichopoulos D, eds. Text of Cancer Epidemiology. 2nd. ed. New York: Oxford University Press; 2008.

82. Schottenfeld D, Fraumeni JF, eds. Cancer Epidemiology and Prevention. 3rd. ed. New York: Oxford University Press; 2006.

83. Blair A, Saracci R, Vineis P, et al. Epidemiology, public health and the rhetoric of false positives. Environ Health Perspect 2009; 117: 1809–1813.

84. Susser MW. Glossary: causality in public health science. J Epidemiol Community Health 2001; 55: 376–378.

85. Bhopal R. Concepts of Epidemiology. An Integrated Introduction to the Ideas, Theories, Principles and Methods of Epidemiology. Oxford: Oxford University Press; 2002.

86. Palmer LJ, Burton PR, Davey Smith G, eds. An Introduction to Genetic Epidemiology. Bristol: The Policy Press, University of Bristol, and University of Chicago Press; 2011.

87. Attia J, Ioannidis JP, Thakkinstian A, et al. How to use an article about genetic association: A. Background concepts. JAMA 2009; 301: 74–81.

88. Attia J, Ioannidis JP, Thakkinstian A, et al. How to use an article about genetic association: B. Are the results of the study valid? JAMA 2009; 301: 191–197.

89. Attia J, Ioannidis JP, Thakkinstian A, et al. How to use an article about genetic association: C. What are the results and will they help me in caring for my patients? JAMA 2009; 301: 304–308.

90. Evans JP, Meslin EM, Marteau TM, et al. Genomics: deflating the genomic bubble. Science 2011; 331: 861–862.

91. Ioannidis JP, Khoury MJ. Improving validation practices in "omics" research. Science 2011; 334:1230–1232.

92. Culyer AJ. The Dictionary of Health Economics. 2nd. ed. Cheltenham: Edward Elgar, 2010.

93. Geyer S, Hemström Ö, Peter R, et al. Education, income, and occupational class cannot be used interchangeably in social epidemiology: empirical evidence against a common practice. J Epidemiol Community Health 2006; 60: 804–810.

94. Greenland S, Robins JM. Conceptual problems in the definition and interpretation of attributable fractions. Am J Epidemiol 1988; 128: 1185–1197.

95. Steenland K, Armstrong B. An overview of methods for calculating the burden of disease due to specific risk factors. Epidemiology 2006; 17: 512–519. Erratum in: Epidemiology 2007; 18: 184.

96. Spasoff RA. Epidemiologic Methods for Health Policy. New York: Oxford University Press; 1999.

97. Jüni P, Egger M. Empirical evidence of attrition bias in clinical trials. Int J Epidemiol 2005; 34: 87-88.

98. Robinson KA, Dennison CR, Wayman DM, et al. Systematic review identifies number of strategies important for retaining study participants. J Clin Epidemiol 2007; 60: 757–765.

99. Kaptchuk TJ. Effect of interpretive bias on research evidence. BMJ 2003; 326: 1453-1455.

100. Greenland S, Pearl J, Robins JM. Causal diagrams for epidemiologic research. Epidemiology 1999; 10: 37–48.

101. Pearl J. Causality: Models, Reasoning and Inference. 2nd. ed. Cambridge: Cambridge University Press; 2009.

102. Robbins NB. Creating More Effective Graphs. Wayne, NJ: Chart House; 2013.

103. Few S. Show Me the Numbers: Designing Tables and Graphs to Enlighten. 2nd. ed. Oakland: Analytics Press; 2012.

104. Tufte ER. The Visual Display of Quantitative Information. 2nd. ed. Cheshire, CT: Graphics Press; 2001.

105. Tufte ER. Envisioning Information. Cheshire, CT: Graphics Press; 1990.

106. Tufte ER. Visual Explanations: Images and Quantities, Evidence and Narrative. Cheshire, CT: Graphics Press; 1997.

107. Clinical Trials Safety Graphics Home Page. https://www.ctspedia.org/do/view/CTSpedia/StatGraphHome

108. Ancker JS, Senathirajah Y, Kukafka R, et al. Design features of graphs in health risk communication: a systematic review. J Am Med Inform Assoc 2006; 13: 608–618.

109. Mann JM, Tarantola DJM, eds. AIDS in the World II. New York: Oxford University Press; 1996. p. 47.

110. Halloran ME, Longini IM, Struchiner CJ. Design and Analysis of Vaccine Studies. New York: Springer; 2010.

111. Etzioni RD, Kadane JB. Bayesian statistical methods in public health and medicine. Annu Rev Public Health 1995; 16: 23–41.

112. Hobbs L, Campbell R, Hildon Z, Michie S. Behaviour change theories across psychology, sociology, anthropology and economics: a systematic review. Psychol Health 2011; 26 (Supplement 1): 31.

113. Ezzati M, Riboli E. Behavioral and dietary risk factors for noncommunicable diseases. N Engl J Med 2013; 369: 954-964.

114. Gellman MD, Turner JR. Encyclopedia of Behavioural Medicine. New York: Springer, 2013.

115. Michie S, Richardson M, Johnston M, et al. The Behaviour Change Technique Taxonomy (v1) of 93 hierarchically-clustered techniques: building an international consensus for the reporting of behavior change interventions. Ann Behav Med 2013; 46: 81–95.

116. Last JM. A Dictionary of Public Health. Oxford: Oxford University Press; 2007.

117. Coughlin SS, Beauchamp TL, Weed DL. Ethics and Epidemiology. 2nd. ed. New York: Oxford University Press; 2009.

118. McKeown RE, Weed DL. Ethics in epidemiology and public health, II. Applied terms. J Epidemiol Community Health 2002; 56: 739–741.

119. Grosse SD, Matte TD, Schwartz J, et al. Economic gains resulting from the reduction in children's exposure to lead in the United States. Environ Health Perspect 2002; 110: 563–569.

120. Grandjean P, Landrigan PJ. Developmental neurotoxicity of industrial chemicals. Lancet 2006; 368: 2167–2178.

121. Espina C, Porta P, Schüz J, et al. Environmental and occupational interventions for primary prevention of cancer: a cross-sectorial policy framework. Environ Health Perspect 2013; 121: 420–426.

122. Gunning-Schepers L. The health benefits of prevention: a simulation approach. Health Policy 1989; 12: 1–255.

123. Stiglitz J, Sen A, Fitoussi JP. Mismeasuring our Lives: Why GDP Doesn't Add Up. The Report by the Commission on the Measurement of Economic Performance and Social Progress. New York: The New Press; 2010.

124. Berkson J. Limitations of the application of fourfold table analysis to hospital data. Biometrics Bull 1946; 2: 47–53.

125. Snoep JD, Morabia A, Hernández-Díaz S, Hernán MA, Vandenbroucke JP. A structural approach to Berkson's fallacy and a guide to a history of opinions about it. Int J Epidemiol 2014 (in press).

126. Flanders WD, Boyle CA, Boring JR. Bias associated with differential hospitalization rates in incident case-control studies. J Clin Epidemiol 1989; 42: 395–401.

127. History and Development of the ICD. ICD-10, Vol. 2, Geneva, Switzerland: WHO; 1993.

128. Holland WW, Olsen J, du V Florey C, eds. The Development of Modern Epidemiology: Personal Reports from Those Who Were There. New York: Oxford University Press; 2007.

129. Arah OA, Chiba Y, Greenland S. Bias formulas for external adjustment and sensitivity analysis of unmeasured confounders. Ann Epidemiol 2008; 18: 637–646.

130. VanderWeele TJ, Arah OA. Bias formulas for sensitivity analysis of unmeasured confounding for general outcomes, treatments, and confounders. Epidemiology 2011; 22: 42-52.

131. Greenland S. Multiple-bias modeling for analysis of observational data (with discussion). J Roy Stat Soc Ser A 2005; 168: 267–308.

132. Garfield E. Citation indexes for science. A new dimension in documentation through association of ideas. Science 1955;122:108–11 (Reprinted: Int J Epidemiol 2006; 35: 1123–1127). http://www.garfield.library.upenn.edu.

133. Porta M. The bibliographic 'impact factor' of the Institute for Scientific Information: how relevant is it really for public health journals?. J Epidemiol Community Health 1996; 50: 606–610.

134. Porta M, Fernandez E, Bolúmar F. The "bibliographic impact factor" and the still uncharted sociology of epidemiology. Int J Epidemiol 2006; 35: 1130–1135.

135. Evans JA. Electronic publication and the narrowing of science and scholarship. Science 2008; 321: 395–399.

136. Ioannidis JP. Contradicted and initially stronger effects in highly cited clinical research. JAMA 2005; 294: 218–228.

137. Tatsioni A, Bonitsis NG, Ioannidis JP. Persistence of contradicted claims in the literature. JAMA 2007; 298: 2517–2526.

138. American Society for Cell Biology. The San Francisco Declaration on Research Assessment (DORA). http://am.ascb.org/dora/

139. Park C, Allaby M. A Dictionary of Environment and Conservation. 2nd. ed. Oxford: Oxford University Press; 2013.

140. Institute of Medicine. Dioxins and Dioxin-like Compounds in the Food Supply: Strategies to Decrease Exposure. Washington, DC: The National Academies Press; 2003.

141. Pike MC, Krailo MD, Henderson BE, et al. "Hormonal" risk factors, "breast tissue age" and the age-incidence of breast cancer. Nature 1983; 303: 767–770.

142. Borkan GA, Norris AH. Assessment of biological age using a profile of physical parameters. J Gerontol 1986; 35: 177–184.

143. Karasik D, Demissie S, Cupples LA, Kiel DP. Disentangling the genetic determinants of human aging: biological age as an alternative to the use of survival measures. J Gerontol A Biol Sci Med Sci 2005; 60: 574–587.

144. Adams J, White M, Forman D. Is the rate of biological aging, as measured by age at diagnosis of cancer, socioeconomically patterned? J Epidemiol Community Health 2005; 59: 146–151.

145. Khoury MJ, Little J, Gwinn M, et al. On the synthesis and interpretation of consistent but weak gene-disease associations in the era of genome-wide association studies. Int J Epidemiol 2007; 36: 439–445.

146. Gallo V, Egger M, McCormack V, et al. STrengthening the Reporting of OBservational studies in Epidemiology–Molecular Epidemiology (STROBE-ME):

an extension of the STROBE statement. PLoS Med 2011; 8 (10): e1001117. www.strobe-statement.org.

147. Thornton JW, McCally M, Houlihan J. Biomonitoring of industrial pollutants: health and policy implications of the chemical body burden. Public Health Rep 2002; 117: 315–323.

148. Toniolo P, Boffetta P, Shuker DEG, et al., eds. Application of Biomarkers in Cancer Epidemiology. IARC Scientific Publications no. 142. Lyon: International Agency for Research on Cancer; 1999.

149. Bingham S, Riboli E. Diet and cancer: the European Prospective Investigation into Cancer and Nutrition. Nat Rev Cancer 2004; 4: 206–215.

150. National Research Council, Committee on Human Biomonitoring for Environmental Toxicants: Human Biomonitoring for Environmental Chemicals. Washington, DC: The National Academies Press; 2006. http://www.nap.edu/catalog/11700.html.

151. Porta M, Puigdomènech E, Ballester F, et al. Monitoring concentrations of persistent organic pollutants in the general population: the international experience. Environ Int 2008; 34: 546–561.

152. Thompson MR, Boekelheide K. Multiple environmental chemical exposures to lead, mercury and polychlorinated biphenyls among childbearing-aged women (NHANES 1999-2004): body burden and risk factors. Environ Res 2013; 121: 23–30.

153. Quinn CL, Wania F. Understanding differences in the body burden-age relationships of bioaccumulating contaminants based on population cross sections versus individuals. Environ Health Perspect 2012; 120: 554–559.

154. Whitlock G, Lewington S, Sherliker P, et al. Body-mass index and cause-specific mortality in 900,000 adults: collaborative analyses of 57 prospective studies. Lancet 2009; 373: 1083–1096.

155. Berrington de Gonzalez A, Hartge P, et al. Body-mass index and mortality among 1.46 million white adults. N Engl J Med 2010; 363: 2211–2219.

156. Finucane MM, Stevens GA, Cowan MJ, et al. National, regional, and global trends in body-mass index since 1980: systematic analysis of health examination surveys and epidemiological studies with 960 country-years and 9.1 million participants. Lancet 2011; 377: 557–567.

157. Pischon T, Boeing H, Hoffmann K, et al. General and abdominal adiposity and risk of death in Europe. N Engl J Med 2008; 359: 2105–2120.

158. Ludwig J, Sanbonmatsu L, Gennetian L, et al. Neighborhoods, obesity, and diabetes—a randomized social experiment. N Engl J Med 2011; 365: 1509–1519.

159. Tukey J. Exploratory Data Analysis. Reading, MA: Addison-Wesley; 1977.

160. Gasull M, Porta M, Pumarega J, et al. The relative influence of diet and serum concentrations of organochlorine compounds on K-ras mutations in exocrine pancreatic cancer. Chemosphere 2010; 79:686–697.

161. Barker DJP. Developmental origins of adult health and disease. J Epidemiol Community Health 2004; 58: 114–115.

162. Ross NA, Wolfson MC, Dunn JR, et al. Relation between income inequality and mortality in Canada and in the United States: cross sectional assessment using census data and vital statistics. BMJ 2000; 320: 898–902.

163. Murray CJL, Vos T, Lozano R, et al. Disability-adjusted life years (DALYs) for 291 diseases and injuries in 21 regions, 1990-2010: a systematic analysis for the Global

Burden of Disease (GBD) Study 2010. Lancet 2012; 380: 2197–2223. All articles in this issue of The Lancet (No. 9859, 15 Dec 2012) report findings of the GBD 2010 Study, pp. 2052–2260.

164. Murray CJ, Lopez AD. Measuring the global burden of disease. N Engl J Med 2013; 369: 448–457.

165. Institute for Health Metrics and Evaluation (IHME). http://www.healthmetric-sandevaluation.org/gbd

166. Lim SS, Vos T, Flaxman AD, et al. A comparative risk assessment of burden of disease and injury attributable to 67 risk factors and risk factor clusters in 21 regions, 1990-2010: a systematic analysis for the Global Burden of Disease Study 2010. Lancet 2012; 380: 2224–2260.

167. Alonso J, Chatterji S, He Y, eds. The Burden of Mental Disorders: Global Perspectives from the WHO World Mental Health Surveys. Cambridge: Cambridge University Press; 2013.

168. World Health Organization. Global Burden of Disease. www.who.int/healthinfo/bodproject/en http://www.who.int/topics/global_burden_of_disease/en/ http://www.who.int/healthinfo/global_burden_disease/estimates_regional/en/index1.html

169. Prüss-Ustün A, Vickers C, Haefliger P, et al. Knowns and unknowns on burden of disease due to chemicals: a systematic review. Environ Health 2011; 10: 9.

170. The Campbell Collaboration. http://www.campbellcollaboration.org

171. Khoury MJ, Lam TK, Ioannidis JP, et al. Transforming epidemiology for 21st century medicine and public health. Cancer Epidemiol Biomarkers Prev 2013; 22: 508-516.

172. Soskolne CL, Andruchow JE, Racioppi F. Developing, Conducting and Disseminating Epidemiological Research: From Theory to Practice. United Nations Development Programme; World Health Organization, European Centre for Environment and Health; and University of Alberta; 2007.

173. Hébert JR, Daguise VG, Hurley DM, et al. Mapping cancer mortality-to-incidence ratios to illustrate racial and sex disparities in a high-risk population. Cancer 2009; 115: 2539–2552.

174. Kauffmann F, Nadif R. Candidate gene-environment interactions. J Epidemiol Community Health 2010; 64: 188–189.

175. Boffetta P, Winn DM, Ioannidis JP, et al. Recommendations and proposed guidelines for assessing the cumulative evidence on joint effects of genes and environments on cancer occurrence in humans. Int J Epidemiol 2012; 41: 686–704.

176. Wittes JT, Colton T, Sidel VW. Capture-recapture methods for assessing the completeness of ascertainment when using multiple information sources. J Chronic Dis 1974; 27: 25–36.

177. Hook EB, Regal RR. Capture-recapture methods in epidemiology: methods and limitations. Epidemiol Rev 1998; 17: 243–264.

178. Lauby-Secretan B, Loomis D, Grosse Y, et al. (International Agency for Research on Cancer Monograph Working Group). Carcinogenicity of polychlorinated biphenyls and polybrominated biphenyls. Lancet Oncol 2013; 14: 287–288.

179. http://monographs.iarc.fr/

180. International Agency for Research on Cancer. Review of Human Carcinogens (Package of 6 volumes A,B,C,D,E,F): IARC Monographs on the Evaluation of Carcinogenic Risks to Humans, Vol. 100. Lyon: International Agency for Research on Cancer; 2012.

181. Demetriou CA, Straif K, Vineis P. From testing to estimation: the problem of false positives in the context of carcinogen evaluation in the IARC monographs. Cancer Epidemiol Biomarkers Prev 2012; 21: 1272–1281.

182. U.S. Department of Health and Human Services, Public Health Service, National Toxicology Program. Report on Carcinogens (RoC). 12th. ed. ; 2011. http://ntp.niehs.nih.gov/?objectid=03C9AF75-E1BF-FF40-DBA9EC0928DF8B15

183. Jirtle RL, Skinner MK. Environmental epigenomics and disease susceptibility. Nat Rev Genet 2007; 8: 253–262.

184. Stein RA. Epigenetics and environmental exposures. J Epidemiol Community Health 2012; 66: 8–13.

185. Henkler F, Luch A. Adverse health effects of environmental chemical agents through non-genotoxic mechanisms. J Epidemiol Community Health 2011; 65: 1–3.

186. Porta M. Human contamination by environmental chemical pollutants: can we assess it more properly?. Prev Med 2012; 55: 560–562.

187. Quinn CL, Wania F, Czub G, et al. Investigating intergenerational differences in human PCB exposure due to variable emissions and reproductive behaviors. Environ Health Perspect 2011; 119: 641–646.

188. Heymann DL, ed. Control of Communicable Diseases Manual. 19th. ed. Washington, DC: United Book Press / American Public Health Association; 2008.

189. Cammack R, Atwood T, Campbell P, et al., eds. Oxford Dictionary of Biochemistry and Molecular Biology. 2nd. ed. Oxford: Oxford University Press; 2006.

190. Concise Medical Dictionary. 8th. ed. Oxford: Oxford University Press; 2010.

191. Gregg MB, ed. Field Epidemiology. 2nd. ed. New York: Oxford University Press; 2002.

192. Kupper LL, McMichael AJ, Spirtas R. A hybrid epidemiologic study design useful in estimating relative risk. J Am Stat Assoc 1975; 70: 524–528.

193. Rosenbaum PR. The case-only odds ratio as a causal parameter. Biometrics 2004; 60: 233–240.

194. Gillespie IA, O'Brien SJ, Frost JA, et. al. A Case-case comparison of *CAMPYLOBACTER* coli and *CAMPYLOBACTER* jejuni infection: a toll for generating hypotheses. Emerg Infect Dis 2002; 8: 937–942.

195. McCarthy N, Giesecke J. Case-case comparison to study causation of common infectious diseases. Int J Epidemiol 1999; 28: 764–768.

196. Giesecke J. Modern Infectious Disease Epidemiology. New York: Arnold; 2002.

197. Vandenbroucke JP, Pearce N. Case-control studies: basic concepts. Int J Epidemiol 2012; 41: 1480–1489. Incidence rates in dynamic populations. Int J Epidemiol 2012; 41: 1472–1479.

198. Maclure M, Mittleman MA. Should we use a case-crossover design? Annu Rev Public Health 2000; 21: 193–221.

199. Hyams KC. Developing case definitions for symptom-based conditions: the problem of specificity. Epidemiol Rev 1998; 20: 148–156.

200. Khoury MJ, Flanders WD. Nontraditional epidemiologic approaches in the analysis of gene-environment interactions: case-control studies with no controls! Am J Epidemiol 1996; 144: 207–213.

201. Vandenbroucke JP. Clinical investigation. In: Lock S, Last JM, Dunea G. The Oxford Companion to Medicine. Oxford: Oxford University Press; 2001.

202. Glasziou P, Vandenbroucke JP, Chalmers I. Assessing the quality of research. BMJ 2004; 328: 39–41.
203. Sackett DL, Haynes RB, Guyatt GH, Tugwell P, Clinical Epidemiology: A Basic Science for Clinical Medicine. 2nd. ed. Boston: Little, Brown; 1991.
204. Zaffanella LE, Savitz DA, Greenland S, et al. The residential case-specular method to study wire codes, magnetic fields and disease. Epidemiology 1998; 9: 16–20.
205. Suissa S. The case-time-control design. Epidemiology 1995; 6: 248–253.
206. Rothman KJ, ed. Causal Inference. Chestnut Hill, MA: Epidemiology Resources; 1988.
207. Susser MW. What is a cause and how do we know one? Am J Epidemiol 1991; 133: 635–648.
208. Geneletti SG, Gallo V, Porta M, et al. Assessing causal relationships in genomics: from Bradford-Hill criteria to complex gene-environment interactions and directed acyclic graphs. Emerging Themes Epidemiol 2011; 8: 5.
209. Hernández-Díaz S, Schisterman EF, Hernán MA. The birth weight "paradox" uncovered? Am J Epidemiol 2006; 164: 1115–1120.
210. Joffe M, Mindell J. Complex causal process diagrams for analyzing the health impacts of policy interventions. Am J Public Health 2006; 96: 473–479.
211. Rose GA. The Strategy of Preventive Medicine. Oxford: Oxford University Press; 1992. (Annotated version edited by Khaw KT, Marmot M. Oxford University Press; 2007).
212. Davey Smith G, Hart C, Hole D, et al. Education and occupational social class: which is the more important indicator of mortality risk? J Epidemiol Community Health 1998; 52: 153–160.
213. McMichael AJ. Globalization, climate change, and human health. N Engl J Med 2013; 368: 1335–1343.
214. McKeown T. The Role of Medicine: Dream, Mirage or Nemesis?. 2nd. ed. London: The Nuffield Provincial Hospitals Trust; 1979.
215. Pearce N. Epidemiology in a changing world: variation, causation and ubiquitous risk factors. Int J Epidemiol 2011; 40: 503–512.
216. Porta M. Epidemiologic plausibility. Am J Epidemiol 1999; 150: 217–218.
217. Krämer A, Kreutzschmar M, Krickeberg K, eds. Modern Infectious Disease Epidemiology: Concepts, Methods, Mathematical Models, and Public Health. New York: Springer; 2010.
218. Nelson KE, Williams CM. Infectious Diseases Epidemiology. 3rd. ed. Burlington, MA: Jones & Bartlett; 2014.
219. Thomas JC, Weber DJ. Epidemiologic Methods for the Study of Infectious Diseases. New York: Oxford University Press; 2001.
220. WHO Growth Standards. http://www.who.int/childgrowth/en/
221. Wendt JK, Symanski E, Du XL. Estimation of asthma incidence among low-income children in Texas: a novel approach using Medicaid claims data. Am J Epidemiol 2012; 176: 744–750.
222. Kuller I. Circular epidemiology. Am J Epidemiol 1999; 150: 897–903.
223. Honderich T, ed. The Oxford Companion to Philosophy. 2nd. ed. Oxford: Oxford University Press; 2005.
224. Feinstein AR. Clinical Epidemiology: The Architecture of Clinical Research. Philadelphia: WB Saunders; 1985.
225. Feinstein AR. Clinimetrics. New Haven: Yale University Press; 1987.

226. All trials. All trials registered and all results reported. http://www.alltrials.net/
227. Spilker B, ed. Quality Assessments in Clinical Trials. New York: Raven Press; 1990.
228. Campbell MK, Piaggio G, Elbourne DR, et al. CONSORT 2010 statement: extension to cluster randomised trials. BMJ 2012; 345: e5661.
229. Higgins JPT, Green S, eds. Cochrane Handbook for Systematic Reviews of Interventions Version 5.1.0. The Cochrane Collaboration; 2011. http://www.cochrane-handbook.org, http://www.cochrane.org and http://www.thecochranelibrary.com
230. Cooper H, Hedges LV, Valentine JC, eds. The Handbook of Research Synthesis and Meta-Analysis. 2nd. ed. New York: Russell Sage Foundation; 2009.
231. Friedrich MJ. The Cochrane Collaboration turns 20 assessing the evidence to inform clinical care. JAMA 2013; 309: 1881–1882.
232. Cochrane AL. Effectiveness and Efficiency: Random Reflections on Health Services. London: Nuffield Provincial Hospitals Trust; 1972. London: British Medical Journal; 1989. London: Royal Society of Medicine Press; 1999.
233. Bosch X, ed. Archie Cochrane: Back to the Front. Barcelona: Institut Català d'Oncologia; 2004.
234. Stevenson A, Lindberg CA, eds. The New Oxford American Dictionary. 3rd. ed. Oxford: Oxford University Press; 2010.
235. Blackburn S. The Oxford Dictionary of Philosophy. 2nd. ed. Oxford: Oxford University Press; 2005.
236. Scott J, Marshall G, eds. A Dictionary of Sociology. 3rd. ed. Oxford: Oxford University Press; 2005.
237. Colman AM. A Dictionary of Psychology. 3rd. ed. Oxford: Oxford University Press; 2009.
238. Susser MW, Watson W, Hopper K. Sociology in Medicine. 3rd. ed. New York: Oxford University Press; 1985.
239. Samet JM, Muñoz A. Evolution of the cohort study. Epidemiol Rev 1998; 20: 1–14.
240. World Health Organization, UNICEF, World Bank. State of the World's Vaccines and Immunization. 3rd. ed. Geneva: World Health Organization; 2009. http://whqlibdoc.who.int/publications/2009/9789241563864_eng.pdf
241. Greenland S, Robins JM, Pearl J. Confounding and collapsibility in causal inference. Stat Sci 1999; 14: 29–46.
242. Greenland S. Quantifying biases in causal models: classical confounding vs. collider-stratification bias. Epidemiology 2003; 14: 300–306.
243. Cole SR, Platt RW, Schisterman EF, et al. Illustrating bias due to conditioning on a collider. Int J Epidemiol 2010; 39: 417–420.
244. Weissberg S. Applied Linear Regression. 3rd. ed. Hoboken: Wiley; 2005.
245. Bjornsson HT, Fallin MD, Feinberg AP. An integrated epigenetic and genetic approach to common human disease. Trends Genet 2004; 20: 350–358.
246. Vineis P. Public health and the common good. J Epidemiol Community Health 2014; 68: 97–100.
247. MacArthur WP, ed. Memoranda on Medical Diseases in Tropical and Subtropical Areas. London: HMSO; 1915; 1946; etc.
248. Anand S, Peter F, Sen A, eds. Public Health, Ethics, and Equity. Oxford: Oxford University Press; 2006.

249. Sen A. Development as Freedom. New York: Random House; 1999.

250. Morris JN. The uses of epidemiology. Br Med J 1955; 2: 395–401.

251. Institute of Medicine (IOM). Initial National Priorities for Comparative Effectiveness Research. Washington, DC: The National Academies Press; 2009.

252. Whitehead M, Petticrew M, Graham H, et al. Evidence for public health policy on inequalities: 2. Assembling the evidence jigsaw. J Epidemiol Community Health 2004; 58: 817–821.

253. Hoffmann K, Heidemann C, Weikert C, Schulze MB, Boeing H. Estimating the proportion of disease due to classes of sufficient causes. Am J Epidemiol 2006; 163: 76–83.

254. Diez Roux AV. A glossary for multilevel analysis. J Epidemiol Community Health 2002; 56: 588–594.

255. Pickett KE, Pearl M. Multilevel analyses of neighbourhood socioeconomic context and health outcomes: a critical review. J Epidemiol Community Health 2001; 55: 111–122.

256. Kakwani NC, Wagstaff A, van Doorslaer E. Socioeconomic inequalities in health: measurement, computation and statistical inference. J Econometrics 1997; 77(1): 87–104.

257. Wagstaff A, van Doorslaer E. Measuring inequalities in health in the presence of multiple-category morbidity indicators. Health Economics 1994; 3: 281–291.

258. Cumming G. Understanding the New Statistics: Effect Sizes, Confidence Intervals, and Meta-Analysis. New York: Routledge; 2012.

259. International Epidemiological Association. General Data Protection Regulation. http://ieaweb.org

260. Bankowski Z, Bryant JH, Last JM, eds. Ethics and Epidemiology: International Guidelines. Geneva: CIOMS/WHO; 1991.

261. Council for International Organizations of Medical Sciences (CIOMS), World Health Organization (WHO). International Ethical Guidelines for Epidemiological Studies. Geneva: CIOMS/WHO; 2008.

262. Council for International Organizations of Medical Sciences (CIOMS), World Health Organization (WHO). International Ethical Guidelines for Biomedical Research Involving Human Subjects. Geneva: CIOMS/WHO; 2002.

263. Fayerweather WE, Higginson J, Beauchamp TL, eds. Ethics in Epidemiology. New York: Pergamon Press; 1991.

264. International Epidemiological Association. Good Epidemiological Practice (GEP). Proper conduct in epidemiologic research. http://ieaweb.org/good-epidemiological-practice-gep/

265. American College of Epidemiology. Ethics guidelines. Ann Epidemiol 2000; 10 (Suppl 1): S1-S103.

266. International Committee of Medical Journal Editors (ICMJE). Uniform Requirements for Manuscripts Submitted to Biomedical Journals. http://www.icmje.org See also www.wame.org/ and www.publicationethics.org.uk

267. Michaels D. Doubt Is Their Product: How Industry's Assault on Science Threatens Your Health. New York: Oxford University Press; 2008.

268. Hernán MA, Hernández-Díaz S, Werler MM, Mitchell AA. Causal knowledge as a prerequisite for confounding evaluation: an application to birth defects epidemiology. Am J Epidemiol 2002; 155: 176–184.

269. Kleinbaum DG, Kupper LL, Morgenstern H. Epidemiologic Research: Principles and Quantitative Methods. Belmont, CA: Lifetime Learning Publications; 1982.

270. Miettinen OS. Theoretical Epidemiology: Principles of Occurrence Research in Medicine. New York: Wiley; 1985.

271. Rubin DB. Causal inference using potential outcomes: design, modeling, decisions. J Am Stat Assoc 2005; 100: 322–331.

272. Porta M. In: Hartzema AG, Porta M, Tilson HH, eds. Pharmacoepidemiology: An Introduction. 3rd. ed. Cincinatti: Harvey Whitney Books; 1998. p. 1–28.

273. Trouble at the lab: unreliable research. The Economist 2013 (Oct 19).

274. Mokkink WLB, Terwee CB, Alonso J, et al. COnsensus-based Standards for the selection of health Measurement INstruments. The COSMIN checklist. http://www.cosmin.nl/

275. Kane RL, Wang J, Garrard J. Reporting in randomized clinical trials improved after adoption of the CONSORT statement. J Clin Epidemiol 2007; 60: 241–249.

276. Sanderson S, Tatt ID, Higgins JPT. Tools for assessing quality and susceptibility to bias in observational studies in epidemiology: a systematic review and annotated bibliography. Int J Epidemiol 2007; 36: 666–676.

277. http://www.consort-statement.org and http://www.cochrane.dk

278. Pan American Health Organization. OSP, CE7, W-15. Washington, DC: PAHO; 1949.

279. Krieger N. Epidemiology and the People's Health: Theory and Context. New York: Oxford University Press; 2011.

280. Mansournia MA, Hernán MA, Greenland S. Matched designs and causal diagrams. Int J Epidemiol 2013; 42: 860–869.

281. Lipsitch M, Tchetgen E, Cohen T. Negative controls: a tool for detecting confounding and bias in observational studies. Epidemiology 2010; 21: 383–388.

282. Tchetgen EJ. The control outcome calibration approach with unobserved confounding. Am J Epidemiol 2014; 179: 633–640.

283. Marriott FHC, Kendall MG, eds. A Dictionary of Statistical Terms. 5th. ed. London: Longman; 1990.

284. Dobson A. The Oxford Dictionary of Statistical Terms. Oxford: Oxford University Press, 2003.

285. Jefferson TO, deMicheli V, Mugford M. Elementary Economic Evaluation in Health Care. 2nd. ed. London: BMJ Books; 2000.

286. Stern N. The Economics of Climate Change: The Stern Review on the Economics of Climate Change. Cambridge: Cambridge University Press; 2007.

287. United Nations Environment Programme (UNEP). Report on the Costs of Inaction on the Sound Management of Chemicals. Nairobi: UNEP; 2013. http://www.unep.org/hazardoussubstances/Portals/9/Mainstreaming/CostOfInaction/Report_Cost_of_Inaction_Feb2013.pdf

288. VanderWeele TJ, Hernán MA. From counterfactuals to sufficient component causes and vice versa. Eur J Epidemiol 2006; 21: 855–858.

289. Clayton D, Hills M. Statistical Models in Epidemiology. Oxford: Oxford University Press; 2013.

290. Marinker M, ed. Constructive Conversations About Health: Policy and Values. Oxford & Seattle: Radcliffe Publishing; 2006.

291. Gravetter FJ, Wallnau LB. Statistics for the Behavioral Sciences. 9th. ed. Belmont, CA: Wadsworth / Cengage; 2013.

292. Janes CR, Stall R, Gifford SM, eds. Anthropology and Epidemiology: Interdisciplinary Approaches to the Study of Health and Disease. Dordrecht: Reidel; 1986.

293. Anonymous. Cross design synthesis: a new strategy for studying medical outcomes? [Editorial]. Lancet 1992; 340: 944–946.

294. Greenland S. Quantitative methods in the review of epidemiologic literature. Epidemiol Rev 1987; 9: 1–30.

295. Greenland S, Robins J. Ecologic studies — Biases, misconceptions and counter-examples. Am J Epidemiol 1994; 139: 747–771.

296. International Statistical Classification of Diseases and Related Health Problems, 10th. rev. (ICD-10), Vol. 2. Geneva: World Health Organization, 1991.

297. Weinstein ND, Klein WM. Resistance of personal risk perceptions to debiasing interventions. Health Psychol 1995; 14: 132–140.

298. Croskerry P. The importance of cognitive errors in diagnosis and strategies to minimize them. Acad Med 2003; 78: 775–780.

299. Croskerry P, Singhal G, Mamede S. Cognitive debiasing, 1: Origins of bias and theory of debiasing. BMJ Qual Saf 2013; 22 (Suppl 2): ii58-ii64.

300. Petitti DB. Meta-Analysis, Decision Analysis and Cost-Effectiveness Analysis: Methods for Quantitative Synthesis in Medicine. 2nd. ed. New York: Oxford University Press; 1999.

301. Li G, Baker S, Langlois J, et al. Are female drivers safer? An application of the decomposition method. Epidemiology 1998; 9: 379–384.

302. World Health Organization. Health Impact Assessment (HIA). Glossary of Terms Used. http://www.who.int/hia/about/glos/en/index1.html

303. Bambra C, Gibson M, Sowden A, et al. Tackling the wider social determinants of health and health inequalities: evidence from systematic reviews. J Epidemiol Community Health 2010; 64: 284–291.

304. Braveman P, Egerter S, Williams DR. The social determinants of health: coming of age. Annu Rev Public Health 2011; 32: 381–398.

305. Mackenbach JP, Stirbu I, Roskam AJ, et al. Socioeconomic inequalities in health in 22 European countries. N Engl J Med 2008; 358:2468-2481.

306. Putnam S, Galea S. Epidemiology and the macrosocial determinants of health. J Public Health Policy 2008; 29: 275–289.

307. Bambra C. Going beyond "The three worlds of welfare capitalism": regime theory and public health research. J Epidemiol Community Health 2007; 61: 1098–1102.

308. Krieger N, Williams DR, Moss NE. Measuring social class in US public health research: concepts, methodologies, and guidelines. Annu Rev Public Health 1997; 18: 341–378.

309. O'Neill MS, McMichael AJ, Schwartz J, et al. Poverty, environment, and health: the role of environmental epidemiology and environmental epidemiologists. Epidemiology 2007; 18: 664–668.

310. McMichael AJ. Prisoners of the proximate: Loosening the constraints on epidemiology in an age of change. Am J Epidemiol 1999; 149: 887-897.

311. Kuh D, Ben-Shlomo Y, eds. A life course approach to chronic disease epidemiology. 2nd. ed. Oxford: Oxford University Press; 2004.

312. De Stavola BL, Nitsch D, Silva ID, et al. Statistical issues in life course epidemiology. Am J Epidemiol 2006; 163: 84–96.

313. Barker DJP. Fetal and Infant Origins of Adult Disease. London: British Medical Journal; 1992.

314. Barker DJP, Gluckman PD, Godfrey KM, et al. Fetal nutrition and cardiovascular disease in adult life. Lancet 1993; 341: 938–941.

315. Victora CG, Adair L, Fall C, et al. Maternal and child undernutrition: consequences for adult health and human capital. Lancet 2008; 371: 340–357.

316. Feinberg AP. Phenotypic plasticity and the epigenetics of human disease. Nature 2007; 447: 433–440.

317. Ozanne SE, Constancia M. Mechanisms of disease: the developmental origins of disease and the role of the epigenotype. Nat Clin Pract Endocrinol Metab 2007; 3: 539–546.

318. Schug TT, Barouki R, Gluckman PD, et al. Environmental stressors in the developmental origins of disease: evidence and mechanisms. Toxicol Sci 2013; 131: 343–350.

319. Barouki R, Gluckman PD, Grandjean P, et al. Developmental origins of noncommunicable disease: implications for research and public health. Environ Health 2012; 11: 42.

320. Burdge GC, Lillycrop KA. Nutrition, epigenetics and developmental plasticity; implications for understanding human disease. Ann Rev Nutr 2010; 30: 315–319.

321. Dolinoy DC, Huang D, Jirtle RL. Maternal nutrient supplementation counteracts bisphenol A-induced DNA hypomethylation in early development. Proc Natl Acad Sci USA 2007; 104:13056–13061.

322. Williamson MA, Snyder LM, eds. Wallach's Interpretation of Diagnostic Tests. 9th. ed. Philadelphia: Lippincott; 2011.

323. Pisano G. Science Business: The Promise, the Reality, and the Future of Biotech. Boston, MA: Harvard Business School Press; 2006.

324. Curtis VA. Dirt, disgust and disease: a natural history of hygiene. J Epidemiol Community health 2007; 61: 660-664.

325. Salathé M, Freifeld CC, Mekaru SR, Tomasulo AF, Brownstein JS. Influenza A (H7N9) and the importance of digital epidemiology. N Engl J Med 2013; 369: 401–404.

326. Blalock HM. Causal Inference in Non-experimental Research. Chapel Hill, NC: University of North Carolina Press; 1964. Blalock HM Jr, ed. Causal Models in the Social Sciences. 2nd. ed. New York: Aldine; 1985. Blalock HM Jr, ed. Causal Models in Experimental Designs. Piscataway, NJ: Aldine; 2007.

327. Arnesen T, Nord E. The value of DALY life: problems with ethics and validity of disability adjusted life years. BMJ 1999; 319: 1423–1425.

328. Mathers CD, Robine JM, Wilkins R. Health expectancy indicators. Recommendations for terminology. In: Mathers CD, Robine JM, McCallum J, eds. Proceedings of Seventh Meeting of the International Network on Health Expectancy (REVES). Canberra: Australian Institute of Health and Welfare; 1994.

329. Pepe MS. The statistical evaluation of medical tests for classification and prediction. Oxford: Oxford University Press; 2003.

330. Pepe MS, Janes H, Longton G, et al. Limitations of the odds ratio in gauging the performance of a diagnostic, prognostic, or screening marker. Am J Epidemiol 2004; 159: 882–890.

331. Pencina MJ, D'Agostino RB, Sr., D'Agostino RB, Jr., et al. Evaluating the added predictive ability of a new marker: From area under the ROC curve to reclassification and beyond. Stat Med 2008; 27: 157–172.

332. Twaddle AC. Sickness and sickness career: some implications. In: Eisenberg L, Kleinman A, eds. The Relevance of Social Science for Medicine. Dordrecht: Reidel; 1981. p. 111–133.

333. Kleinman A. The Illness Narratives: Suffering, Healing, and the Human Condition. New York: Basic Books; 1988.

334. Coe RM. Sociology of Medicine. New York: McGraw-Hill; 1970. p. 89–115.

335. Eisenberg L. The subjective in medicine. Perspect Biol Med 1983; 1: 40–48.

336. Kleinman A, Eisenberg L, Good B. Culture, illness and care: clinical lessons from anthropologic and cross-cultural research. Ann Inter Med 1978; 88: 251–258.

337. Moynihan R, Dora E, Henry D. Disease mongering is now part of the global health debate. PLoS Med 2008; 5 (5): 684–686.

338. Payer L. Disease-Mongers: How Doctors, Drug Companies, and Insurers Are Making You Feel Sick. New York: Wiley; 1992.

339. Porta M, Hernández-Aguado I, Lumbreras B, et al. "Omics" research, monetization of intellectual property and fragmentation of knowledge: can clinical epidemiology strengthen integrative research? J Clin Epidemiol 2007; 60: 1220–1225.

340. Whiting P, Rutjes AWS, Reitsma JB, et al. The development of QUADAS: a tool for the quality assessment of studies of diagnostic accuracy included in systematic reviews. BMC Med Res Methodol 2003; 3: 25. http://www.bris.ac.uk/quadas/.

341. Soto-Ramírez N, Ziyab AH, Karmaus W, et al. Epidemiologic methods of assessing asthma and wheezing episodes in longitudinal studies: measures of change and stability. J Epidemiol 2013; 23: 399–410.

342. Vandenberg LN, Colborn T, Hayes TB, et al. Hormones and endocrine-disrupting chemicals: low-dose effects and nonmonotonic dose responses. Endocr Rev 2012; 33: 378–455.

343. Lyytinen HK, Dyba T, Ylikorkala O, et al. A case-control study on hormone therapy as a risk factor for breast cancer in Finland: intrauterine system carries a risk as well. Int J Cancer 2010; 126: 483–489.

344. Doll R, Peto R. Mortality in relation to smoking: 20 years' observations on male British doctors. Br Med J 1976; 2: 1525–1536.

345. Bang H, Robins JM. Doubly robust estimation in missing data and causal inference models. Biometrics 2005; 61: 962–973.

346. Funk MJ, Westreich D, Wiesen C, et al. Doubly robust estimation of causal effects. Am J Epidemiol 2011; 173: 761–767.

347. United States National Center for Infectious Diseases, Division of Parasitic Diseases, 2004. http://www.cdc.gov/malaria/glossary.htm.

348. Raviglione MC, Smith IM. XDR tuberculosis: implications for global public health. N Engl J Med 2007; 356: 656–659.

349. Khoury MJ, Burke W, Thomson EJ. Genetics and Public Health in the 21st Century: Using Genetic Information to Improve Health and Prevent Disease. New York: Oxford University Press; 2000.

350. Susser M, Susser E. Choosing a future for epidemiology: I. Eras and paradigms. Am J Public Health 1996; 86: 668–673.

351. Susser M, Susser E. Choosing a future for epidemiology: II. From black box to Chinese boxes and eco-epidemiology. Am J Public Health 1996; 86: 674–677.

352. Porta M, Alvarez-Dardet C. Epidemiology: bridges over (and across) roaring levels [Editorial]. J Epidemiol Community Health 1998; 52: 605.

353. Drummond MF, Sculpher MJ, Torrance GW, et al. Methods for the Economic Evaluation of Health Care Programmes. 3rd. ed. Oxford: Oxford University Press, 2005.

354. Palmer S, Torgerson DJ. Economic notes: definitions of efficiency. BMJ 1999; 318: 1136.

355. Krugman P, Wells R. Microeconomics. 3rd. ed. New York: Worth, 2013.

356. Torrance GW. The measurement of health status utilities for economic appraisal: a review. J Health Economics 1986; 5: 1-30.

357. Krieger N. A glossary for social epidemiology. J Epidemiol Community Health 2001; 55: 693-700.

358. Eikemo TA, Bambra C. The welfare state: a glossary for public health. J Epidemiol Community Health 2008; 62: 3–6.

359. Martens P, McMichael AJ, eds. Environmental Change, Climate and Health. Cambridge: Cambridge University Press; 2003.

360. White F, Stallones L, Last J. Global Public Health: Ecological Foundations. New York: Oxford University Press; 2013.

361. Kavanagh AM, Broom DH. Embodied risk: my body, myself? Soc Sci Med 1998; 46: 437–444.

362. Krieger N. Embodiment: a conceptual glossary for epidemiology. J Epidemiol Community Health 2005; 59:350–355.

363. Everett M. The social life of genes: privacy, property and the new genetics. Soc Sci Med 2003; 56: 53–65.

364. Hall E. Spaces and networks of genetic knowledge making: the "geneticisation" of heart disease. Health Place 2004; 10: 311–318.

365. Scheper-Hughes N, Wacquant L, eds. Commodifying Bodies. London: Sage; 2006.

366. Fielding JE, Teutsch SM. Public Health Practice: What Works. New York: Oxford University Press; 2012.

367. Jones KE, Patel NG, Levy MA, et al. Global trends in emerging infectious diseases. Nature 2008; 451: 990–993.

368. Wolfe ND, Dunavan CP, Diamond J. Origins of major human infectious diseases. Nature 2007; 447: 279–283.

369. Benach J, Muntaner C, Santana V. Employment Conditions Knowledge Network (EMCONET). Employment Conditions and Health Inequalities: Final report to the WHO Commission on Social Determinants of Health (CSDH). Geneva: World Health Organization; 2007. http://www.who.int/social_determinants/resources/articles/emconet_who_report.pdf

370. International Labour Organization. Decent Work. http://www.ilo.org/global/topics/decent-work/lang--en/index.htm

371. Banta JE. Treating the traveler: a brief guide to emporiatrics. Postgrad Med 1973; 53: 53–58.

372. Kelly-Hope LA, McKenzie FE. The multiplicity of malaria transmission: a review of entomological inoculation rate measurements and methods across sub-Saharan Africa. Malar J 2009; 8: 19.

373. Shaukat AM, Breman JG, McKenzie FE. Using the entomological inoculation rate to assess the impact of vector control on malaria parasite transmission and elimination. Malar J 2010; 9: 122.

374. Everitt BS. Statistics in the Medical Sciences. Cambridge: Cambridge University Press; 1995.

375. Brown P. Race, class and environmental health: a review and systematization of the literature. Environ Res 1995; 69: 15-30.
376. Cohen JE. How Many People Can the Earth Support? New York: Norton; 1995. p. 13.
377. Nieuwenhuijsen MJ. Exposure Assessment in Occupational and Environmental Epidemiology. Oxford: Oxford University Press; 2003.
378. Herbst AL, Ulfelder H, Poskanzer DC. Adenocarcinoma of the vagina: association of maternal stilbestrol therapy with tumor appearance in young women. N Engl J Med 1971; 284: 878–881.
379. Centers for Disease Control: Pneumocystis pneumonia–Los Angeles. MMWR 1981; 30: 250–252.
380. European Centre for Disease Prevention and Control (ECDC). Epidemic Intelligence. www.ecdc.eu.int/Activities/Epidemic_Intelligence.html.
381. World Health Organization. Epidemic and Pandemic Alert and Response (EPR). http://www.who.int/csr/alertresponse/epidemicintelligence/en/index.html.
382. Rosen G. A History of Public Health. New York: MD Publications; 1958.
383. Hecker JFK. Der grossen Volkskrankheiten des Mittelalters (Epidemics of the Middle Ages). Berlin: Enslin, 1865 (English translation published by the Sydenham Society, London, 1883).
384. Creighton C. A History of Epidemics in Britain. 2 vols. Cambridge: Cambridge University Press; 1891–1994.
385. Fine PEM. Herd immunity: history, theory, practice. Epidemiol Rev 1993; 15: 265–302.
386. McNeill W. Plagues and Peoples. New York: Doubleday; 1976.
387. McKeown T. The Origins of Human Disease. Oxford: Blackwell; 1988.
388. Pusey WA. The History and Epidemiology of Syphilis. Springfield, IL: Thomas; 1933.
389. Dubos R, Dubos J. The White Plague: Tuberculosis, Man and Society. Boston: Little, Brown; 1952.
390. Hopkins DR. The Greatest Killer: Smallpox in History. Chicago: The University of Chicago Press; 2002.
391. Zinsser H. Rats, Lice and History. Boston: Little, Brown; 1935.
392. Grmek MD. History of AIDS: Emergence and Origin of a Modern Pandemic. Princeton: Princeton University Press; 1990.
393. Grmek MD. Les Maladies à l'Aube de la Civilisation Occidentale. Paris: Payot; 1983.
394. Grmek MD. Diseases in the Ancient Greek World. Baltimore: Johns Hopkins University Press; 1991.
395. Evans AS. Causation and Disease: A Chronological Journey. New York: Plenum; 1993.
396. Omran AR. The epidemiologic transition; a theory of the epidemiology of population change. Milbank Mem Fund Quart 1971; 49: 509–538 (Reprinted: Bull World Health Org 2001; 79: 161–170).
397. Mackenbach JP. The epidemiologic transition theory. J Epidemiol Community Health 1994; 48: 329–332.
398. Amsterdamska O. Demarcating epidemiology. Science Technol Human Values 2005; 30: 17–51.
399. Porta M, Vandenbroucke JP, Ioannidis JPA, et al. Trends in citations to books on epidemiological and statistical methods in the biomedical literature. PLoS One 2013; 8(5): e61837.
400. Willett W, Greenland S, MacMahon B, et al. The discipline of epidemiology. Science 1995; 269: 1325–1326.

401. Trichopoulos D. Accomplishments and prospects of epidemiology. Prev Med 1996; 25: 4–6.

402. MacMahon B. Strengths and limitations of epidemiology. In: The National Research Council in 1979. Washington, DC: National Academy of Sciences; 1979.

403. Shy CM. The failure of academic epidemiology: witness for the prosecution. Am J Epidemiol 1997; 145: 479–484.

404. Wing S. Limits of epidemiology. Med Global Surv 1994; 1: 74–86.

405. Samet JM. Epidemiology and policy: the pump handle meets the new millennium. Epidemiol Rev 2000; 22: 145–154.

406. Krieger N. Epidemiology and the web of causation: has anyone seen the spider? Soc Sci Med 1994; 39: 887–903.

407. Bambra C. Changing the world? Reflections on the interface between social science, epidemiology and public health. J Epidemiol Community Health 2009; 63: 867–868.

408. Vandenbroucke JP. Is "The causes of cancer" a miasma theory for the end of the twentieth century? Int J Epidemiol 1988; 17: 708–709.

409. Jablonka E. Epigenetic epidemiology. Int J Epidemiol 2004; 33: 929–935.

410. Feinberg AP, Tycko B. The history of cancer epigenetics. Nat Rev Cancer 2004; 4: 143–153.

411. Jaenisch R, Bird A. Epigenetic regulation of gene expression: how the genome integrates intrinsic and environmental signals. Nat Genet 2003; 33Supl: 245–254.

412. Vercelli D. Genetics, epigenetics, and the environment: switching, buffering, releasing. J Allergy Clin Immunol 2004; 113: 381–386.

413. Thayer ZM, Kuzawa CW. Biological memories of past environments: epigenetic pathways to health disparities. Epigenetics 2011; 6: 798–803.

414. Herman JG, Baylin SB. Gene silencing in cancer in association with promoter hypermethylation. N Engl J Med 2003; 349: 2042–2054.

415. Poirier MC. Chemical-induced DNA damage and human cancer risk. Nat Rev Cancer 2004; 4: 630–637.

416. Luch A. Nature and nurture: lessons from chemical carcinogenesis. Nat Rev Cancer 2005; 5: 113–125.

417. Ting AH, McGarvey KM, Baylin SB. The cancer epigenome: components and functional correlates. Genes Dev 2006; 20: 3215–3231.

418. www.cdc.gov/epiinfo.

419. Knorr-Cetina K. Epistemic cultures. In: Restivo S, ed. Science, Technology, and Society: An Encyclopedia. Oxford: Oxford University Press; 2005.

420. Carpiano RM, Daley DM. A guide and glossary on postpositivist theory building for population health. J Epidemiol Community Health 2006; 60: 564–570.

421. Miettinen OS. Epidemiology: quo vadis? Eur J Epidemiol 2004; 19: 713–718.

422. Bolúmar F, Porta M. Epidemiologic methods: beyond clinical medicine, beyond epidemiology. Eur J Epidemiol 2004; 19: 733–735.

423. Enhancing the Quality and Transparency of Health Research (EQUATOR). http://www.equator-network.org

424. White M, Adams J, Heywood P. How and why do interventions that increase health overall widen inequalities within populations? In: Babones SJ, ed. Social Inequality and Public Health. Bristol: Policy Press; 2012. p. 65–81.

425. Lorenc T, Petticrew M, Welch V, et al. What types of interventions generate inequalities? Evidence from systematic reviews. J Epidemiol Community Health 2013; 67: 190–193.

426. Benach J, Malmusi D, Yasui Y, et al. A new typology of policies to tackle health inequalities and scenarios of impact based on Rose's population approach. J Epidemiol Community Health 2013; 67: 286–291.

427. Taket A. Health Equity, Social Justice and Human Rights. Abingdon: Routledge; 2012.

428. Machin D, Day S, Green S, eds. Textbook of Clinical Trials. Hoboken, NJ: Wiley; 2004.

429. Schwartz S, Carpenter KM. The right answer to the wrong question: consequences of type III error for public health research. Am J Public Health 1999; 89: 1175–1180.

430. Bhopal R. Glossary of terms relating to ethnicity and race: for reflection and debate. J Epidemiol Community Health 2004; 58: 441–445.

431. Tajima K, Sonoda S. Ethnoepidemiology, a new paradigm for studying cancer risk factors and prevention strategy. In: Tajima K, Sonoda S, eds. Ethnoepidemiology of Cancer. Tokyo: Japan Scientific Societies Press; 1996.

432. Black N, Neuhauser D. Books that have changed health services and health care policy. J Health Serv Res Policy 2006; 11: 180–183.

433. Evans AS. Causation and disease: the Henle-Koch postulates revisited. Yale J Biol Med 1976; 49: 175–195.

434. Ransohoff DF. Rules of evidence for cancer molecular-marker discovery and validation. Nat Rev Cancer 2004; 4: 309–314.

435. Ransohoff DF. How to improve reliability and efficiency of research about molecular markers: roles of phases, guidelines, and study design. J Clin Epidemiol 2007; 60: 1205–1219.

436. Brownson RC, Gurney JG, Land G. Evidence-based decision making in public health. J Pub Health Management Pract 1999; 5: 86–97.

437. Rychetnik L, Frommer M, Hawe P, Shiell A. Criteria for evaluating evidence on public health interventions. J Epidemiol Community Health 2002; 56: 119–127.

438. Rychetnik L, Hawe P, Waters E, et al. A glossary for evidence based public health. J Epidemiol Community Health 2004; 58: 538–545.

439. Rodríguez-Artalejo F. La salud pública basada en la evidencia. Gac Sanit 1997; 11: 201–203.

440. Browson RC, Baker EA, Lee TL, et al. Evidence-Based Public Health. 2nd. ed. New York: Oxford University Press; 2011.

441. Oxman AD, Lavis JN, Lewin S, et al. SUPPORT Tools for evidence-informed health Policymaking (STP) 1: what is evidence-informed policymaking? Health Res Policy Syst 2009; 7(Suppl 1): S1.

442. Kramer JM. The rising pandemic of mental disorders and associated chronic diseases and disabilities. Acta Psychiatr Scand 1980; 62 (suppl 285): 382–397.

443. Thorpe KE, Zwarenstein M, Oxman AD, et al. A pragmatic-explanatory continuum indicator summary (PRECIS): a tool to help trial designers. J Clin Epidemiol 2009; 62: 464–475.

444. Schwartz D, Lellouch J. Explanatory and pragmatic attitudes in therapeutic trials. J Chron Dis 1967; 20: 637–648.

445. Schwartz D, Flamant L, Lellouch J. L'Essai Thérapeutique Chez l'Homme. 2nd. ed. Paris: Flammarion; 1981.

446. Wild CP. Complementing the genome with an "exposome": the outstanding challenge of environmental exposure measurement in molecular epidemiology. Cancer Epidemiol Biomarkers Prev 2005; 14: 1847–1850.

447. Wild CP. The exposome: from concept to utility. Int J Epidemiol 2012; 41: 24–32.

448. Centers for Disease Control and Prevention (2012). Exposome and Exposomics. http://www.cdc.gov/niosh/topics/exposome.

449. White E, Saracci R, Armstrong BK. Principles of Exposure Measurement in Epidemiology. 2nd. ed. Oxford: Oxford University Press; 2008.

450. Duffus JH, Nordberg M, Templeton DM, eds. (for the International Union of Pure and Applied Chemistry). Glossary of terms used in toxicology. 2nd. ed. (IUPAC Recommendations 2007). Pure Appl Chem 2007; 79: 1153–1344. http://sis.nlm.nih.gov/enviro/iupacglossary/frontmatter.html

451. Kazandjian VA. The extremal quotient in small area variation analysis. Health Serv Res 1989; 24: 665–684.

452. Benjamini Y, Hochberg Y. Controlling the false discovery rate: a practical and powerful approach to multiple testing. J Royal Stat Soc Series B (Methodological) 1995; 57: 289–300.

453. Strimmer K. A unified approach to false discovery rate estimation. BMC Bioinformatics 2008; 9: 303.

454. Khoury MJ, Bedrosian SR, Gwinn M, et al., eds. Human Genome Epidemiology: Building the Evidence for Using Genetics Information to Improve Health and Prevent Disease. 2nd. ed. New York: Oxford University Press; 2010.

455. Ondaatje M. Running in the Family. London: Bloomsbury; 1993. p. 47–48, 86–87.

456. Camus A. Le Premier Homme. Paris: Gallimard; 1994.

457. Yoon PW, Scheuner MT, Khoury MJ. Research priorities for evaluating family history in the prevention of common chronic diseases. Am J Prev Med 2003; 24: 128–135.

458. ICD-10. Vol. 1: Report of the International Conference for the Tenth Revision of the International Classification of Diseases. Geneva: WHO; 1993. p. 9–28.

459. Madden R, Sykes C, Ustun TB, for the World Health Organization. Family of International Classifications: Definition, Scope and Purpose. 2007. http://www.who.int/classifications/en/FamilyDocument2007.pdf

460. Farr W. Vital Statistics. A Memorial Volume of Selections from the Reports and Writings of William Farr. Edited by Noel Humphries. London: Stanford; 1985.

461. Goodman RA, Munson JW, Dammers K, et al. Forensic epidemiology: law at the intersection of public health and criminal investigations. J Law Med Ethics 2003; 31: 684–700. http://www.publichealthlaw.info.

462. Independent UK Panel on Breast Cancer Screening. The benefits and harms of breast cancer screening: an independent review. Lancet 2012; 380: 1778–1786.

463. Goldberger AL, West BJ. Fractals in physiology and medicine. Yale J Biol Med 1987; 60: 421–435.

464. Abramson JH, Abramson ZH. Making Sense of Data: A Self-Instruction Manual of the Interpretation of Epidemiological Data. 3rd. ed. New York: Oxford University Press; 2001.

465. Egger M, Smith GD, Schneider M, et al. Bias in meta-analysis detected by a simple, graphical test. BMJ 1997; 315: 629–634.

466. Peters JL, Sutton AJ, Jones DR, et al. Contour-enhanced meta-analysis funnel plots help distinguish publication bias from other causes of asymmetry. J Clin Epidemiol 2008; 61: 991–996.

467. Song F, Parekh S, Hooper L, et al. Dissemination and publication of research findings: an updated review of related biases. Health Technol Assess 2010; 14: iii-xi, 1–193.

468. Shiri R, Karppinen J, Leino-Arjas P, et al. The association between obesity and low back pain: a meta-analysis. Am J Epidemiol 2010; 171: 135–154.

469. Borrell C, Muntaner C, Benach J, et al. Social class and self-reported health status among men and women: what is the role of work organisation, household material standards and household labour? Soc Sci Med 2004; 58: 1869–1887.

470. Morange M. The Misunderstood Gene. Cambridge, MA: Harvard University Press; 2001.

471. Anonymous. Coping with complexity [editorial]. Nature 2006; 441: 383–384.

472. ENCODE Project Consortium. Identification and analysis of functional elements in 1% of the human genome by the ENCODE pilot project. Nature 2007; 447: 799–816.

473. Hunter DJ. Gene-environment interactions in human diseases. Nat Rev Genet 2005; 6: 287–298.

474. Rothman KJ, Gallacher JE, Hatch EE, et al. Why representativeness should be avoided. Int J Epidemiol 2013; 42: 1012–1028.

475. Khoury MJ, Beaty TH, Cohen BH. Fundamentals of Genetic Epidemiology. New York: Oxford University Press; 1993.

476. Adelman DE. The false promise of the genomics revolution for environmental law. Harvard Environ Law Rev 2005; 29: 117–177.

477. Davey Smith G, Ebrahim S, Lewis S, et al. Genetic epidemiology and public health: hope, hype, and future prospects. Lancet 2005; 366: 1484–1498.

478. Vineis P, Schulte P, McMichael AJ. Misconceptions about the use of genetic tests in populations. Lancet 2001; 357: 709–12.

479. Vainio H. Genetic biomarkers and occupational epidemiology: recollections, reflections and reconsiderations. Scand J Work Environ Health 2004; 30: 1–3.

480. Caporaso NE. Why have we failed to find the low penetrance genetic constituents of common cancers? Cancer Epidemiol Biomarkers Prev 2002; 11: 1544–1549.

481. Shostak S. Locating gene-environment interaction: at the intersections of genetics and public health. Social Sci Med 2003; 56: 2327–2342.

482. Porta M. The genome sequence is a jazz score. Int J Epidemiol 2003; 32: 29–31.

483. Menashe I, Figueroa JD, Garcia-Closas M, et al. Large-scale pathway-based analysis of bladder cancer genome-wide association data from five studies of European background. PLoS One 2012; 7(1): e29396.

484. Manolio TA, Collins FS, Cox NJ, et al. Finding the missing heritability of complex diseases. Nature 2009; 461: 747–753.

485. Zintzaras E, Lau J. Synthesis of genetic association studies for pertinent gene-disease associations requires appropriate methodological and statistical approaches. J Clin Epidemiol 2008; 61: 634–645.

486. www.gis.com.

487. Robins JM. The analysis of randomized and non-randomized AIDS treatment trials using a new approach to causal inference in longitudinal studies: health service research methodology: a focus on AIDS. In: Sechrest L, Freeman H, Mulley A, eds. Washington, DC: U.S. Public Health Service, National Center for Health Services Research; 1989. p. 113–159.

488. Robins JM. Marginal structural models versus structural nested models as tools for causal inference. In: Halloran ME, Berry D, eds. Statistical Models in Epidemiology: The Environment and Clinical Trials. New York: Springer; 1999.

489. Robins JM, Hernán MA. Estimation of the causal effects of time-varying exposures. In: Fitzmaurice G, Davidian M, Verbeke G, et al., eds. Advances in Longitudinal Data Analysis. New York: Chapman and Hall/CRC Press; 2009. p. 553–559.

490. Gini C. Measurement of inequality of incomes. Economic Journal 1921; 31 (No. 121): 124–126.

491. De Maio FG. Income inequality measures. J Epidemiol Community Health 2007; 61: 849–852.

492. Koplan JP, Bond T, Merson M, et al. Towards a common definition of global health. Lancet 2009; 373: 1993–1995.

493. Campbell RM, Pleic M, Connolly H. The importance of a common global health definition: how Canada's definition influences its strategic direction in global health. J Glob Health 2012; 2: 10301.

494. World Health Organization. Trade, Foreign Policy, Diplomacy and Health: Glossary of Globalization, Trade and Health Terms. http://www.who.int/trade/glossary/en/

495. Kawachi I. Globalization and workers' health. Industr Health 2008; 46: 421–423.

496. Smith R. Globalization: the key challenge facing health economics in the 21st century. Health Economics 2008; 17: 1–3.

497. Smith RD, Chanda R, Tangcharoensathien V. Trade and health: 4. Trade in health-related services. Lancet 2009; 373: 593–601.

498. Labonte R, Mohindra K, Schrecker T. The growing impact of globalization for health and public health practice. Annu Rev Public Health 2001; 32: 263–283.

499. www.ich.org.

500. www.wma.net/e/policy/b3.htm.

501. www.emea.europa.eu/Inspections/GCPgeneral.html.

502. www.fda.gov/oc/gcp/default.htm.

503. http://apps.who.int/medicinedocs/pdf/whozip13e/whozip13e.pdf

504. Guyatt G, Oxman AD, Akl EA, et al. GRADE guidelines: 1. Introduction. GRADE evidence profiles and summary of findings tables. J Clin Epidemiol 2011; 64: 383-394.

505. Stafoggia M, Lallo A, Fusco D, et al. Spie charts, target plots, and radar plots for displaying comparative outcomes of health care. J Clin Epidemiol 2011; 64: 770–778.

506. McDonald CJ, Overhage JM. Guidelines you can follow and can trust: an ideal and an example. JAMA 1994; 271: 872–873.

507. Mayo E. The Social Problems of an Industrial Civilization. London: Routledge; 1949.

508. Wickström G, Bendix T. The "Hawthorne effect": what did the original Hawthorne studies actually show? Scand J Work Environ Health 2000; 26: 363–367.

509. Leonard K, Masatu MC. Outpatient process quality evaluation and the Hawthorne effect. Soc Sci Med 2006; 63: 2330–2340.

510. Stokes J, 3rd., Noren JJ, Shindell S. Definition of terms and concepts applicable to clinical preventive medicine. J Commun Health 1982; 8: 33–41.

511. Becker MH, ed. The Health Belief Model and Personal Health Behavior. Thorofare, NJ: Slack; 1974.

512. Robine JM, Mathers CD, Bucquet D. Distinguishing health expectancies and health-adjusted life expectancies. Am J Public Health 1993; 83: 797–798.

513. European Observatory on Health Systems and Policies. Research Topics: Health Impact Assessment. www.euro.who.int/observatory.

514. Ståhl T, Wismar M, Ollila E, et al. Health in All Policies: Prospects and Potentials. Helsinki: Ministry of Social Affairs and Health; 2006.

515. Freiler A, Muntaner C, Shankardass K, et al. Glossary for the implementation of Health in All Policies (HiAP). J Epidemiol Community Health 2013; 67: 1068–1072.

516. World Health Organization. Ottawa Charter for Health Promotion. Geneva: WHO; 1986.

517. Donabedian A. A Guide to Medical Care Administration, Vol. 2. New York: American Public Health Association; 1969.

518. Korn EL, Graubard BI. Analysis of Health Surveys. New York: Wiley; 1999.

519. Aday LA. Designing and Conducting Health Surveys: A Comprehensive Guide. 2nd. ed. San Francisco: Jossey-Bass; 2006.

520. World Health Organization. The World Health Report 2000: Health Systems: Improving Performance. Geneva: World Health Organization; 2000.

521. Varkevisser CN, Pathmanathan I, Brownlee A. Designing and Conducting Health Systems Research Projects. Geneva: International Development Research Centre and World Health Organization; 1991.

522. Milio N. Public Health in the Market: Facing Managed Care, Lean Government, and Health Disparities. Ann Arbor, MI: The University of Michigan Press; 2000.

523. McMichael AJ, Spirtas R, Kupper LL. An epidemiologic study of mortality within a cohort of rubber workers, 1964-72. J Occup Med 1974; 16: 458–464.

524. Mehrez A, Gafni A. Quality adjusted life years, utility theory and healthy years equivalents. Med Decis Making 1989; 9: 142–149.

525. Hyder AA, Rotllant G, Morrow RH. Measuring the burden of disease: healthy life years. Am J Pub Health 1998; 88: 196–202.

526. Allaby M. A Dictionary of Zoology. Oxford: Oxford University Press; 2009.

527. Fox JP, Elveback L, Scott W, et al. Herd immunity: basic concept and relevance to public health immunization practices. Am J Epidemiol 1971; 94: 179-189.

528. Müller-Wille S, Rheinberger HJ, editors. Heredity Produced: At the Crossroads of Biology, Politics, and Culture, 1500-1870. Cambridge, MA: The MIT Press; 2007.

529. Cobb M. Heredity before genetics: a history. Nat Rev Genetics 2006; 7: 953–958.

530. Vineis P, Pearce NE. Genome-wide association studies may be misinterpreted: genes versus heritability. Carcinogenesis 2011; 32: 1295–1298.

531. Canadian Task Force on the Periodic Health Examination. The Canadian Guide to Clinical Preventive Health Care. Ottawa; 1994.

532. U.S. Preventive Services Task Force. Guide to Clinical Preventive Services 2006. Baltimore, MD: Williams & Wilkins, 2006.

533. Hill AB. The environment and disease: association or causation. Proc R Soc Med 1965; 58: 295–300.

534. Calabrese EJ. Hormesis: a revolution in toxicology, risk assessment and medicine. EMBO Rep 2004; 5(Suppl 1): S37–S40.

535. Calabrese EJ, Baldwin LA. Toxicology rethinks its central belief. Nature 2003; 421: 691–692.

536. www.cdc.gov/genomics/hugenet

537. Popper K. The Logic of Scientific Discovery. 11th. ed. London: Hutchinson; 1983.

538. Buck C. Popper's philosophy for epidemiologists. Int J Epidemiol 1975; 4: 159–168.

539. Gifford SM. The meaning of lumps: A case study of the ambiguities of risk. In: Janes CR, Stall R, Gifford SM, eds. Anthropology and Epidemiology: Interdisciplinary Approaches to the Study of Health and Disease. Dordrecht: Reidel; 1986. p. 213–246.

540. Last JM. The iceberg. Lancet 1963; 2: 28–31.

541. Van der Vaart AW. Asymptotic Statistics. New York: Cambridge Univ Press; 1998.

542. www.ieaweb.org and http://ije.oxfordjournals.org

543. Suissa S, Ernst P. Bias in observational study of the effectiveness of nasal cortico-steroids in asthma. J Allergy Clin Immunol 2005; 115: 714–719.

544. Baker JL. Evaluating the Impact of Development Projects on Poverty: A Handbook for Practitioners. Washington, DC: The World Bank; 2000. http://siteresources.worldbank.org/INTISPMA/Resources/handbook.pdf

545. Gertler PJ, Martinez S, Premand P, et al. Impact Evaluation in Practice. Washington, DC, USA: The International Bank for Reconstruction and Development/The World Bank, 2011.

546. Heller RF, Dobson AJ, Attia J, et al. Impact numbers: measures of risk factor impact on the whole population from case-control and cohort studies. J Epidemiol Community Health 2002; 56: 606–610.

547. National Institutes of Health. Implementation Science Information and Resources. http://www.fic.nih.gov/researchtopics/pages/implementationscience.aspx

548. Ioannidis JP, Schully SD, Lam TK, et al. Knowledge integration in cancer: current landscape and future prospects. Cancer Epidemiol Biomarkers Prev 2013; 22: 3–10.

549. King RC, Stansfield WD, Mulligan PK. A Dictionary of Genetics. Oxford: Oxford University Press; 2007.

550. Eysenbach G. Infodemiology and infoveillance: framework for an emerging set of public health informatics methods to analyze search, communication and publication behavior on the internet. J Med Internet Res 2009; 11(1): e11.

551. Illner AK, Freisling H, Boeing H, et al. Review and evaluation of innovative technologies for measuring diet in nutritional epidemiology. Int J Epidemiol 2012; 41:1187-1203.

552. Relman AS. The Ingelfinger rule. N Engl J Med 1981; 305: 824-826.

553. Angell M, Kassirer JP. The Ingelfinger rule revisited. N Engl J Med 1991; 325: 1371–1373.

554. Altman LK. The Ingelfinger rule, embargoes, and journal peer review. Part 1. Lancet 1996; 347: 1382-1386. Part 2. Lancet 1996; 347: 1459–1463.

555. Cavallis L, Feldman MW. Models for cultural inheritance: 1. Group mean and within group variation. Theoretical Population Biology 1973; 4: 42–55.

556. Baker SP, O'Neill B, Ginsburg MJ, et al., eds. The injury fact book. New York: Oxford University Press; 1992.

557. Hernán MA, Robins JM. Instruments for causal inference: an epidemiologist's dream? Epidemiology 2006; 17: 360–372.

558. http://www.who.int/classifications/icf/en/

559. Classification Committee of the World Organization of National Colleges, Academies, and Academic Associations of General Practitioners/Family Physicians (WONCA). International Classification of Primary Care (ICPC-2). 2nd. ed. Oxford: Oxford

University Press; 1998. http://www.globalfamilydoctor.com and http://www.woncaeurope.org.

560. Classification Committee of the World Organization of National Colleges, Academies, and Academic Associations of General Practitioners/Family Physicians (WONCA). International Classification of Primary Care (ICPC-2-R). 2nd. ed, revised. Oxford: Oxford University Press; 2005.

561. Horton R. The rhetoric of research. BMJ 1995; 310: 985–987.

562. Vandenbroucke JP. Medical journals and the shaping of medical knowledge. Lancet 1998; 352: 2001-2006.

563. Gould SJ. The Hedgehog, the Fox and the Magister's Pox: Mending and Minding the Misconceived Gap Between Science and the Humanities. London: Vintage; 2004. p. 102-104, 113-116.

564. Rothenburg R, Ford ES, Vaitianen R. Ischemic heart disease: estimating the impact of interventions. J Clin Epidemiol 1992; 45: 21–29.

565. Tudor Hart J. The inverse care law. Lancet 1971; 1: 405–412.

566. Hernán MA, Robins JM. Estimating causal effects from epidemiological data. J Epidemiol Community Health 2006; 60; 578–586.

567. http://www.cancer.fi/syoparekisteri/en/

568. Tanaka K, Hirohata T, Takeshita S, et al. Hepatitis B virus, cigarette smoking and alcohol consumption in the development of hepatocellular carcinoma: a case-control study in Fukuoka, Japan. Int J Cancer 1992; 51: 509–514.

569. The James Lind Library. http://www.jameslindlibrary.org

570. Jarman B. Identification of underprivileged areas. Br Med J 1983; 286: 1705–1709.

571. García AM, Checkoway H. A glossary for research in occupational health. J Epidemiol Community Health 2003; 57; 7–10.

572. Egan M, Bambra C, Thomas S, et al. The psychosocial and health effects of workplace reorganisation: 1. A systematic review of organisational-level interventions that aim to increase employee control. J Epidemiol Community Health 2007; 61: 945–954.

573. Kakwani NC. Measurement of tax progressivity: an international comparison. Economic Journal 1977; 87: 71–80.

574. Kaplan EL, Meier P. Non-parametric estimation for incomplete observations. J Am Stat Assoc 1958; 53: 457–481.

575. Guggenmoos-Holzman I. The meaning of kappa: probabilistic concepts of reliability and validity revisited. J Clin Epidemiol 1996; 49: 775–782.

576. Hoehler FK. Bias and prevalence effects on kappa viewed in terms of sensitivity and specificity. J Clin Epidemiol 2000; 53: 499–503.

577. Kraemer HC, Periyakoil VS, Noda A. Kappa coefficients in medical research. Stat Med 2002; 21: 2109–2129.

578. Bithell JF. An application of density estimation to geographical epidemiology. Stat Med 1990; 9: 691–701.

579. Merz M. Knowledge construction. In: Restivo S, ed. Science, Technology, and Society: An Encyclopedia. Oxford: Oxford University Press; 2005.

580. Cancer Epidemiology Matters Blog. National Cancer Institute. http://blog-epi.grants.cancer.gov/2012/10/16/how-can-we-use-epidemiology-to-integrate-knowledge-emerging-from-basic-clinical-and-population-sciences/

581. Carrat F, Valleron AJ. Epidemiologic mapping using the "Kriging" method: application to an influenza-like illness in France. Am J Epidemiol 1992; 135: 1293–1300.

582. Frankel S, Davison C, Davey Smith G. Lay epidemiology and the rationality of responses to health education. Br J General Practice 1991; 41: 428–430.

583. Ledermann S. Alcool, Alcoolisme et Alcoolisation. Paris: Presses Universitaires de France; 1956.

584. Goodman RA, Loue S, Shaw FE. Epidemiology and the law. In: Brownson RC, Petitti DB, eds. Applied Epidemiology: Theory to Practice. Oxford: Oxford University Press; 2006.

585. Holmes TH, Rahe RH. The social readjustment rating scale. J Psychosom Res 1967; 1: 213–218.

586. Michie S, van Stralen MM, West R: The behaviour change wheel: a new method for characterising and designing behaviour change interventions. Implement Sci 2011; 6: 42.

587. Anselin L. Local Indicators of Spatial Association – LISA. Geographical Analysis 1995; 27: 93–115.

588. Bland JM, Altman DG. The logrank test. BMJ 2004; 328: 1073.

589. Lorenz MO. Methods of measuring the concentration of wealth. Publications of the American Statistical Association 1905; 9 (70): 209–219.

590. Kurose K, Hiratsuka K, Ishiwata K, et al. Genome-wide association study of SSRI / SNRI-induced sexual dysfunction in a Japanese cohort with major depression. Psychiatry Res 2012; 198: 424–429.

591. Mantel N, Haenszel W. Statistical aspects of the analysis of data from retrospective studies of disease. J Natl Cancer Inst 1959; 22: 719–748.

592. Robins JM, Hernán MA, Brumback B. Marginal structural models and causal inference in epidemiology. Epidemiology 2000; 11: 550–560.

593. Bator FM. The anatomy of market failure. Quarterly Journal of Economics 1958; 72 (3): 351–379.

594. Arrow KJ. Uncertainty and the welfare economics of medical care. Am Economic Rev 1963; 53 (5): 941–973.

595. Hamra G, MacLehose R, Richardson D. Markov chain Monte Carlo: an introduction for epidemiologists. Int J Epidemiol 2013; 42: 627–634.

596. Hamer W. Epidemic disease in England. Lancet 1906; 1: 733–739.

597. Meade MS, Emch M. Medical Geography. 3rd. ed. New York: Guilford; 2010.

598. Pacione M, ed. Medical Geography: Progress and Prospect. London: Taylor & Francis; 2013.

599. Wennberg JH. Tracking Medicine: A Researcher's Quest to Understand Health Care. Oxford: Oxford University Press, 2010.

600. Clarke AE, Shim JK, Mamo L, et al. Biomedicalization: Technoscientific transformations of health, illness, and US biomedicine. Am Sociol Rev 2003; 68: 161-194.

601. Davey Smith G, Ebrahim S. "Mendelian randomization": can genetic epidemiology contribute to understanding environmental determinants of disease? Int J Epidemiol 2003; 32: 1–22.

602. Avise JC. Evolving genomic metaphors: a new look at the language of DNA. Science 2001; 294: 86–87.

603. Brashers DE. Communication and uncertainty management. J Communicat 2001; 51: 477–497.

604. Egger M, Davey Smith G, Sterne JAC, et al. Systematic reviews and meta-analysis. In: Detels R, McEwen J, Beaglehole R, et al., eds. Oxford Textbook of Public Health. 4th. ed. Vol. 2. New York: Oxford University Press; 2002. p. 655–676.

605. www.undp.org/mdg/basics.shtml.

606. Jaeschke R Singer J, Guyatt GH. Measurement of health status: Ascertaining the minimal clinically important difference. Contr Clin Trials 1989; 10: 407–415.

607. Revicki D, Hays RD, Cella D, et al. Recommended methods for determining responsiveness and minimally important differences for patient-reported outcomes. J Clin Epidemiol 2008; 61: 102–109.

608. Little RJ, Rubin DB. Statistical Analysis with Missing Data. 2nd. ed. New York: Wiley; 2002.

609. Sterne JA, White IR, Carlin JB, et al. Multiple imputation for missing data in epidemiological and clinical research: potential and pitfalls. BMJ 2009; 338: b2393.

610. Gehlke C, Biehl K. Certain effects of grouping upon the size of the correlation coefficient in census tract material. J Am Stat Assoc 1934; 29.(Suppl): 169–170.

611. Jackson AL, Davies CA, Leyland AH. Do differences in the administrative structure of populations confound comparisons of geographic health inequalities? BMC Med Res Methodol 2010; 10: 74.

612. Wild C, Vineis P, Garte S, eds. Molecular Epidemiology of Chronic Diseases. Chichester: Wiley; 2008.

613. Schulte PA, Perera FP. Molecular Epidemiology: Principles and Practices. Orlando, FL: Academic Press; 1993.

614. Carrington M, Hoelzel R. Molecular Epidemiology. New York: Oxford University Press; 2001.

615. Rebbeck TR, Ambrosone CB, Shields PG, eds. Molecular Epidemiology: Applications in Cancer and Other Human Diseases. New York: Informa, 2008.

616. Einav L, Finkelstein A, Ryan SP, et al. Selection on moral hazard in health insurance. Am Econ Rev 2013; 103: 178–219.

617. Diez-Roux A. Bringing context back into epidemiology: variables and fallacies in multilevel analysis. Am J Public Health 1998; 88: 216–222.

618. Von Engelhardt D. Causality and conditionality in medicine around 1900. In: Delkeskamp-Hayes C, Cutter MAG, eds. Science, Technology, and the Art of Medicine. Dordrecht: Kluwer; 1993. p. 75–104.

619. Robins J, Sued M, Lei-Gomez Q, et al. Comment: performance of double-robust estimators when "inverse probability" weights are highly variable. Stat Sci 2007; 22: 544-559.

620. Vansteelandt S, VanderWeele TJ, Tchetgen EJ, et al. Multiply robust inference for statistical interactions. J Am Stat Assoc 2008; 103: 1693–1704.

621. Snow J. On the Mode of Communication of Cholera. London; 1855.

622. Culyer AJ. Need: the idea won't do–but we still need it. Soc Sci Med 1995; 40: 727–730.

623. Wright J, Williams R, Wilkinson JR. Development and importance of health needs assessment. BMJ 1998; 316: 1310–1313.

624. Cavanagh S, Chadwick K. Health Needs Assessment: A Practical Guide. London: National Institute for Health & Clinical Excellence (NICE); 2005. http://www.nice.org.uk/media/150/35/Health_Needs_Assessment_A_Practical_Guide.pdf

625. Stevens A, Mant J, Raftery J, et al. Health Care Needs Assessment: The Epidemiological Based Needs Assessment Reviews. Oxford: Radcliffe; 2004.

626. Fanelli D. Negative results are disappearing from most disciplines and countries. Scientometrics 2012; 90: 891–904.

627. Lawn JE, Cousens S, Zupan J. Neonatal survival: 4 million neonatal deaths: when? where? why? Lancet 2005; 365: 891–900.

628. Caldarelli G, Catanzaro M. Networks: A Very Short Introduction. Oxford: Oxford University Press; 2012.

629. Guyatt G, Sackett D, Taylor DW, et al. Determining optimal therapy: randomized trials in individual patients. N Engl J Med 1986; 314: 889–892.

630. McLeod RS, Taylor DW, Cohen Z, et al. Single-patient randomised clinical trial: use in determining optimum treatment for patient with inflammation of Kock continent ileostomy reservoir. Lancet 1986; 1: 726–728.

631. Porta M. The search for more clinically meaningful research designs: single patient clinical trials [Editorial]. J Gen Intern Med 1986; 1: 418–419.

632. Rosenbaum R. Nomograms for rates per 1000. Br Med J 1963; 1:169–170.

633. Rosenbaum L, Lamas D. Facing a "slow-motion disaster": the UN meeting on noncommunicable diseases. N Engl J Med 2011; 365: 2345–2348.

634. World Health Organization. The Global Status Report on Noncommunicable Diseases 2010. Geneva: World Health Organization; 2011. http://www.who.int/nmh/publications/ncd_report2010/en/

635. Shackelford RE, Kaufmann WK, Paules RS. Cell cycle control, checkpoint mechanisms, and genotoxic stress. Environ Health Perspect 1999; 107 (Supl 1): 5–24.

636. Faber K. Nosography in Modern Internal Medicine. New York: Hoeber; 1923.

637. Laupacis A, Sackett DL, Roberts RS. An assessment of clinically useful measurements of the consequences of treatment. N Engl J Med 1988; 318: 1728–1733.

638. Chatellier G, Zapletal E, Lemaitre D, et al. The number needed to treat: a clinically useful nomogram in its proper context. BMJ 1996; 312: 426–429.

639. Hill AB. Observation and experiment. N Engl J Med 1953; 248: 995–1001.

640. Vandenbroucke JP. Observational research, randomised trials, and two views of medical science. PLoS Med 2008; 5: 339–343.

641. Hernán MA, Alonso A, Logan R, et al. Observational studies analyzed like randomized experiments: an application to postmenopausal hormone therapy and coronary heart disease. Epidemiology 2008; 19: 766–779.

642. World Health Organization - Regional Office for the Eastern Mediterranean. Occupational Health: A Manual for Primary Health Care Workers. 2001. WHO-EM/OCH/85/E/L. http://whqlibdoc.who.int/emro/2001/WHO-EM_OCH_85_E_L.pdf

643. Checkoway H, Pearce N, Kriebel D. Research Methods in Occupational Epidemiology. 2nd. ed. New York: Oxford University Press; 2004.

644. Monson RR. Occupational Epidemiology. 2nd. ed. Boca Raton, FL: CRC Press; 1990.

645. European Centre for Disease Prevention and Control. Definition of a Pandemic. http://ecdc.europa.eu/en/healthtopics/pandemic_preparedness/basic_facts/Pages/definition_of_pandemic.aspx

646. Doshi P. The elusive definition of pandemic influenza. Bull World Health Org 2011; 89: 532–538.

647. Nicoll A. Planning for uncertainty: a European approach to informing responses to the severity of influenza epidemics and pandemics. Bull World Health Org 2011; 89: 542–544.

648. Kuhn T. The Structure of Scientific Revolutions. Chicago: University of Chicago Press; 1962.

649. Nieto FJ. Understanding the pathophysiology of poverty. Int J Epidemiol 2009; 38:787–790.

650. Cappelleri JC, Zou KH, Bushmakin AG, et al. Patient-Reported Outcomes: Measurement, Implementation and Interpretation. New York: Chapman & Hall / CRC; 2013.

651. Fayers P, Machin D. Quality of Life: The Assessment, Analysis and Interpretation of Patient-reported Outcomes. 2nd. ed. Chichester: Wiley; 2007.

652. World Health Organization. Neonatal and Perinatal Mortality: Country, Regional and Global Estimates. Geneva: World Health Organization; 2006. http://apps.who.int/iris/handle/10665/43800

653. Buzunov VA, Strapko NP, Pirogova EA, et al. Epidemiological survey of the medical consequences of the Chernobyl accident in Ukraine. World Health Stat Q 1996; 49: 4–6.

654. Strom BL, Kimmel SE, Hennessy S, eds. Pharmacoepidemiology. 5th. ed. Chichester: Wiley; 2012.

655. Porta M, Carné X. Pharmacoepidemiology. In: Trichopoulos D, Olsen J, eds. Teaching of Epidemiology. 1st. ed. Oxford: Oxford University Press; 1992. p. 285–304.

656. Silman AJ, Croft PR. Musculoskeletal diseases. In: Detels R, Holland WW, McEwen J, Omenn G, eds. Oxford Textbook of Public Health. 3rd. ed. Vol. 3. New York: Oxford University Press; 1997. p. 1175.

657. Sivakumaran S, Agakov F, Theodoratou E, et al. Abundant pleiotropy in human complex diseases and traits. Am J Hum Genet 2011; 89: 607–618.

658. Rajabi F. Evidence-informed health policy making: the role of policy brief. Int J Prev Med 2012; 3: 596–598.

659. http://global.evipnet.org

660. Franco A, Álvarez-Dardet C, Ruiz MT. Effect of democracy on health: ecological study. BMJ 2004; 329: 1421–1424.

661. Mackenbach JP. Politics is nothing but medicine at a larger scale: reflections on public health's biggest idea. J Epidemiol Community Health 2009; 63: 181–184.

662. Rothman KJ, Adami HO, Trichopoulos D. Should the mission of epidemiology include the eradication of poverty? Lancet 1998; 352: 810–813.

663. Rothman KJ, Stein Z, Susser M. Rebuilding bridges: what is the real role of social class in disease occurrence? Eur J Epidemiol 2011; 26: 431–432.

664. Morgan LM. Political economy of health. In: Restivo S, ed. Science, Technology, and Society: An Encyclopedia. Oxford: Oxford University Press; 2005.

665. Bambra C, Fox D, Scott-Samuel A. A politics of health glossary. J Epidemiol Community Health 2007; 61: 571–574.

666. Vineis P, Malats N, Lang M, et al., eds. Metabolic polymorphisms and susceptibility to cancer. IARC Scientific publications, no. 148. Lyon: International Agency for Research on Cancer; 1999.

667. Brown P. Popular epidemiology and toxic waste contamination: lay and professional ways of knowing. J Health Social Behaviour 1992; 33: 267–281.

668. MacMahon B, Pugh TF. Epidemiology: Principles and Methods. Boston: Little, Brown; 1970.

669. Cole P, MacMahon B. Attributable risk percent in case-control studies. Br J Prev Soc Med 1971; 25: 242–244.

670. Young TK. Population Health: Concepts and Methods. New York: Oxford University Press; 1998.

671. Westreich D, Cole SR. Positivity in practice. Am J Epidemiol 2010; 171: 674–681.

672. Petersen ML, Porter KE, Gruber S, Wang Y, van der Laan MJ. Diagnosing and responding to violations in the positivity assumption. Stat Methods Med Res 2010; 21: 31–54.

673. Birn AE, Pillay Y, Holtz TH. Textbook of International Health: Global Health in a Dynamic World. 3rd. ed. New York: Oxford University Press; 2009.

674. Calhoun C, ed. Dictionary of the Social Sciences. Oxford: Oxford University Press; 2002.

675. Aronsson G, Gustafsson K. Sickness presenteeism: prevalence, attendance-pressure factors, and an outline of a model for research. J Occup Environ Med 2005; 47: 958–966.

676. Agudelo-Suárez AA, Benavides FG, Felt E, et al. Sickness presenteeism in Spanish-born and immigrant workers in Spain. BMC Public Health 2010; 10: 791.

677. Prasad V, Jena AB. Prespecified falsification end points: can they validate true observational associations? JAMA 2013; 309: 241–242.

678. Beaglehole R, Bonita R, Kjellström T. Basic Epidemiology. Geneva: WHO; 1993. p. 85–88.

679. Bentzen N, ed. WONCA Dictionary of General / Family Practice. Copenhagen: Laegeforeningens Forlag; 2003.

680. Hannaford PC, Smith BH, Elliott AM. Primary care epidemiology: its scope and purpose. Family Practice 2006; 23: 1–7.

681. Starfield B. Primary Care: Concept, Evaluation and Policy. New York: Oxford University Press; 1992.

682. World Health Organization. Glossary of Terms Used in the Health for All Series No. 1–8. Geneva: WHO; 1984.

683. Preferred Reporting Items for Systematic Reviews and Meta-Analyses. http://www.prisma-statement.org

684. Moher D, Liberati A, Tetzlaff J, et al. Preferred reporting items for systematic reviews and meta-analyses: The PRISMA Statement. J Clin Epidemiol 2009; 62: 1006–1012.

685. Weed LL. Medical records that guide and teach. N Engl J Med 1968; 278: 593–600 and 652-657.

686. Lucas A. Programming by Early Nutrition in Man: Ciba Foundation Symposium 156. The Childhood Environment and Adult Disease. Chichester: Wiley, 1991.

687. Feinstein AR. Clinical biostatistics: LVII. A glossary of neologisms in quantitative clinical science. Clin Pharmacol Ther 1981; 30: 564–577.

688. D'Agostino RB Jr. Propensity score methods for bias reduction in the comparison of a treatment to a non-randomized control group. Stat Med 1998; 17: 2265–2281.

689. Whiting PF, Rutjes AW, Westwood ME, et al. QUADAS-2: a revised tool for the quality assessment of diagnostic accuracy studies. Ann Intern Med 2011; 155: 529–536.

690. Schwandt TA. Qualitative Inquiry: A Dictionary of Terms. Thousand Oaks, CA: Sage Publications; 1997.

691. Moher D, Cook DJ, Eastwood S, et al. Improving the quality of reports of meta-analyses of randomised controlled trials: the QUOROM statement. Lancet 1999; 354: 1896–1900.

692. Martin E, Hine R, eds. Oxford Dictionary of Biology. 6th. ed. Oxford: Oxford University Press; 2008.

693. Omi M, Winant H. On the theoretical status of the concept of race. In: McCarthy C, Crichlow W, eds. Race, Identity and Representation. New York: Routledge; 1993. p. 1–9.

694. Rapid epidemiological assessment. Int J Epidemiol 1989; 18 (Suppl 2): S1-S67.

695. Burón A, Vernet M, Roman M, et al. Can the Gail model increase the predictive value of a positive mammogram in a European population screening setting? Results from a Spanish cohort. Breast 2013; 22: 83–88.

696. Newcombe HB. Handbook of Record Linkage. Oxford, England: Oxford Medical Publications; 1988.

697. Dunn HL. Record linkage. Am J Public Health 1946; 36: 1412.

698. Lambert ML, Hasker E, Van Deun A, et al. Recurrence in tuberculosis: relapse or reinfection? Lancet Infect Dis 2003; 3: 282–287.

699. Wilcox AJ. The analysis of recurrence risk as an epidemiological tool. Paediatr Perinat Epidemiol 2007; 21 (Suppl 1): 4-7.

700. Flynn JA, Choi MJ, Wooster LD, eds. Oxford American Handbook of Clinical Medicine. 2nd. ed. New York: Oxford University Press; 2013.

701. Goldberg J, Gelfand HM, Levy PS. Registry evaluation methods. Epidemiol Rev 1980; 2: 210–220.

702. World Health Organization, International Union against Tuberculosis and lung disease, Royal Netherlands Tuberculosis Association: revised international definitions in tuberculosis control. Int J Tuberc Lun Dis 2001; 5: 213–215.

703. Verver S, Warren RM, Beyers N, et al. Rate of reinfection tuberculosis after successful treatmet is higher than rate of new tuberculosis. Am J Resp Crit Med Care Med 2005; 17: 1430–1435.

704. Suissa S. Relative excess risk: an alternative measure of comparative risk. Am J Epidemiol 1999; 150: 279–282.

705. Mackenbach JP, Kunst AE. Measuring the magnitude of socio-economic inequalities in health: an overview of available measures illustrated with two examples from Europe. Soc Sci Med 1997; 44: 757–771.

706. Sergeant JC, Firth D. Relative index of inequality: definition, estimation, and inference. Biostatistics 2006; 7: 213–224.

707. Patrick DL, Erickson P. Health Status and Health Policy: Allocating Resources to Health Care. New York: Oxford University Press; 1993.

708. Beaton DE, Bombardier C, Katz JN, et al. A taxonomy for responsiveness. J Clin Epidemiol 2001; 54: 1204–1217.

709. Husted JA, Cook RJ, Farewell VT, et al. Methods for assessing responsiveness: a critical review and recommendations. J Clin Epidemiol 2000; 53: 459–468.

710. VanderWeele TJ. Re: "Religious service attendance and major depression: a case of reverse causality?" Am J Epidemiol 2013; 177: 275–276.

711. Bross IDJ. How to use ridit analysis. Biometrics 1958; 14(1): 18–38.

712. Slovic P. Perception of risk. Science 1987; 236: 280–285.

713. Burns WJ, Peters E, Slovic P. Risk perception and the economic crisis: a longitudinal study of the trajectory of perceived risk. Risk Anal 2012; 32: 659–677.

714. Douglas M. Risk and Blame: Essays in Cultural Theory; Collected Works, Volume XII. Abingdon: Routledge; 2003.

715. Beck U. World at Risk. Cambridge: Polity Press; 2007.

716. Mythen G, Walkate S, eds. Beyond the Risk Society: Critical Reflections on Risk and Human Security. Maidenhead: Open University Press; 2006.

717. Tulloch JC, Zinn JO. Risk, health and the media. Health Risk Soc 2011; 13: 1–16.

718. Fischhoff B, Kadvany J. Risk: A Very Short Introduction. New York: Oxford University Press; 2011.

719. Dawber TR, Kannel WB, Revotskie N, et al. Some factors associated with the development of coronary heart disease: Six years' follow-up experience in the Framingham study. Am J Public Health 1959; 49: 1349–1356.

720. Bailey JE. Lessons from metabolic engineering for functional genomics and drug discovery. Nature Biotechnol. 1999; 17: 616–618.

721. Feinstein AR. The Santayana Syndrome. I: Errors in getting and interpreting evidence. Perspect Biol Med 1997; 41: 45–57.

722. Feinstein AR. The Santayana Syndrome. II: Problems in reasoning and learning about error. Perspect Biol Med 1997; 41: 73–85.

723. Santayana G. Reason in common sense. In: The Life of Reason, Vol. 1. New York: C. Scribner's Sons; 1905 (Amherst, NY: Prometheus Books; 1998).

724. Sartwell PE. The incubation period of infectious diseases. Am J Hygiene 1950; 51: 310–318.

725. Ostfeld RS, Glass GE, Keesing F. Spatial epidemiology: an emerging (or re-emerging) discipline. Trends Ecol Evol 2005; 20: 328–336.

726. Lilienfeld DE, Stolley PD. Foundations of Epidemiology. 3rd. ed. New York: Oxford University Press; 1994.

727. Brouwer JJ, Schreuder RF. Scenarios and Other Methods to Support Long Term Health Planning. Utrecht: Jan van Arkel; 1988.

728. Medawar P. Pluto's Republic: The Art of the Soluble; Induction and Intuition in Scientific Thought. Oxford: Oxford University Press; 1984.

729. Raffle AE, Gray M. Screening: Evidence and Practice. Oxford: Oxford University Press; 2007.

730. Hernán MA, Hernández-Díaz S, Robins JM. A structural approach to selection bias. Epidemiology 2004; 15: 615–625.

731. Olson SH, Voigt LF, Begg CB, et al. Reporting participation in case-control studies. Epidemiology 2002; 13: 123–126.

732. Kunzli N, Tager IB. The semi-individual study in air pollution epidemiology: a valid design as compared to ecologic studies. Environ Health Perspect 1997; 105: 1078-1083.

733. Schneeweiss S. Sensitivity analysis and external adjustment for unmeasured confounders in epidemiologic database studies of therapeutics. Pharmacoepidemiol Drug Safety 2006; 15: 291–303.

734. Iman RL, Helton JC. An investigation of uncertainty and sensitivity analysis techniques for computer-models. Risk Analysis 1988; 8: 71–90.

735. www.fda.gov/Safety/FDAsSentinelInitiative.

736. Marmot M, Feeney A, Shipley M, et al. Sickness absence as a measure of health status and functioning: from the UK Whitehall II study. J Epidemiol Community Health 1995; 49: 124–130.

737. Benavides FG. Ill health, social protection, labour relations, and sickness absence. Occup Envir Med 2006; 63: 228–229.

738. Simpson EH. The interpretation of interaction in contingency tables. J R Stat Soc Ser B 1951; 13: 238–241.

739. Hernán MA, Clayton D, Keiding N. The Simpson's paradox unraveled. Int J Epidemiol 2011; 40: 780–785.

740. Blyth CR. On Simpson's paradox and the sure-thing principle. J Am Stat Assoc 1972; 67: 364–366.

741. Berkman LF, Kawachi I. Social Epidemiology. New York: Oxford University Press; 2000.

742. Lin N. Building a network theory of social capital. Connections 1999; 22: 28–51.

743. Bourdieu P. Le capital social: notes provisoires. Actes de la Recherche en Sciencies Sociales 1980; 31: 2–3.

744. Coleman JS. Foundations of Social Theory. Cambridge, MA: Harvard University Press; 1990.

745. Kawachi I, Kim DJ, Coutts A, Subramanian SV. Reconciling the three accounts of social capital. Int J Epidemiol 2004; 33: 682–690.

746. Marmot M, Wilkinson RG. Social Determinants of Health. 2nd. ed. New York: Oxford University Press; 2005.

747. Galobardes B, Lynch J, Davey-Smith G. Measuring socioeconomic position in health research. Br Med Bull 2007; 81-82: 21–37.

748. Braveman PA, Cubbin C, Egerter S, et al. Socioeconomic status in health research: one size does not fit all. JAMA 2005; 294: 2879–2888.

749. Krieger N. Sticky webs, hungry spiders, buzzing flies, and fractal metaphors: on the misleading juxtaposition of "risk factor" versus "social" epidemiology. J Epidemiol Community Health 1999; 53: 678–680.

750. Galea S, Link BG. Six paths for the future of social epidemiology. Am J Epidemiol 2013; 178: 843–849.

751. Kotler RN, Roberto N, Lee N. Social Marketing: Improving Quality of Life. 2nd. ed. London: Sage; 2002.

752. Alexander F. Estimation of sojourn time distributions and false negative rates in screening programmes which use two modalities. Stat Med 1989; 8: 743–755.

753. Lloyd CD. Local Models for Spatial Analysis. 2nd. ed. Boca Raton, FL: CRC Press; 2011.

754. Ransohoff DF, Feinstein AR. Problems of spectrum and bias in evaluating the efficacy of diagnostic tests. N Engl J Med 1978; 299: 926–930.

755. Mulherin SA, Miller WC. Spectrum bias or spectrum effect? Subgroup variation in diagnostic test evaluation. Ann Intern Med 2002; 137: 598–602.

756. Bossuyt PM, Reitsma JB, Bruns DE, et al. Towards complete and accurate reporting of studies of diagnostic accuracy: the STARD initiative. BMJ 2003; 326: 41–44.

757. Leeflang M, Reitsma J, Scholten R, et al. Impact of adjustment for quality on results of metaanalyses of diagnostic accuracy. Clin Chem 2007; 53: 164–172.

758. Diamond I, Jefferies J. Beginning Statistics: An Introduction for Social Scientists. London: Sage; 2001.

759. Kotz D, Spigt M, Arts ICW, et al. Use of the stepped wedge design cannot be recommended: a critical appraisal and comparison with the classic cluster randomized controlled trial design. J Clin Epidemiol 2012; 65:1249–1252.

760. Saltman RB, Ferroussier-Davis O. The concept of stewardship in health policy. Bull World Health Organ 2000; 78: 732–739.

761. Von Elm E, Altman D, Egger M, et al. Strengthening the reporting of observational studies in epidemiology: the STROBE statement. Prev Med 2007; 45: 247–251. http://www.strobe-statement.org

762. Kamel F. Epidemiology: paths from pesticides to Parkinson's. Science 2013; 341: 722–723.

763. Centers for Disease Control. Comprehensive Plan for Epidemiologic Surveillance. Atlanta, GA: CDC; 1996.

764. Sarfati D, Blakely T, Pearce N. Measuring cancer survival in populations: relative survival vs cancer-specific survival. Int J Epidemiol 2010; 39: 598–610.

765. Estève J, Benhamou E, Croasdale M, et al. Relative survival and the estimation of net survival: elements for further discussion. Stat Med 1990; 9: 529–538.

766. Vineis P. Individual susceptibility to carcinogens. Oncogene 2004; 23: 6477–6483.

767. Zolg W. The proteomic search for diagnostic biomarkers: lost in translation? Mol Cell Proteomics 2006; 5: 1720–1726.

768. United Nations, World Commission on Environment and Development's (the Brundtland Commission). Report: Our Common Future. General Assembly Resolution 42/187, 11 December 1987.

769. Merriam-Webster Dictionary. http://www.merriam-webster.com/dictionary/system

770. Bambra C. Real world reviews: a beginner's guide to undertaking systematic reviews of public health policy interventions. J Epidemiol Community Health 2011; 65: 14–19.

771. Hales CN, Barker DJP. Type 2 (non-insulin-dependent) diabetes mellitus: the thrifty phenotype hypothesis. Diabetologia 1992; 35: 595–601.

772. Arons AM, Krabbe PF, Schölzel-Dorenbos CJ, et al. Thurstone scaling revealed systematic health-state valuation differences between patients with dementia and proxies. J Clin Epidemiol 2012; 65: 897–905.

773. Krabbe PF. Thurstone scaling as a measurement method to quantify subjective health outcomes. Med Care 2008; 46: 357–365.

774. Townsend P, Phillimore P, Beattie A. Health and Deprivation: Inequality and the North. London: Croom Helm; 1988.

775. Kessner DM, Snow CK, Singer J. Assessment of Medical Care for Children. Washington, DC: National Academy of Sciences, Institute of Medicine; 1974.

776. Transdisciplinarity. Stimulating synergies, integrating knowledge. Paris: UNESCO; 1998. http://unesdoc.unesco.org/images/0011/001146/114694eo.pdf.

777. Leggat PA, Goldsmid JM, eds. Primer of Travel Medicine. 3rd. ed. Brisbane, Australia: ACTM Publications, 2002.

778. Des Jarlais DC, Lyles C, Crepaz N. TREND Group. Improving the reporting quality of nonrandomized evaluations of behavioral and public health interventions: the TREND statement. Am J Public Health 2004; 94: 361–366.

779. Centers for Disease Control and Prevention. Tuberculosis Fact Sheet. http://www.cdc.gov/tb/publications/factsheets/testing/skintesting.htm

780. www.who.int/mediacentre/factsheets/fs104/en.

781. Porter JDH, McAdam KPWJ. The re-emergence of tuberculosis. Annu Rev Public Health 1994; 15: 303–323.

782. World Health Organization. Global Tuberculosis Report 2013. http://www.who.int/tb/publications/global_report/en/index.html

783. Webb EJ, Campbell DT, Schwartz RD, et al. Unobtrusive Measures. Chicago: Rand McNally; 1966.

784. Chandramohan D, Maude GH, Rodriques LC, et al. Verbal autopsies for adult deaths: issues in their development and validation. Int J Epidemiol 1994; 23: 213–230.

785. WHO Global Consultation on Violence and Health. Violence: A Public Health Priority. Geneva: World Health Organization; 1996.

786. Von Neumann J, Morgenstern O. Theory of Games and Economic Behavior. Princeton: Princeton University Press; 1944.

787. Hartnell NR, Wilson JP. Replication of the Weber effect using post-marketing adverse event reports voluntarily submitted to the United States Food and Drug Administration. Pharmacotherapy 2004; 24: 743–749.

788. Stephenson WP, Hauben M. Data mining for signals in spontaneous reporting databases: proceed with caution. Pharmacoepidemiol Drug Saf 2007; 16: 359–365.

789. MacMahon B, Pugh TF, Ipsen J. Epidemiologic Methods. Boston: Little, Brown; 1960.

790. Zelen M. The randomization and stratification of patients to clinical trials. J Chron Dis 1974; 27: 365–373.

791. Richiardi L, Bellocco R, Zugna D. Mediation analysis in epidemiology: methods, interpretation and bias. Int J Epidemiol 2013; 42: 1511–1519.

792. Gunasekara FI, Richardson K, Carter K, et al. Fixed effects analysis of repeated measures data. Int J Epidemiol 2014; 43: 264–269.

793. Taylor P. Standardized mortality ratios. Int J Epidemiol 2013; 42: 1882–1890.

794. Andersen PK, Geskus RB, de Witte T, et al. Competing risks in epidemiology: possibilities and pitfalls. Int J Epidemiol 2012; 41: 861–870.

795. Pearce N. Classification of epidemiological study designs. Int J Epidemiol 2012; 41: 393–397.

796. Steyerberg EW, Vickers AJ, Cook NR, et al. Assessing the performance of prediction models: a framework for traditional and novel measures. Epidemiology 2010; 21: 128–138.

797. Schneeweiss S, Rassen JA, Glynn RJ, et al. High-dimensional propensity score adjustment in studies of treatment effects using health care claims data. Epidemiology 2009; 20: 512–522.

798. VanderWeele TJ. Sufficient cause interactions and statistical interactions. Epidemiology 2009; 20: 6–13.

799. Vineis P, Stringhini S, Porta M. The environmental roots of non-communicable diseases and the epigenetic impacts of globalization. Environmental Research 2014.

800. Hernán MA, Hernández-Díaz S, Robins JM. Randomized trials analyzed as observational studies. Ann Intern Med 2013; 159: 560–562.